MEDLINE on CD-ROM

**National Library of Medicine
Evaluation Forum**

**Bethesda, Maryland
September 23, 1988**

Editors:
Rose Marie Woodsmall
Becky Lyon-Hartmann
Elliot R. Siegel

Consulting Editor:
Pauline A. Cochrane

Learned Information, Inc.
1989

National Library of Medicine Cataloging in Publication

Z
699.5.M39
M491
1988

MEDLINE on CD-ROM: National Library of Medicine
evaluation forum, September 23, 1988, Bethesda,
Maryland / editors, Rose Marie Woodsmall, Becky Lyon-
Hartmann, Elliot R. Siegel ; consulting editor, Pauline A.
Cochrane.—Medford, N.J., U.S.A. ; Learned Information,
1989. Includes index.

1. MEDLARS-MEDLINE Information System - congresses.
2. Video Recording - congresses. I. Woodsmall, Rose Marie.
II. Lyon-Hartmann, Becky. III. Siegel, Elliot R. IV. National
Library of Medicine (U.S.)

PREFACE

On September 23, 1988, over 250 members of the health science library community gathered at the National Library of Medicine for an Evaluation Forum entitled "MEDLINE on CD-ROM." This audience far exceeded the capacity of the Lister Hill Center Auditorium, so satellite rooms and closed circuit television had to be arranged. Not only did the topic hold such great interest but many people came because the planners of the forum had prepared an unusual opportunity for all participants to see and hear about a collaborative evaluation project which involved seven products evaluated at twenty-one different sites. There were evaluation reports from the various sites, some in clinical settings, which collected data either formally by means of a questionnaire, or informally by direct observation, regarding performance and user acceptance. The producers of the CD-ROM versions of MEDLINE, who had cooperated during the evaluation period which spread out over several months, were on hand on September 23 to exhibit and discuss the effort.

This was an unusual gathering and it is for this reason that this volume was produced—to record more than the "proceedings." Besides the transcription of what proceeded at the forum, this volume includes all the evaluation project reports which were presented only in abbreviated form at the forum, a summary report of the nationwide evaluation, a checklist of CD-ROM features, a bibliography on the subject of CD-ROM and an index.

It is hoped that this evaluation effort will make a positive contribution to the knowledge and understanding of all who must make decisions about new technologies in the health science library.

P. Cochrane

ACKNOWLEDGMENTS

The forum organizers want to give special thanks to Carolyn Tilley for the exhibits, Alvin J. Barnes for the bibliography, Joyce E. B. Backus for the features checklist, Barbara Rapp who helped tremendously at the last minute, and the Friends of the National Library of Medicine for the reception.

CONTENTS

PART III. APPENDIXES

PART I

Evaluation Forum

INTRODUCTION TO EVALUATION FORUM

Elliot R. Siegel
Assistant Director for Planning and Evaluation
National Library of Medicine

Nearly three years ago, the National Library of Medicine signed its first experimental CD-ROM agreement with Cambridge Scientific Abstracts. It provided for the first development of this new technology using the MEDLINE database. We have certainly come a long way in a fairly short period of time. Since that beginning, a dozen other firms have come to the National Library of Medicine for the same purpose, to work with us on these products. Another seven MEDLINE on CD-ROM Systems have been produced and are operating very successfully.

An essential element of this collaboration with the private sector has been the field testing and evaluation of the systems at twenty-one health science libraries and clinical sites around the country—three separate sites per system.

We estimate that upwards of 4,000 health professionals and students have searched MEDLINE using one of these CD-ROM products during a coordinated two to three month period earlier this year—ten months in the case of Columbia University and the University of Washington. About half of these persons also completed a post-search questionnaire which asked comparable questions at each of the test sites. We provided the sites with what we called a "generic questionnaire". They had an opportunity to modify it and adapt it to their own needs. We gave all the sites a free hand to develop their own evaluation studies that happened to fit the circumstances of their own institution.

Today's forum is really a culmination of that process. We have brought all the participants together: the vendors, the evaluators, the users, the prospective users. They are here to share their data, share their experiences and their insights. We at the National Library of Medicine like to think we're a catalyst in all this, and I can tell you we're very pleased with the goodwill, the cooperation, and the hard work that's been shown by everyone.

We have structured panel sessions to report research findings. We also have hands-on demonstrations of all seven systems outside in the lobby. We did add an eighth system, Med-Base, which came on the market after our evaluation began, and in the interest of completeness, Med-Base is here as well.

You may want to take a minute now to look at your registration packet. It contains materials we think you will find helpful. In it is a bibliography of nearly four hundred references pertinent to CD-ROM technology.* Then there's a "Features Checklist"* which displays, in a handy comparison format, the pres-

---

* Included in the appendices of this volume

ence of a wide variety of system features and capabilities which we think would be of interest to organizations contemplating the purchase of a CD-ROM system. We don't tell you how well they work nor do we indicate whether more features are necessarily better than fewer. You'll have to work that out for yourself. We've also given you a card for picking up a commemorative poster which we have had commissioned.

Finally, I should tell you, the entire program is being videotaped. It will be available on loan from the National Library of Medicine and from the Regional Medical Libraries after the conference.**

**Z699.5.M39 VC no. 4.1 to no. 4.7 1988. Issued in both 3/4" and 1/2" formats.

OPENING REMARKS

Donald A. B. Lindberg
Director, National Library of Medicine

It is my pleasure to welcome you to the CD-ROM conference. I want to thank Elliot Siegel, Rose Marie Woodsmall and Becky Lyon-Hartmann on the NLM staff, and the many others who helped by performing the studies reported here and who helped put the conference together. This evaluation forum offered a unique opportunity for the National Library of Medicine to work with a number of firms from the private sector—an opportunity we don't always have. It worked out very well and we look forward to more such opportunities. The idea of a forum also gave us the opportunity to organize a nationwide evaluation project in which member libraries in the Regional Medical Library Network could share the results of their investigations.

In the past few years we have all been excited about this new medium. Just twenty years ago this medium would have appeared to be absolutely miraculous, even unimaginable. But like all good things, once you have it in hand, you can think of many uses for it. At the same time, of course, you become aware of its limitations and want even higher storage densities, more information at ever greater speeds, and all at lower cost.

Although we will hear today about some of these limitations, most users seem to remain enthusiastic, on balance. The vendors, the library institutions and the users have dealt with those limitations in different ways. This diversity of solutions is of great interest to me: if you can only put one full year of MEDLINE on one diskette, then the interesting questions are what to do, how to store, how to subset, how to repackage, how to combine with other complementary products. We will hear how different people have responded in different ways to meet the needs of a non-homogeneous audience. The on-site first-hand knowledge of a range of health care professionals who have used MEDLINE on several CD-ROM versions will provide invaluable information to which we will give great attention.

I have spent a lot of time in medical education, and it is wonderful to think that students can learn how to search the literature using these CD-ROM products. Yet at times when I consider this new medium, two prospects send chills down my spine:

(1) the possibility that somebody is telling a poor medical student that all he or she has to do is search one year of MEDLINE as guide to action. I don't believe that is happening at all, of course, but it still concerns me.

(2) It also horrifies me to think that the world is filling up with outdated

CD-ROMs. We have talked to the various vendor companies about this and the policies for keeping up to date vary. I hope we hear a discussion on that matter during the forum.

My guess as to the size of the MEDLINE CD-ROM market is that it is very large. I am not talking about the present small number of online users of medical bibliographic information services divided among twenty or so vendors of MEDLINE CD-ROM products. The present knowledgeable, consistent users of medical bibliographic services in the U.S. is a very small percent of those who would potentially benefit from MEDLINE CD-ROM use. That market is probably at least an order of magnitude greater. I believe there is plenty of room for CD-ROM, plenty of room for online, and plenty of room for a combination of the two. I'm confident that this new technology would help to bring in a host of new users of information services and I'm also confident that they will benefit from that experience. Outside the U.S. I think the market for MEDLINE CD-ROM products will explode and you could multiply all the above predictions by at least two.

One area of future concentration is even more clever packaging of MEDLINE with other related databases. All of us can also look forward to better search software. NLM has spent a lot of time and effort in recent years perfecting its own retrieval software systems. But even combining the cleverness that you will see in the exhibits in the lobby, there is plenty of room for even smarter and better adapted search software systems. Ways will also be found to increase the volume of local storage; certainly a year of MEDLINE is not enough, but is five years too much?

Two final points that may also be a part of the future improvements and developments. One is better indexing and accessing methods. Through our project called the Unified Medical Language System (UMLS), NLM is developing a distributed national experiment with researchers at eight universities. It is a major long term project—5 to 10 years—to improve the extent to which computer-based systems can understand the search requests that users formulate and to map these onto existing systems, including NLM's own MeSH. Since the project is being developed with 100% federal money, the product will be 100% in the public domain. We have taken pains to be sure that the individual projects within UMLS will develop sequentially and that we will not have to wait 10 years for a usable final product. There will be a number of partial solutions that will be available starting this year in the form of software and resources.

This evaluation forum provided us with a chance to work closely with several commercial firms. We would welcome another opportunity to work even more closely with these companies. One of the things I would like to see developed is GRATEFUL MED integrated into CD-ROM versions of MEDLINE. This would give the user the assurance that he/she could get complete information if the circumstances warrant. If the CD-ROM version provides 1, 2, 3, 4, or 5 years and that's ample for the immediate need, fine. But I would like to see a combination of the two available so that the user could decide how much information was necessary and then get as complete a search as needed. But that's the subject of another forum. For this one, welcome, and thank you for coming.

MEDLINE ON CD-ROM: SUMMARY REPORT OF A NATIONWIDE EVALUATION

Barbara A. Rapp, Elliot R. Siegel, Rose Marie Woodsmall
and Becky Lyon-Hartmann
National Library of Medicine, 8600 Rockville Pike
Bethesda, MD 20894

Introduction

In the past three years, we have seen a tremendous growth in the development of CD-ROM as a new and important access medium for bibliographic databases. This comes just fifteen years after the introduction of online information storage and retrieval systems, and just two years after the introduction of search assistance programs that facilitate end user searching. CD-ROM technology promises to bring database searching even closer to the end user community.

The first CD-ROM version of the National Library of Medicine's (NLM's) MEDLINE® database appeared in early 1987, and the number grew to eight by mid-1988. The MEDLINE database includes citations to nearly 6,000,000 articles from 1966 forward and covers approximately 3,400 journals in the fields of medicine, nursing, dentistry, veterinary medicine, and the preclinical sciences. Each of the CD-ROM products derived from the MEDLINE database was produced by an independent company in the private sector, but NLM has been actively involved in the development and testing stages. As part of its evaluation program, NLM launched a series of independent field tests for seven of the CD-ROM MEDLINE products. The purpose of the field tests was to assess the performance and acceptance of the CD-ROM products in a variety of settings, but not to compare systems with each other.

Feedback provided to the vendors as a result of this collaboration was useful to them in the refinement of later versions of their CD-ROM products. At the end of the evaluation period, study participants and CD-ROM vendors participated in a forum hosted by NLM in order to share information with each other and present the study findings to an audience of approximately 250 people.

In this paper we present an overview of the nationwide evaluation of MEDLINE products on CD-ROM. The results of each specific study are presented and discussed in individual reports included in Part II of this volume. Here we provide the general background and methodology for the evaluation project and summarize in a general way the composite results of the separate studies.

Background

In 1985, NLM signed its first CD-ROM agreement with Cambridge Scientific Abstracts, after Cambridge requested approval by NLM to mount portions of the MEDLINE database on compact disc. This experimental agreement provided for a limited cost-free lease of the MEDLINE database by Cambridge leading to the development, with input from NLM, of the first use of this important new technology as an access medium for MEDLINE. Since that time, NLM continued to execute similar agreements with other companies. Currently there are eight different companies marketing a MEDLINE CD-ROM product.

When NLM provided its MEDLINE tapes at no charge to companies intending to develop CD-ROM products, it embarked on a unique collaborative effort with the private sector. An essential element of this collaboration was the requirement that NLM review and evaluate the products as they moved from the prototype stage to the marketplace. The terms of the lease agreement with each company provided that the company would furnish NLM with three turnkey systems which NLM would arrange to have field tested at health science libraries and clinical sites of its choosing.

As the number of CD-ROM MEDLINE products increased, NLM put in place a plan to launch a coordinated evaluation project involving field tests at a variety of user sites throughout the country. This evaluation project included seven of the eight CD-ROM MEDLINE products. The eighth product was released to the marketplace after the field tests were well underway.

The name of each of the CD-ROM MEDLINE products evaluated, product coverage at the time of the field tests, and the name and address of each of the vendors are given in Table 1. Products not included in the field test are also listed in Table 1, but are so noted. Changes in product coverage since the time of the field test are also noted.

The Evaluation Studies

The evaluation project was designed so that each of the seven CD-ROM MEDLINE systems was evaluated in three locations, resulting in twenty-one separate evaluations throughout the country. Six of the Regional Medical Libraries were included as test sites; the additional sites were selected in order to represent a variety of library sizes, types, and geographic locations. At five of the test sites, the CD-ROM system was evaluated in a clinical setting as well as a library setting. At the sixteen other sites, the CD-ROM system was installed in the medical library only. NLM served as the coordinator of the field tests, but the individual evaluations were carried out independently.

Most of the evaluations were carried out during a coordinated 2-4 month test period in 1988. The Compact Cambridge product, however, was tested over a 10-month period since it was the first to be developed and testing was already underway when the series of simultaneous evaluation studies began.

Each of the twenty-one test sites was assigned one of the seven CD-ROM systems to evaluate. Some test sites in fact evaluated more than one system, since in some cases they already had purchased one of the other systems or they made separate arrangements with other CD-ROM vendors to acquire their products for testing. The names of the twenty-one test sites, the product they were asked to evaluate, and any additional products evaluated are listed in Table 2. Four of the test sites also compared the CD-ROM system with an in-house system for searching MEDLINE. In-house systems included miniMEDLINE at the Medical University of South Carolina and George Washington University; CLIO MEDLINE at Columbia University; and MELVYL MEDLINE at UCLA.

Site Setup

There was great variety across the test sites in the placement of the CD-ROM workstations and the management of access to the systems. Some sites placed the work station within view of the reference desk, so that the reference librarian could maintain some control over the system and be available to offer assistance when needed. Others placed the work station in a location apart from the reference desk, allowing users to work completely on their own. Some sites required users to obtain the disks at the circulation desk, while others had the disks freely available at the work stations. Except for the clinical settings, which are discussed later, the investigators were generally satisfied with whatever setting they had in place.

At sites where controlled and supervised access to the CD-ROM workstation was implemented, investigators reported that they had been concerned about two issues: availability of a librarian to provide assistance, and prevention of theft or damage to equipment. These sites found that the availability of librarians to provide assistance was in fact important to the success of the CD-ROM system. Sites with less control, however, did not cite lack of assistance from librarians as a shortcoming. Although several sites reported difficulties surrounding machine maintenance and system "lock-ups," none reported any problem with theft or vandalism of disks or equipment.

Data Collection

There was some variety in the data collection methods and instruments, but most asked each user to fill out a post-search questionnaire after every search, throughout the entire test period. At one site the questionnaires were administered on 11 sample days rather than every day throughout the test period. At another site, where data collection was automated, a substantial portion of the data collected was lost due to computer problems, so that the results reflect activity during only the latter part of the evaluation period. The post-search questionnaire contained comparable questions at each test site. Sites were provided with a "generic" questionnaire from NLM to use as a model, included here as Appendix A. Otherwise they had a free hand to design their evaluations according to the particular needs and circumstances of their institutions. The papers reporting their results indicate these variations from the instrument provided by NLM.

Composite Results

Almost 2000 questionnaires were collected during the course of the evaluation studies, but the questionnaires alone do not reflect the total amount of use. We estimate that over 4000 health professionals and students searched MEDLINE using one of the CD-ROM products during the course of the studies.

In this section we summarize the results from the questionnaires in a general way, aggregating data from all the test sites. Although answers to several questions ranged widely across the diverse test sites, and there is some variation in the questions that were included on the questionnaire, results given here reflect the general patterns reported. We first discuss users and uses in the health science library setting, then in the clinical care setting.

CD-ROM in the Health Sciences Library

The post-search questionnaire solicited information on user character-istics; types of searches performed and reasons for doing the search; user satisfaction with their searches and the search systems, including preferred access method; and reactions to product features and costs. These areas will be discussed in turn.

User characteristics

Contrary to speculation by many information professionals, CD-ROM is not just for students. In general, about one third of the users were students; about one third physicians, faculty, or researchers; and the remaining third a mixture of other classes of users. At one site it was noted that, although students made up the largest single group of CD-ROM users, their level of use was proportional to their numbers within that library's setting. As this observation points out, in order to accurately assess the audience for CD-ROM databases, it is important to consider user statistics in the context of the general user population at a particular setting. Although most test sites did not specifically compare the user characteristics in this way, the general impression is that the distribution of users of the CD-ROM system did not differ markedly from that of users of other MEDLINE sources.

Whenever a new access medium is introduced, one expects and hopes that the technology will reach new user populations. The CD-ROM technology did attract new users to MEDLINE. Generalizing across all test sites, an average of about 25% of those who had completed a questionnaire had not previously conducted or requested a MEDLINE search, although many had used *Index Medicus,* the printed counterpart to MEDLINE. At one site, however, none of the users were new to MEDLINE; all had previously requested a mediated search through the hospital library carrying out the evaluation.

The evaluation studies suggest that the CD-ROM products also attract users who have had previous experience with MEDLINE searching, either as end users or as requestors of mediated searches. Again generalizing across all test sites, about half of the CD-ROM users who responded to the questionnaire had requested mediated searches in the past, and about 25% were already performing their own online searches as end users.

Search characteristics

As most studies of online searching reveal, including a recent survey of individual users conducted by NLM (1), the overwhelming majority of searches performed were subject searches. Use of the MeSH vocabulary for subject searching varied across test sites, and appeared to depend on librarian involvement as well as the particular CD-ROM system used, since the implementation of MeSH varies across systems.

The concept of search complexity was not consistently or directly addressed in the study reports, but the clear impression is that users did simple searches of one or two words. Although the duration of searches was not reported directly, at most sites where users were restricted to specified time slots, scheduling of half-hour search sessions was sufficient for orderly pacing of CD-ROM use. One site, however, found it necessary to schedule search sessions in one-hour segments.

User satisfaction

User satisfaction and enthusiasm for searching MEDLINE on CD-ROM was high at all but one test site. At this site, a hospital library, users were satisfied with the mediated search service available to them and expressed little interest in changing to the CD-ROM system in order to perform their own searches.

There were differences in the level of enthusiasm between new users and those who were already end users of MEDLINE. Among those CD-ROM users who were not current users of MEDLINE online, CD-ROM was preferred overwhelmingly to the printed *Index Medicus* and to librarian-mediated searching. They appear to be happy to have a computerized system they can use themselves, without having to express their search topic to someone else and, to a certain extent, without having to pay for it. On the other hand, among CD-ROM users who were also end users of online databases, online searching was generally preferred, presumably due to their familiarity with the online system as well as the greater convenience, flexibility, and wider coverage of that access medium.

Product features and costs

A detailed analysis of features and capabilities was not done as part of the field test and evaluation at the twenty-one test sites. However, each system underwent testing by NLM staff during the development process to assure minimal standards of performance prior to release of the product. NLM also prepared a features checklist indicating the presence of a wide range of features, as of August 1988, for the seven field-tested products plus the eighth product that was not included in the evaluation project. The features checklist is included in this volume in an appendix. A product review by Kittle (2) is an additional source of comparative information on product features for six of the MEDLINE CD-ROM products.

In the evaluation studies, the post-search questionnaires generally included questions regarding the number of CD-ROM disks used, ease of changing disks, quality of online instructions and user manuals, system response time, product coverage, and overall ease of use. The individual study reports vary widely in their treatment of user reactions to product features and capabilities; the products themselves differ substantially from each other; and each of the products was evaluated at only three sites. It is therefore difficult to summarize reactions to specific product features in an overview paper, but certain general impressions can be captured.

Users did find CD-ROM products easy to use overall, and, as already mentioned, were generally satisfied with their search results. When users did encounter difficulty, they tended not to use the on-screen or printed documentation provided by the vendors, but rather requested assistance from available library staff. At some sites library staff compiled short handouts instructing users in the basics of the system, and these appeared to be the most useful of any types of documentation.

Users were split in their opinions about coverage of the CD-ROM MEDLINE versions, but generally indicated that it is desirable to include as many years and journals as possible. When faced with having to change disks in order to search the older literature, however, many users felt it was too cumbersome. As a group, researchers were more concerned about comprehensive coverage than were other users, especially with respect to the number of journals covered and the research focus of the journals.

Cost, or lack thereof, was consistently cited as an important factor in the decision to use a CD-ROM system. At the test institutions, as is the case in most settings where MEDLINE on CD-ROM is offered, no charge was imposed for use of the CD-ROM system. However, most users indicated they would be willing to pay $1.00-$5.00 for a search.

Management issues and concerns

While a few of the test sites expressed tremendous excitement about CD-ROM, enthusiasm of librarians was somewhat tempered by logistical and budget concerns, and in some cases by preference for local subsets of MEDLINE. At virtually all of the test sites, the librarians believe that CD-ROM is a valuable alternative to other modes of access to MEDLINE information, but they vary in their eagerness to embrace and promote it. By the end of the evaluation period, however, over half of the test sites had made the decision to purchase one of the CD-ROM MEDLINE systems.

Management issues were addressed in varying levels of detail and included staff time to support and train new users; equipment placement, security and maintenance (as already discussed); and the costs of supporting print, online, and CD-ROM products. A recent article by Halperin (3) addresses the cost aspects of online, CD-ROM, and inhouse search systems.

Most sites reported the need for a significant amount of staff support in helping users get started and in helping them recover from errors that resulted in the system freezing up. This prompted suggestions that some type of user training is needed, as well as better documentation. Users, however, made little use of on-screen or printed documentation. At some sites, librarians prepared one- or two-page handouts instructing users in the basics of system use; these seemed to be the most useful of any of the documentation provided. A few sites offered training sessions, but most did not. The amount of staff time devoted to assisting with the actual process of searching varied across sites according to policies that had been established. Librarians from several of the test sites felt that the users should not be "left alone" with the system, and expect to make it available only during the hours that the reference desk is staffed.

Most sites seemed willing to make the adjustment to duty schedules in order to accommodate the added demands of CD-ROM, partly because they believe CD-ROM to be an important addition to the library's resources and partly because it has time savings advantages that at least partially balance its demands. For example, several sites reported that CD-ROM relieved the volume of reference inquiries somewhat. The CD-ROM databases were also reported to be useful for performing simple and routine searches, bibliographic verification, and pre-search trials of search strategies to be run against online databases. At least one site reported that they are considering the use of CD-ROM systems as a replacement for little-used printed indexes and online searches for certain databases.

The evaluation reports also raise an area of concern that is not directly related to its impact on the management of library services. Several reports suggest that the CD-ROM systems may be deceptively easy to use, or that they are being operated on too simple a level that does not take full advantage of the power that is there. Since CD-ROM systems are designed for end user access, the concern is that less experienced users may be satisfied with searches that yielded less than optimal results. This concern, of course, is not limited to CD-ROM systems, but has been expressed in connection with any system targeted to the end user community. It is interesting to note that the concern dates back as far as 1915 (4), with a controversy over allowing library patrons to have "end user access" to the *Readers' Guide to Periodical Literature*.

Impact on online searching

One question of particular interest to the information community is how CD-ROM products will affect the searching of online databases. A recent article in Anders and Jackson (5) addresses this topic directly, and reports results similar to those found in the evaluation studies of MEDLINE on CD-ROM.

For the limited time period of the evaluations, the overall volume of online searches requested at the test sites did not decrease. There was one exception to this, where the online usage did decrease, but this was consistent with a gradual decreasing trend seen over the past year, and was not attributed to the availability of the CD-ROM product. CD-ROM appears to be finding its own niche and generally does not detract from online searching of MEDLINE. Study results suggest that it is an important supplement to online MEDLINE, but certainly not a replacement. In addition, there is some support for the suggestion that CD-ROM systems could in fact increase the overall volume of online searching by virtue of exposing and introducing new user groups to the benefits of computerized database searching.

As stated earlier, end users of online databases who also searched MEDLINE on CD-ROM tended to prefer the online database over CD-ROM. In addition, some of the users of mediated search services also preferred online databases, albeit in smaller numbers. Reasons cited in the study reports for a continuing preference by current users for doing online searches include:

- end users prefer the convenience and flexibility of doing searches from their home or office at any time of day;
- end users are already familiar with the system they are currently using and are unwilling to change;
- users prefer the wider coverage of the online databases and are unwilling to sacrifice coverage even for a free system;
- users of mediated search services are accustomed to the convenience of the online services provided by the library and do not have the time or interest to do searches on their own;
- ignorance about product distinctions, resulting in duplicate searches on CD-ROM systems and online databases;
- name and product recognition (one site reported that online MEDLINE and GRATEFUL MED were considered "prestigious").

Among end users of online databases, convenience is probably the most important reason for preferring online searching. CD-ROM systems as they exist today are stand-alone systems accessible from a single fixed location by only one user at a time. Some libraries suggested the possibility of networking CD-ROM systems, thereby making them widely available across campus and more convenient to use. Some of the CD-ROM vendors are in fact exploring the development of products for a networked environment.

CD-ROM technology is still very new. Levels of use are certain to increase as its availability becomes more widely known, and patterns of use are certain to change as well. Although some users expressed a preference for online searching, a substantial number did prefer the CD-ROM system. The number who prefer CD-ROM may very well increase as CD-ROM databases become more widespread and word of mouth increases awareness.

A negative impact on online searching can also come from use of CD-ROM by library staff. Several reports mentioned that librarians are using CD-ROM instead of the online database for simple searches and for pre-search testing. In the future, this could account for some decrease in online searching, although the volume of this type of search would be tempered in part by the use of the CD-ROM system by library patrons, since a typical CD-ROM workstation can be used by only one person at a time. As previously mentioned, CD-ROM databases are also under consideration as substitutes for print product subscriptions and online searching of certain databases. This type of use by libraries could have a more pronounced impact on the information industry.

CD-ROM in the Clinical Setting*

Since CD-ROM technology is especially targeted for use directly by end users, part of the evaluation project was designed to gain information about its use outside the library setting. At five of the test sites, investigators were also asked to place the CD-ROM workstation in a clinical practice setting for part of the evaluation period. The test sites participating in this clinical evaluation were the VA Medical Center in Biloxi, MS; St. Louis University; University of Utah; University of Nevada; and the University of Illinois Medical Center at Rockford. In addition to these five sites, three CD-ROM products were installed for two week periods in the emergency room at Suburban Hospital in Bethesda, MD.

The CD-ROM systems were installed in a variety of settings, including an internal medicine conference room, an operating room area, the office of the head nurse in a neurology unit, a patient floor, two ambulatory care clinics, and an emergency room. At each of the sites, little or no assistance or training was available from the library, and there was generally no system for monitoring the level of use that MEDLINE on CD-ROM was receiving.

Response to the post-search questionnaire was quite low in the clinical settings, but data collection was supplemented by focus groups and interviews with the investigators. At one site, the investigator reviewed transaction logs that were automatically captured at the time of each search. The results of these various data gathering mechanisms suggest that the systems received a low to moderate level of use. At the high end, approximately 60 searches over a seven week period were performed at the University of Nevada's clinical site, and 57 searches over an eight week period were performed at the University of Illinois clinical site. At the low end, only one search over a two week period was performed in the internal medicine department at the VA Medical Center in Biloxi. However, when the system was moved to the VA's ambulatory care clinic for a second two week period, almost all of the 14 physicians performed at least one search.

Reasons suggested for relatively low usage included: the environment was not conducive to searching; the need for factual rather than bibliographic information in some circumstances, e.g., in the emergency room; lack of time or

---

* A composite report of the Evaluation Forum panel discussion on clinical uses of MEDLINE on CD-ROM has been prepared by its moderator, Dr. Prudence Dalrymple, and appears in this volume as a separate paper. In addition to capturing the essence of the issues addressed by the panel, the paper describes each of the clinical settings and summarizes the results that were reported.

lack of information need during the test period; lack of assistance from a librarian; and, in the case where the system was located in the office of the head nurse, limited access to the system.

Most users were satisfied with the searches they did and with the journal coverage and time span of the products used. Users were generally in favor of having MEDLINE on CD-ROM available at the clinical site, mainly because of its convenience and availability during late hours. However, those who delegated their searching to an assistant generally indicated that proximity to the system was not important to them. There did appear to be a consensus that someone should be available to assist with system use when needed.

Several issues concerning CD-ROM in clinical settings were raised in the evaluation reports, some extending beyond the characteristics of CD-ROM as the particular database access medium. The questions raised include: Who should be responsible for training and attending to users' questions and technical problems in a clinical setting? What is the quality of the searches performed? What type of information is needed by clinicians, and what is the immediacy of the information need? When and where do clinicians prefer to do their MEDLINE searching? These and other questions were addressed at the Evaluation Forum during the panel discussion of the clinical setting experiences.

The Evaluation Forum

The Evaluation Forum held September 23, 1988, was a culmination of the evaluation process. With the National Library of Medicine as the catalyst, it provided an opportunity for all participants — vendors, evaluators, current users, and prospective users — to come together for the purpose of sharing data, experiences, and insights. The Forum consisted of a full day of panel sessions as well as hands-on exhibits of all the vendors' systems, and was attended by over 250 people.

The panel sessions were designed to explore the key issues of:

Who are the users of MEDLINE on CD-ROM?

What is the role of CD-ROM in biomedical information transfer at libraries and other potential points of use, here and abroad?

What are the favored system features, capabilities, and database contents for MEDLINE on CD-ROM?

What impact will this technology have on library services, management, and costs?

What does the future hold for this new information technology?

Although NLM had already heard from the study participants carrying out the evaluations, by way of their formal evaluation reports, the Evaluation Forum was an especially important opportunity to hear from the CD-ROM vendors. From their perspective, the evaluation period was useful to them, and improvements have been made to each of the products as a result.

In looking forward, the vendors expect greater use of data compression techniques and more multi-slot readers in the near future. This is in response to the real inconvenience of having to change disks when moving from one database year to the next. Multi-user access via local area networks is being explored by some of the vendors, as is the integration of graphics. We can also expect to see further blurring of the distinction between CD-ROM and online systems, e.g., with dial-up capabilities to retrieve very old or very recent references from online databases. In this regard, NLM announced at the Evaluation Forum that it will make available to interested CD-ROM vendors the Grateful Med search engine which will permit dial-up access to MEDLINE on NLM's computers.

Conclusion

The evaluation studies proved to be valuable for the participating libraries, the CD-ROM vendors, and the National Library of Medicine. A large number of libraries, not always large in size, had the opportunity to gain firsthand experience in carrying out a formal evaluation having national implications. Their feedback regarding product coverage, product features, and user acceptance was important in shaping the products as they are today. As one of the vendors stated during the Evaluation Forum, the evaluative and competitive environment created by NLM encouraged the CD-ROM vendors to produce for the biomedical community the very best products possible.

References

1. Wallingford, Karen T.; Selinger, Nancy E.; Humphreys, Betsy L.; and Siegel, Elliot R. *Survey of individual users of MEDLINE on the NLM system*. Bethesda, Md.: U.S. Dept. of Health and Human Services, Public Health Service, National Institutes of Health, National Library of Medicine, 1988 Nov. 130p. (Technical Report No. NLM-MED-88-04; NTIS Order No. PB89-133722).

2. Kittle, Paul. Medline on CD-ROM: A review of six products. *Laserdisk Professional* 1988 Sep;1(3):18-28.

3. Halperin, Michael and Renfro, Patricia. Online vs CD-ROM vs onsite: high volume searching — considering the alternatives. *Online* 1988 Nov;12(6):36-42.

4. Bacon, Corinne. The Readers' Guide: why not let the reader use it. *The Wilson Bulletin* 1915 May;1(3):40-42.

5. Anders, Vicki and Jackson, Kathy M. Online vs CD-ROM: the impact of CD-ROM databases upon a large online searching program. *Online* 1988 Nov;12(6):24-32.

TABLE 1
PRODUCT NAMES, MEDLINE COVERAGE, AND VENDORS

Product Name and Coverage at Time of Field Test	Vendor Name and Address

MEDLINE Knowledge Finder
   Core Product:
   220 MEDLINE Clinical Journals*
   1984-1988
   Five years/disk
   Comprehensive Product:
   All MEDLINE Journals
   1983-1988**
   One year/disk
	Aries Systems Corporation
	1 Dundee Park
	Andover, MA 01810
	Phone: 508-475-7200

BRS/COLLEAGUE Disc
   All MEDLINE English
   Language Journals
   1985-1988
   One year/disk
	BRS Information Technologies
	1200 Route 7
	Latham, NY 12110
	Phone: 518-783-1161

Compact Cambridge MEDLINE
   All MEDLINE Journals
   1982-1988**
   One year/disk
	Cambridge Scientific Abstracts
	7200 Wisconsin Avenue
	Bethesda, MD 20814
	Phone: 301-961-6700

DIALOG OnDisc MEDLINE
   All MEDLINE Journals
   1984-1988
   One year/disk
	Dialog Information Services, Inc.
	3460 Hillview Avenue
	Palo Alto, CA 94034
	Phone: 415-858-4058 or 800-334-2564

BiblioMed
   500 MEDLINE English
   Language Journals
   1985-1988
   Three years/disk
	Digital Diagnostics
	601 University Avenue
	Sacramento, CA 95825
	Phone: 916-921-6629

MEDLINE/EBSCO CD-ROM
   Core Product:
   Abridged Index Medicus,
   Nursing, Dentistry Journals*
   1985-1988
   Three years/disk
   Comprehensive Product:***
   All MEDLINE Journals
   1986-present
   One year/disk
	EBSCO Electronic Information, Inc.
	P.O. Box 13787
	Torrence, CA 90503
	Phone: 213-530-7533

SilverPlatter MEDLINE
   All MEDLINE Journals
   1983-1988**
   One year/disk
	SilverPlatter Information, Inc.
	37 Walnut Street
	Wellesley Hills, MA 02181
	Phone: 617-239-0306

Compact Med-Base***
   All MEDLINE Journals
   1966-present
   Entire database on 8 disks
	Online Research Systems, Inc.
	951 Amsterdam Avenue, Suite 2C
	New York, NY 10025
	Phone: 212-932-1481 or 212-408-3311

*   Journal coverage has been enhanced since the field test
** The 1989 product will cover additional MEDLINE back files
*** Not included in field tests

TABLE 2
TEST SITES AND CD-ROM SYSTEMS EVALUATED

Test Site	Assigned MEDLINE CD-ROM System	Other CD-ROM Systems Evaluated
Oregon Health Sciences Univ.	BiblioMed	None
Univ. of Nevada School of Medicine @	BiblioMed	None
Univ. of California, Davis	BiblioMed	None
St. Louis Univ. @	BRS/Colleague Disc	MICROMEDEX
Univ. of North Carolina at Chapel Hill	BRS/Colleague Disc	None
School of Medicine and Dentistry, Univ. Rochester	BRS/Colleague Disc	None
Columbia Univ. *	Compact Cambridge	Not Named in Report
Univ. of Washington	Compact Cambridge	None
Tufts Univ.	Compact Cambridge	None
New York Academy of Medicine	DIALOG OnDisc	None
Univ. of Nebraska Medical Center	DIALOG OnDisc	BRS/Colleague Disc Compact Cambridge Ebsco CD-ROM SilverPlatter
Univ. of Texas Southwestern Medical Center	DIALOG OnDisc	None
Univ. of Utah @	Ebsco CD-ROM	SilverPlatter
VA Medical Center Biloxi, MS @	Ebsco CD-ROM	None
Univ. of Illinois at Chicago	Ebsco CD-ROM	None
Univ. of Illinois College of Medicine at Rockford @	Knowledge Finder	None
Good Samaritan Medical Center, Phoenix, AR	Knowledge Finder	None
Medical University of South Carolina **	Knowledge Finder	Ebsco CD-ROM
George Washington Univ. Medical Center **	SilverPlatter	BRS/Colleague Disc Compact Cambridge
UCLA ***	SilverPlatter	None
Meharry Medical College	SilverPlatter	Compact Cambridge

@ Test sites participating in clinical evaluations

* At this site CD-ROM system was compared with in-house system, CLIO

** At these sites CD-ROM systems were also compared with in-house system, miniMEDLINE

*** At this site CD-ROM system was compared with in-house system, MELVYL MEDLINE

"GENERIC" MEDLINE CD-ROM EVALUATION QUESTIONNAIRE
(JANUARY 1988)

Instructions

This MEDLINE CD-ROM (Product Name) system is being tested by
the (site name). We would like you to fill out this
questionnaire in order to help us find out who is using the
system, and how useful it is to you. Thank you!
(Note: Provide users with details on how answers are to be
recorded; to whom questionnaires should be returned, etc.)

1.   My primary affiliations is:

     a. Medicine   d. Public Health

     b. Dentistry   e. Occupational/Physical Therapy

     c. Nursing   f. Other

     Enter ONE only:

2.   My profession is:

     a. physician

     b. nurse

     c. dentist

     d. other health care professional

     e. educator

     f. scientist/researcher

     g. student

     h. librarian

     i. other

     Enter ALL that apply:

3.   I was looking for articles:

     a. by an author

     b. under a title

c. on a subject

d. in a journal

e. other

Enter ALL that apply:

4. I needed the information for:

a. patient care

b. a paper or report

c. a research project

d. keeping current

e. to check a reference

f. teaching/planning a course

g. not needed, just curious

h. other

Enter ALL that apply

5. The information I found was:

a. what I was looking for

b. more than I needed

c. some of what I needed

d. not useful

e. other

Enter ONE only:

6. Have you used any of the printed publications produced from the MEDLINE system (e.g. INDEX MEDICUS, the INTERNATIONAL NURSING INDEX, the INDEX TO DENTAL LITERATURE, or the HOSPITAL LITERATURE INDEX)?

a. yes

b. no

c. don't know

Enter ONE only:

7.   If yes, you've used printed versions, how do they
      compare to (Product Name) MEDLINE?

      a. easier to use

      b. harder to use

      c. about the same to use

      d. other

      Enter ONE only:

8.   Have you used an online version of MEDLINE (either
      yourself or by having a librarian process a search
      for you)?

      a. yes, by myself

      b. yes, librarian search

      c. no

      d. don't know

      Enter ALL that apply:

9.   If yes, you've used online MEDLINE, which system do you
      prefer?

      a. online, own search

      b. (Product Name) MEDLINE

      c. online, librarian search

      d. don't know

      Enter ONE only:

10.   If this MEDLINE CD-ROM system had not been available
      today, what would you have done?

      a. used a printed version

b. used an online version

c. asked a library staff member

d. asked a friend or colleague

e. browsed through the stacks

f. nothing

g. other

Enter ALL that apply:

11. Next time you need this sort of information, what will you do?

a. try (Product Name) MEDLINE

b. try a printed version

c. try an online version

d. try another source

Enter ALL that apply:

12. (Product Name) MEDLINE is provided free of charge to library users. How important a consideration was this in your decision to use this system, instead of an online version of MEDLINE?

a. very important

b. somewhat important

c. relatively unimportant

d. would not have used an online version of MEDLINE

Enter ONE only:

13. How often have you used (Product Name) MEDLINE

a. first time

b. once before

c. 3-5 times

d. 6 or more times

14. (Product Name) MEDLINE contains material on (blank)
     discs covering (blank) years. How many discs did you
     use today?

     a. 1 disc

     b. 2 discs

     c. 3 discs

     d. (number as many discs as applicable)

15. Instructions on (Product Name) MEDLINE screens were
     sufficient for my use.

Enter ONE only (on the following 5 point scale) for
questions 15 through 20.

SCALE: A   B   C   D   E
        Strongly   Strongly
         Agree   Agree   Neutral   Disagree   Disagree

16. The rate at which the computer responds is
     satisfactory.

17. The (Product Name) MEDLINE manual helped me to use the
     system.

18. Changing (Product Name) MEDLINE discs is easy.

19. The time span covered by (Product Name) MEDLINE was
     sufficient for my needs.

20. Overall, I found (Product Name) MEDLINE easy to use.

CLINICAL USES OF MEDLINE ON CD-ROM
A Composite Report of a Panel Discussion on Five Sites

Prudence Ward Dalrymple
Library of the Health Sciences
University of Illinois College of Medicine at Rockford
1601 Parkview Ave., Rockford, IL 61107

This article summarizes findings from six clinical sites in which a MED-LINE CD-ROM system was made available to health care practitioners (see Table 1). Five of these clinical studies were conducted in conjunction with formal, library-based evaluations in which data were collected, analyzed and reported as part of the National Library of Medicine's CD-ROM MEDLINE Evaluation Forum. The sixth consisted of short evaluations conducted entirely in the Emergency Room of a community hospital in Bethesda, Maryland. Compared to the library-based studies, the clinical evaluations were much more informal in nature, and while the reports are derived mostly from anecdotal information, they provide numerous insights about the assessment of information systems in clinical settings, and about the process of clinical information gathering itself.

Initially, clinical settings were defined as those in which the CD-ROM system was made available at the point of health care delivery, such as an ambulatory care clinic, emergency room, nursing station, or departmental conference room. In reviewing sites for inclusion in the panel session, however, this definition of a clinical setting was expanded to include hospital libraries since these are common access points for transfer of biomedical literature to practitioners. Furthermore, despite wide variations among hospital libraries in terms of collections, services, and accessibility, most hospital librarians regard the delivery of clinical information to health care professionals as a primary objective. The clinical sites included both urban and rural environments and both teaching and non-teaching settings.

While typical biomedical information support services such as mediated MEDLINE searching, document delivery, and reference services were available to practitioners at all sites, not all sites provided end-user information retrieval systems such as Grateful Med or PaperChase. In all cases, placing the CD-ROM in a clinical area represented an additional enhancement to information access.

The descriptive findings presented in this paper were gleaned from reviewing the clinical reports of the six evaluation sites. Pertinent data regarding the sites, the systems, and the evaluation are summarized in Table 1; additional information is presented below. To the extent possible in such an exploratory study, common findings across sites are discussed. Additionally, the discussion questions developed by the author in consultation with the investigators are presented, together with the panelists' response to them at the Evaluation Forum.

I. Clinical Evaluation Sites

At the Veterans Administration Medical Center in Biloxi, Mississippi, the EBSCO system was placed in the internal medicine department for two weeks and in the ambulatory care department for two weeks. In the outpatient setting, the system was used only once, but in the internal medicine department, most physicians used the system at least once. Biloxi VA had not previously provided end-user searching.

The St. Louis University Medical Center is an urban teaching hospital with a wide range of library services, including a program of clinician end-user searching (Grateful Med) initiated by the pathology department that met with varying degrees of success. In both Biloxi and St. Louis, the decision to place the CD-ROM MEDLINE in the internal medicine department conference room was made partly in response to a request from the departmental chair. Although only nine users filled out questionnaires, the calls for assistance in searching suggests that considerably more searching took place.

Clinicians at the University of Utah's teaching hospital have access to biomedical literature both through a clinical library located at the hospital and through the Spencer S. Eccles Health Sciences Library. The latter is currently engaged in development and implementation of the IAIMS (Integrated Academic Information Management System) program in conjunction with the National Library of Medicine. Both mediated online searches and end-user access to Grateful Med and BRS Colleague are available in the clinical library. The CD-ROM MEDLINE system was located in the head nurse's office on the neurology unit, and the head nurse and her assistant conducted searches in response to requests from nurses and other health professionals.

In Nevada, two clinical evaluations of BiblioMed were conducted at teaching sites of the University of Nevada. In one of the settings, the clinical library, the system was accessible primarily to library staff, who logged more than half of the 60 searches recorded. At the VA hospital, the system was located on the third floor of the hospital, whereas the library's CD-ROM system was located in a building adjacent to the hospital. All 57 of these searches were conducted by residents, clerks and clinical faculty.

The Aries System's Knowledge Finder, the only CD-ROM MEDLINE available for Macintosh, was placed in an ambulatory care clinic at the Office for Family Practice at the University of Illinois College of Medicine at Rockford. A transaction log captured data about the process of searching the system, as well as providing an unobtrusive measure of the amount of searching that was done (26 searches in two months). No other end-user searching is available in Rockford.

At Suburban Hospital in Bethesda, Maryland, three CD-ROM systems were rotated through the Emergency Room for a period of two weeks each. Dr. Robert Rothstein, Chairman of the Department of Emergency Medicine, reported his observations of the ways in which these systems were used by health care professionals throughout the six weeks they were available.

Even though each evaluation had a character all its own, some things were experienced in common.

• Most non-library clinical settings had little or no assistance of any kind available for searchers on site. Searchers were given neither training prior to nor coaching during their search sessions.

• There appeared to be no correlation between whether clinical departments themselves had initiated the request for a CD-ROM and the level of use or satisfaction observed. Departments that were eager for the system evidenced some of the lowest use, leading to speculations that there may have been other motives for requesting the equipment, such as status, or personal, non-MEDLINE related uses such as word processing.

• Where mechanical problems occurred, none proved insurmountable, either to the users or the librarian evaluators. During this study, at least, risk factors such as damage or loss were not a problem.

• As might be expected, obtaining responses to questionnaires in unmonitored sites was very difficult. The preferred methods of data collection were logs, interviews, and personal observation.

II. Evaluation Questions and Issues

In order to synthesize the findings of the clinical evaluations, it was decided to structure the panel around a set of common issues and questions. Some of these questions were derived from the list provided by the National Library of Medicine, while others emerged from conversations among the panelists and author during the preparation of the panel presentation. Still others were suggested by the growing body of literature on information transfer in the clinical medical setting. A tentative set of questions was sent to the panelists for their consideration. Each panelist was asked to think about the questions and to rank them in importance and relevance to their experience. The author also interviewed each evaluator and from these discussions, proposed a final set of questions that were to form the basis of the panel presentation. The questions are:

• Who are the users of MEDLINE on CD-ROM in the clinical setting?

• What factors predict the successful use of CD-ROM in a clinical setting?

• What are the problems associated with the evaluation of results of information retrieval in a clinical setting?

• What is the role of CD-ROM MEDLINE in urban and rural settings, or in developing countries?

• In clinical settings what are users' preferences for the delivery of biomedical information via CD-ROM?

• What enhancements should vendors consider in designing CD-ROM products for clinical settings?

III. Who Are the Users of CD-ROM MEDLINE?

Clinical settings in which there is a commitment to teaching generally had the highest level of use. Students are avid users of CD-ROM MEDLINE. In part, this may be attributable to the lack of an access fee. Another factor is the continual need in medical school to stay abreast of recent developments and to review the literature from an academic perspective. Residents comprise another heavy user group for similar reasons. In hospitals, third and fourth year medical students are frequent users, while in academic medical libraries, first and second year students are the heaviest users. When the systems were placed in areas accessible to nurses and other health personnel, these groups were more likely to use the CD-ROM.

There may be many reasons that account for this pattern. Physicians who are in private practice in a community hospital are much more likely to know their patients, to know how to treat their hospitalized patients, and to feel more pressure to run back to their primary offices. If these clinicians have the need to search for information, they are used to delegating that responsibility, just as they delegate many other aspects of patient care. For this group, physical proximity to the information source is less an issue than it is for staff based in the hospital, such as nurses. That is, a faculty member or clinician based in his or her home office will send a secretary over to the library to retrieve information, while a nurse is more likely to access an information system only if it is physically proximate to the primary office, usually located on the patient care floor. Area of specialization may also predict use of CD-ROM MEDLINE. One panelist suggested that physicians in primary care specialties such as internal medicine are more likely than those in surgery or emergency medicine to search the literature and therefore to use MEDLINE in whatever form it is provided.

Location of the CD-ROM also determines to a large extent the user population. If the system is introduced on the nursing unit, nurses will be the heaviest users; if placed in a department of medicine, clinical faculty and residents will be heaviest users. If the CD-ROM is located in the library, the most frequent use will be by those who either have the time to visit the library or whose need to know is sufficient to motivate them to overcome other barriers to convenience. In most instances, the user population will also be more heterogeneous in a library than in a clinical setting. For example, when the CD-ROM was located in a nursing area, other nurses from adjacent floors tended to use it because they regarded it as belonging to nurses in general, as distinct from students or doctors.

These findings suggest another perspective on the general assumption that physical proximity of the information source is a strong determinant of information use. That is, proximity is inversely correlated with ability to delegate information searching. When delegation is an option, physical proximity no longer matters; when delegation is impossible, physical proximity becomes an issue. Additionally, interest in the technology of the system and personal motivation to seek information led to system use. If interest and motivation were absent, even having the system in the office next door would not entice individuals to use it.

IV. Factors Contributing to Successful Use of CD-ROM

From the panel's discussions, several dimensions of successful implementation of CD-ROM MEDLINE were identified. One dimension is locating and sponsoring the system within the clinical setting. It is important to have an understanding of the sociology of the institution, particularly those who act as its gatekeepers, as well as an ability to enlist the support of these individuals.

At the University of Nevada, enthusiasm on the part of the person initially requesting the system contributed to the successful integration of CD-ROM MEDLINE into the teaching program. The requestor, a clinical faculty member, used it as a tool for learning in the clinical setting. Many of the clerks and residents who used the system had already had experience with computers and did not find it intimidating in any way. In fact, they usually regarded searching CD-ROM as fun. At St. Louis University, there was strong support and interest from the departmental chair, who publicized it and made it available in the conference room. At the University of Utah hospital, having an individual to promote and manage the system was a contributing factor to its successful adoption on the neurology nursing unit.

The level of responsibility and involvement these sponsors were prepared to deliver differed across sites, as did their apparent motives for becoming involved. Some were motivated by a sense of control, wanting the system to be available only to their group or department so that they would not have to compete for access as they might in a library. Being able to retreat to an office or conference late at night where they could work uninterrupted was appealing to this group. In another instance, the sponsor provided instruction and assistance partly in return for having the system located adjacent to an office and partly to maintain control. While many health care staff expressed curiosity about the CD-ROM, they often felt as if access was being controlled by the sponsor or gatekeeper. Additionally, the presence of technical equipment in the unit enhanced the status of the staff who worked there.

Another dimension is a realistic approach to providing support to users of the system. The willingness or ability of gatekeepers to provide the necessary instruction or back-up support varied. While one head nurse was willing and able to provide assistance (even mediated searches) for health care personnel, clinical faculty in another institution complained bitterly that the department chair insisted on providing instruction, the quality of which was questionable. Reports of such experiences led the panel to speculate as to whether initial instruction and ongoing support are needed in a clinical setting and if so, who should provide them.

In one of the evaluations (Jones), instruction was given a high priority. During the library evaluation, formal training classes were given. It was found that the subjects that were given the training were more comfortable with complex subject searching and appeared to be more satisfied with their search results. Whether the effect was due to the actual training or resulted from increased self-confidence was unclear. In the clinical evaluation, however, classes were given to groups of fourteen physicians at a medical staff meeting. There was no "hands on" instruction prior to the clinical evaluation, whereas there was considerable "hands on" time during the library classes.

Searching support from library staff was available by telephone in another site (Plutchak). The most frequent difficulty that searchers had was not with the technique of searching on CD-ROM, but on the intellectual formulation of a search and how to select terms. Because the clinical setting was physically remote from the library, users were not willing to take the time to contact the reference librarian. How to provide effective, accessible support to users located in a clinical setting and who should provide that support remains an important issue not only for planning but also for evaluation of CD-ROM MEDLINE.

Initial enthusiasm was often accompanied by a lack of understanding of the system's capabilities, however. When the systems actually arrived and turned out not to meet expectations, sometimes they were not used. For example, one ambulatory care practitioner was disappointed that the system gave her a bibliographic citation instead of a complete answer. While users at some sites found the journal coverage of their system's database less than adequate in both size and scope, others appreciated the limited scope. For example, Zenan reported that one of the reasons BiblioMed was so successful was that it covers 500 English language journals for a three year period. Almost everything that users found was available either in the hospital library or at other local libraries. Document delivery even within the institution was a major factor in the success of CD-ROM MEDLINE in Mississippi (Jones). What users wanted was "one stop shopping" where they can go to one place and get everything they need. Where that source was located was less important than the comprehensiveness of the service.

VI. Evaluation of Search Results in a Clinical Setting

Most evaluators attempted to get a sense of how satisfied users were with the results they received, and unanimously, they reported that users were very satisfied with the CD-ROM MEDLINE. Not every evaluator was willing to take this observation at face value, however. At one site, the evaluator (Plutchak) reported,

"As we got further into the study, we became more and more concerned about the reliability of using the idea of satisfaction and what it really meant when somebody said that they were satisfied. Most everybody loved the system. They liked using it. It's fun. They get in and they get something out, but we can tell from our observations that a lot of them are not using the system terribly well and perhaps not getting what they think that they're getting. This is a real concern for us. I had an extreme example of a woman who never got the hang of combining terms. So she would go in with a couple of search terms and she would print out her citations and then she would put in the next term and print out her citations. Then she would walk out with her two printouts, really happy, really satisfied. She loved the system. She was there a couple of times a week. "

The evaluator went on to express concern that in the clinical setting it was more difficult to identify users who were having difficulty, partly because they could not be observed while they were searching, and were unlikely to call or visit the library. In order to convey the relationship of aptitude with satisfaction, he described the matrix that appears in Figure 1.

FIGURE 1

```
                    Satisfaction
              Low           High
      High
                    |        |
                    |        |
                    A        B
   Aptitude  _____

      Low          |   C    |   D
```

The four quadrants describe four user experiences. Those who are inept at searching and also dissatisfied will present themselves for assistance (Quadrant C). Those who are good searchers but dissatisfied with their results will also present themselves in order to complain about the system (Quadrant A). The third group are competent searchers who are satisfied with their results (Quadrant B). They present themselves only to obtain additional access. The fourth group is comprised of those inept searchers who are satisfied with their results. Individuals of this type rarely present themselves because they are happy with whatever they have retrieved. This is the group described by Plutchak. The question of responsibility for and obligation to this group of searchers is important to librarians who are working in clinical settings. That is, if a system is paid for by a clinical department for its own use, should the library care whether it is used effectively? Further, what is the role of the library vis `a vis the flow of information within the institution?

Other panelists had a different perspective. From her interviews with a cardiologist, Dougherty observed that while he does not exploit their full capabilities, he still finds very useful information for his practice from both CD-ROM MEDLINE and BRS Colleague. From his point of view, then, he is being successful, even though he may not be finding the "right" things, or may not be obtaining full retrieval. Dougherty also suggested that another way of enhancing success is by tailoring the coverage of the CD-ROM to a particular group. In a MEDLINE subset that emphasized nursing literature, nurses were more satisfied with their results.

VII. The Role of CD-ROM MEDLINE in Urban and Rural Settings and Developing Countries

The clinical evaluations took place in a variety of settings, both urban and rural. Those working in rural settings, however, expressed their belief that CD-ROM has great potential utility in areas where telecommunications can be problematic. The ability to plug the system into an electrical outlet and not worry about modems and telephone connection is appealing to staff who are busy with patient care. Most systems were designed to be directly accessible by end-users and were relatively trouble-free. As the search interfaces improve as they almost certainly will, CD-ROM technology presents a very viable way for health care practitioners to obtain biomedical information. A clinical subset of MEDLINE, including abstracts, where available, is a particularly attractive product.

VIII. Clinicians' Preferences for Delivery of Biomedical Information in a Clinical Setting

The majority of the CD-ROM evaluations were conducted in libraries by librarians, but in the clinical evaluations, questions were raised about how information is best delivered to health care professionals, and whether the library has a role in and responsibility for insuring that adequate, accurate information is made available in the clinic. The easy installation of a CD-ROM MEDLINE and the freedom from maintaining records of connect time charges or restricting database access has made CD-ROM a very appealing technology for non-library settings. Just what information should be available on the CD-ROM and in what form is another question. Some panelists (Rothstein and Jones) suggested that the capabilities of CD-ROM MEDLINE may be more useful in an inpatient setting than in an out-patient setting. In an Emergency Room, the need for information may be so acute that a clinician has neither the time nor the desire to look at a recent article on a given topic. All that matters is what the disease is, and how to treat it. Textbook-like material together with a brief bibliography may be more helpful. The bibliography provides the incentive to go to MEDLINE later on to look at more recent literature. In teaching hospitals, the availability of MEDLINE at all times so that both faculty and students can seek out the most recent articles for use in both patient care and in preparing rounds is highly desirable.

IX. Desired Enhancements for CD-ROM MEDLINE in the Clinical Setting

Overall, both users and evaluators liked the systems. The ability to tailor MEDLINE subsets to user groups would be desirable, however. Clinicians do not require immediate access to basic research literature, and reducing the size of the files often eliminates the need to switch disks. The experience of having MEDLINE on CD-ROM in clinics and hospitals prompted some users to wish for MEDLINE on their local network, along with patient information. Users of other information systems such as MicroMedex or EmergIndex would like to be able to move from that system immediately into MEDLINE, either on-line or on CD-ROM. Users would like a single access to information in multiple systems and in varied formats such as textbook, abstract, or bibliographic citation. The varied information needs of clinicians suggests that while MEDLINE CD-ROM does not replace technologies already available, it occupies an important place in the spectrum of information systems currently available.

TABLE 1
CLINICAL SITES FOR MEDLINE CD-ROM EVALUATION

Location	Site	CD-ROM System	Duration	Subjects	Data Collected From:	Investigator
Internal Medicine Ambulatory Care	VA Medical Center Biloxi, MS	EBSCO	2 weeks	1 M.D. 14 M.D.'s	Focus groups	Jones
Internal Medicine Conference Room	St. Louis University Medical Center, St. Louis, MO	BRS	4 weeks	9 M.D.'s	Question- naires, observation	Plutchak
Neurology Unit Nursing Station	University of Utah Hospital	EBSCO	8 weeks	Nurses	Interviews	Dougherty
Clinical Library	University Medical Center, Las Vegas, NV	BiblioMed	7 weeks	M.D.'s students health profession- als, library staff (60)	User log	Zenan
Patient floor	VA Hospital Reno, NV	BiblioMed	8 weeks	M.D.'s Clerks, residents (57)	User log, interviews	Zenan
Ambulatory Care Clinic	University of Illinois Office for Family Practice, Rockford	Knowledge Finder	8 weeks	Residents	Transaction logs, nterviews	Dalrymple
Emergency Room	Suburban Hospital Bethesda, MD	EBSCO, Silver Platter Cambridge	2 weeks each	M.D.'s	Observation	Rothstein

ASSESSING THE COSTS DURING BUDGET PLANNING FOR MEDLINE ON CD-ROM

by Paul B. Kantor
Tantalus, Inc.
3257 Ormond Road,
Cleveland, Ohio 44118

When I heard Dr. Rothstein of Suburban Hospital in Bethesda talking this morning about the pressures of emergency room work, I thought that preparing this economic report is much like emergency room work. I had to get some answers together in a hurry in order to get the "patient" up in the ward where you can really take care of him. I put together a short list of questions whose answers would help to define a concrete cost model for the CD-ROM operation in a library. The idea is this: it's pretty clear that any technology that permits unlimited use with no *per use* charge will eventually become very cost effective. If you prepare a standard budget, showing cost per use, you can easily persuade your boss that this is a good buy. You will soon have the equipment and begin the service. Unfortunately, because it really was a good choice, use grows. You get into that familiar but paradoxical situation where the (unit) cost is very low but you are spending quite a large amount. There are some growth and support factors you may have failed to identify as costs in your first budget.

These factors seem to be relevant. At least, when I talked to librarians involved in this project they agreed with me about considering them (but some went on to say that they didn't have time to look into it). When I talked to the CD-ROM vendors they said, "That's the kind of information that is important, but it's probably proprietary."

I visualize the cost model for CD-ROM use as being broken into three columns and four rows (See Figure 1). The columns are hardware, software, and

Figure 1
Cost model for CD-ROM

	Hardware	Software	Staff
Fixed			
Month-ized			
Time-based			
Use-based			

peopleware (or staff). The costs are *fixed month-ized* (i.e., costs in terms of months), *time-based* (i.e., costs incurred per month or per year whether or not anyone is using the service) and finally *use-based* costs which will grow as the use grows. The four shaded squares represent the most difficult parts of the cost model to figure out (e.g., hardware costs, time-based and all use-based costs).

Other costs can give trouble. In the first row (fixed costs), the hardware cost is difficult to estimate because maintenance costs are never known at the beginning. It's cost related to the hardware that occurs over time because the equipment does not work. One estimate I obtained from a vendor is that 2% of the units which had been out in the field for about a year have had problems. Over a five-year time span that means that about ten percent will have problems. I am cautious about using this estimate because when I bring together people who have been selling CD-ROM equipment for about two years, hardly anybody would report having had any trouble. Yet we all listened to the talks this morning and we have heard things as extreme as one maintenance call per day needed to keep things working. A lot of factors go into making this number elusive: the vendors can only report what comes to their attention; anything that was fixable in the library didn't come to their attention. Those vendors who don't provide maintenance support or hardware support don't find out about the problems.

Many conversations with manufacturers of computer equipment prompt me to say that when they quote a figure of five years as the mean time between failures what they really mean is "for our equipment that works."

When you take equipment out of the box you don't know whether you got one of the ones that works. Most likely, high performance reflects experience *after* the first month, which may not count in the reported performance statistics.

In summary, I think it's probably reasonable to suppose that you will have one *major* problem just about every year. That means you will incur some cost that is extremely hard to calculate. There's a direct cost. You will have to pay for a maintenance call or for a maintenance contract. Also, you should estimate the cost of lost service for the few days you are without the equipment. Even your in-house maintenance repairs will incur some loss of service, and lost service should be considered even if it is for only a three- or four-hour period.

Before making such a purchase it would be a good idea to talk to a lot of people who have CD-ROMs and ask about them about their experiences with breakdowns and maintenance. Even better than this informal data collection would be some kind of formal sharing of information among people who are moving ahead in this field. I think that it is important to go into any new service with our eyes open about such costs.

An easier cost to compute is the cost of hardware (See Figure 2). The pur-

Figure 2

HARDWARE: $\quad \dfrac{2500}{5 \times 12} = \$41.67/\text{mo.}$

chase cost may be divided by sixty months to get some kind of monthly figure. I use five years as the lifetime for a piece of equipment because it probably will last five years if it is "one of the ones that works." You may not be *satisfied* with it for five years, but you might not be satisfied with it after three years. I don't know how to factor that in as a hard economic fact.

Similarly there are *software* or database costs (See Figure 3). Under the

Figure 3

SOFTWARE:

Current   **Back**

$$750/\text{yr.} + 4 \times 500 = 2750/\text{yr.}$$

$$\frac{2750}{12} = \$230/\text{mo.}$$

lease basis by which MEDLINE is available, those costs can easily be expressed in terms of a cost per year or cost per month. As I understand it, you buy in a year at a time, but you must remain current in order to prevent outdated information from getting to your patrons.

There is a box in the upper right hand corner which is fixed cost related to staff. That's where you would put, at least initially, the cost required for training the staff. The people whom I surveyed by telephone downplayed that cost and suggested that it might be no more than four hours training time. The more detailed reports that we heard this morning suggest figures like thirty hours of staff training time. Again, all I can say is "talk to people who really have been responsible for handling that training to get a realistic number."

As we have heard several times the prior computer experience of the people involved is a determining factor. If you are going to use this occasion to upgrade the computer literacy of particular individuals it will cost more than if you take the less expensive route and only train computer-literate people who can learn the CD-ROM system without any help.

Now we are ready to worry about the much more difficult problems of use-based costs (See Figure 4). There are two kinds of users: new and old. Each of

Figure 4

	Uses Month	Use Time Month	Support Time Month
New Users			
Old Users			

these types will, as time goes by, represent some number of uses a month. There will be, let's say, 200 uses a month. Perhaps 30 of them are by new users and 170 are by old users. They affect the library differently in two ways. One way is the *use time* that they generate as they occupy the equipment, which is one-person unit (See Figure 5). It seems clear that *per use,* new users will take more time than old users. It is not clear which total will be more important per month.

Figure 5

$$\frac{\text{Use time}}{\text{Month}} = (\text{New Users}) \text{ X } (\text{New Use Time})$$

$$+ (\text{Old Users}) \text{X} (\text{Old Use Time})$$

The other factor that is important is the support time. This is the time of your staff that has to be put into helping these people. Again it seems clear that there will be more support time per person required for new users. Even if they do not represent a very large fraction of the total number of users this is a cost which should be included (See Figure 6). This equation is very easy to

Figure 6

$$\frac{\text{Support time}}{\text{Month}} = (\text{New Users}) \text{ X } (\text{Start Up Time})$$

$$+ (\text{Old Users}) \text{ X } (\text{Fraction Needing Help})$$

$$\text{X } (\text{Help Time})$$

understand. The total support time per month is just two terms; first, the number of new user events per month multiplied by however long it takes to get them launched on the system. We heard this morning that it might take two hours to launch them, one hour during which you're teaching them and helping them to do their first search and then the second hour when you watch and guide them as they do it. The second part of the equation is a little more complicated. Experienced users come back because they like the system. They'll need a certain amount of help per event. But not all need help. I don't have a solid estimate of the fraction needing help, but I'd guess that among the old users, it's less than half but probably more than 10%. That leaves a wide range for the estimate of support time needed. The help time that they require is probably between five and ten minutes. It's hard to have a helpful conversation without losing five minutes of work time. On the other hand, you will probably be able to solve any problem in ten.

Estimates of support time also depend on whether you consider your users so computer literate that they are self-starting, or whether you think they will take thirty minutes to get trained. I would estimate on the conservative side and say thirty minutes support time.

You can turn the support time into support cost by multiplying it by whatever your staff costs. A figure of $25,000 per year might bring tears to some people's eyes, but let's use it. It's custom in turning time into cost to recognize that about 25% of anyone's time disappears into the cracks, so we use 1,500 hours for what you might call a good or productive work-year, which works out to close to 30 cents a minute. A thirty minute training session will cost about ten dollars (excluding overhead).

Figure 7

$$\frac{\text{Support Cost}}{\text{Month}} = \frac{\text{Support time}}{\text{Month}} \times \frac{\text{Cost}}{\text{Unit Time}}$$

Figure 8

$$\text{WAGE} = 25,000/\text{yr.}$$

$$= \frac{25,000}{1500} /\text{good hour} = \$.28/\text{min.}$$

CONGESTION OF FACILITIES.

There is another troubling factor about MEDLINE on CD-ROM. As a new tool in the library, and possibly in the clinical setting, its use will grow. At some point the amount of use is going to be more than the equipment is able to handle. The use time per month—that is, how many new users you have per month multiplied by however much time they use it, plus the old users' per month multiplied by their time of use, is going to have to be compared with how many hours the equipment is available.

If you are using a time slice method, where people sign up, you can limit and regulate the use time. If the service is available the whole time the library is open, more people can use it but you can't regulate their access to specific hours. I was interested to note that a number of people here this morning either began with the sign-up system or moved to a sign-up system because of congestion.

If a service permits users to arrive randomly the inconvenience will grow very quickly as the use grows. Roughly speaking, if your machine is in use half of the time then your users will spend half their time waiting to use it. If it's in use two-thirds of the time they will roughly spend two-thirds of their time waiting. This could be a very serious problem in some situations. (You might lend them beepers, and leave them free to use the library until the CD-ROM is free.)

I have tried various ways to put together projections to show growth in use and support need. Figure 9 is just one rough model with a rough path. As the number

Figure 9

Growth in Use and Support Need

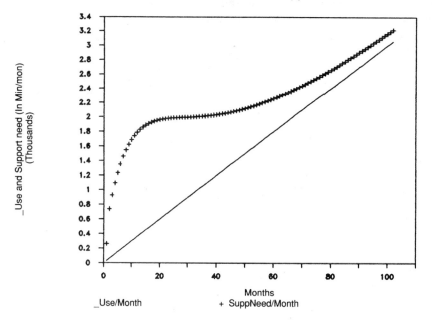

Figure 10

Growth in Use and Support Need

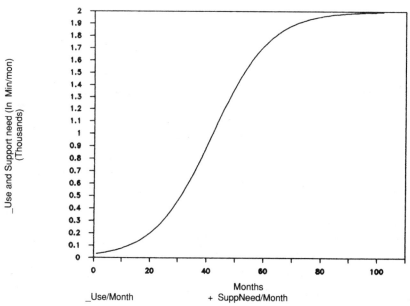

of people using the system grows the environment changes and your support time requirement is a curve that will grow quickly at first but then it will begin to level off. That's one possible projection into the future.

Another model that I tried to work with in a little more detail is based on the familiar S-shaped curve for growth in cost. First let's consider the support requirements. Figure 10 shows growth over 100 months with a projected final level of 2,000 uses per month. This is way over what anybody is reporting, but it gives the idea. The two key questions about this curve are:

(1) How high is it going to go; what is the eventual level of use per month? I think at this point we can't begin to project, but we can say something about who is the most important user population. It seems they will be students, residents in a teaching situation, and researchers. In your library you can get a total of those whom you serve, but we don't know yet how frequently each person will make use of such a tool. Whether it's once every week, once a month, once a semester, I don't know. Again, data can be gathered for projections by asking the users when was the last time they used the service.

(2) What is the maximum rate of adoption? This curve starts off slowly. Then it kind of "takes off" and somewhere in the middle, halfway to that final plateau, you may add new users faster than you ever did before. If we look at cost we see that when that happens we get two parts to the cost. The one which traces the shape of the original curve is the cost of supporting the experienced users. It

Figure 11

Growth in Use and Support Need

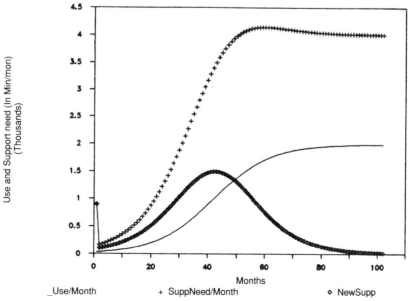

just traces the number of users. The cost that bumps up and then goes down is the cost of training new users, a cost which is higher per person. When you add these support costs together you get a cost curve that slightly overshoots the final projected figure.

HARDWARE REQUIREMENTS UNDER GROWTH.

As the use curve grows, unless you have a sufficiently small population or provide very poor service, the curve will cross the point at which you have to add an additional piece of hardware, and/or an additional subscription. There might be two such points along the way. Those are the surprises that you have to prepare for in advance because those are going to be sudden jumps. The projected cost is going to look something like that in Figure 12.

In Figure 11 we saw a fairly well behaved growth in support cost, but in Figure 12 the hardware cost which stays comfortably constant for some period at your original budget (the figure that you persuaded your institution to give you) is no longer adequate because of increased use. In this projection we see that the total cost (the broken curve of zeros), which is the sum of all costs, at first grows smoothly, then jumps up, then grows smoothly and then jumps up again.

If you go back through the equations I talked about you can see how to build these things together. If you can make a reasonable estimate of how much time each user needs at the workstation, you can make a reasonable estimate of

Figure 12

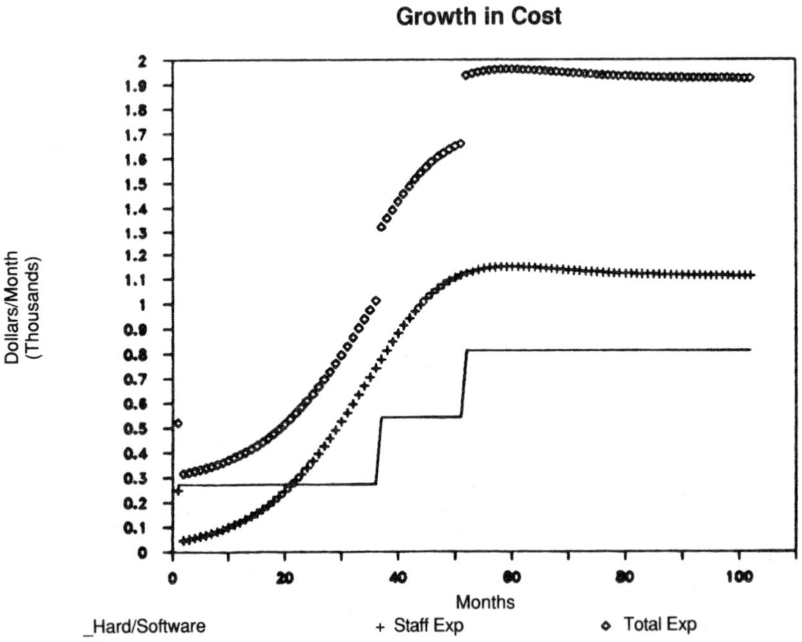

Growth in Cost

_Hard/Software   + Staff Exp   ◇ Total Exp

42

when this use level is going to hit a point where you have to have a new work-station.

That is all that I have to say about assessing costs as you are planning a budget for MEDLINE on CD-ROM. I hope that what I have said will help cut down the surprises you have in store.

QUESTIONS TO DR. KANTOR: I would like to add a couple of comments which would refer to costs in an academic setting. New users and new user costs will never go down to zero. We have a new group of students coming in every year, and the other thing we're seeing in our setting is that as the number of experienced users goes up, the support cost, the support time that we're required to put out, goes down because there is more likely to be an experienced user around who is happy to help somebody out.

KANTOR: That is the best argument that I have ever heard for buying one fewer terminal than you will need. That way there are always people standing around who can help. That's a very good point.

QUESTION: Can you construct an economic argument to persuade the medical journal publishers to publish their journals on CD-ROM to reduce cost to libraries?

KANTOR: One of the things you learn as an economic researcher is that you can hardly ever persuade anyone in business to do anything.

LESSONS LEARNED AND FUTURE PLANS
A Panel Discussion of Participating Vendors

Moderator: W. DAVID PENNIMAN
AT&T Bell Laboratories

Panelists:

LYNDON HOLMES, President, Aries Systems Corp.
MEDLINE Knowledge Finder

BETTE BRUNELLE, BRS Information Technologies
BRS Colleague Disc

JANE KELLY, Cambridge Scientific Abstracts
Compact Cambridge MEDLINE

WESLEY TAOKA, DIALOG Information Services, Inc.
DIALOG OnDisc MEDLINE

RICHARD WERTZ, Digital Diagnostics, Inc.
BiblioMed

JEANNE SPALA, EBSCO Electronic Information, Inc.
MEDLINE/EBSCO CD-ROM

RON RIETDYK, SilverPlatter Information, Inc.
SilverPlatter MEDLINE

MARK NELSON, Online Research Systems, Inc.
Compact Med-Base

PENNIMAN: There are two questions that I would like you to focus on.

The first one has to do with your experience with the technology thus far and your reaction to the variation in systems. If you want to talk about having the technology evaluated, I would say that is fair game. A related and important topic for this audience would be what are your projections about where this technology is going.

The second question has to do with international aspects of this type of product. What can you tell us about overseas implementations and what do you think about a subset of overseas implementations that have to do with developing countries. Then come back to the United States and take a look at areas within the United States where information systems are thin and this kind of technology could represent significant change.

LYNDON HOLMES (MEDLINE Knowledge Finder): The first question we have today is where is the technology going? To answer this question we first have to remember that we are dealing with a number of technologies. The obvious one is CD-ROM, but I think there are probably some more fundamental and more long-term technologies that we should try to focus on as well. We must look at the user interface and how the user interacts with the technology. That interface itself is technology and it is a very sophisticated and complex technology. I see the CD-ROM storage technology as being a somewhat transitory technology. The CD-ROM is a technology that fits the need today. I think we are going to see applications that move into the sphere of applicability of CD-ROM. We are going to see applications and parts of MEDLINE which move out of the sphere of applicability of CD-ROM. CD-ROM is, I think, a static technology today. It's not going to change much in the next five years. I hear announcements about density doubling, tripling, quadrupling, but I am going to wait for the next generation to come along. I don't think that is going to happen. From the hardware vendors you get the message that the current quantitative characteristics of CD-ROM are going to be pretty static for the next 3 or 4 years, so don't wait around for that technology to evolve. We are seeing other optical storage technologies of all kinds, like CD-I, DVI, Write-Once Read Multiple, and erasable optical. I hear people saying they will wait for one of those to come along and maybe it would be a better product.

CD-ROM is a very suitable technology for what we are trying to do today. We are going to see it evolve into network installations as people get frustrated by single-user workstations. We are showing here a network version of our system. It allows multiple users at workstations to search a single CD-ROM database. That arrangement is going to be a very important way to deal with the queing problems that we have heard about today.

Are we going to see the geographical access problem solved by networking? As most users aren't going to come to the library to do their searching, they will want to do it in their place of work and that is the way access will be accomplished by networking.

As we move into broader based distribution environments we need to consider "biomedical knowledge access and dissemination" in a broader sense. We are going to see CD-ROM superceded in some cases by more traditional technologies. We are going to see parts of a CD-ROM database being copied on to magnetic storage so that it will run faster, and the question of whether we should be focusing on CD-ROM will become less of an issue. CD-ROM will become one of the technologies that we have in our bag of tools to provide a solution to the knowledge access and dissemination problems.

I encourage you when looking at the CD-ROM technology to look beyond CD-ROM and look toward our objective of trying to provide as much of knowledge to as many people as we can, as quickly as possible and at the lowest possible cost. I think that if we do that then we will see CD-ROM taking its rightful place.

BETTE BRUNELLE (BRS Colleague Disc): I would first like to respond very quickly to what it's like to be evaluated. The presentations this morning have been wonderful learning sessions. I think a forum like this is a great way to learn new things. Obviously, when it comes to CD-ROM technology and its use the vendors are not the experts. If we were the experts there would not be so many of us at this table. In terms of the technology, we at BRS are still dealing with some of the larger issues. For one thing, we are still trying to find out how CD-ROM fits into the entire medical information system. Along with the librarians we heard from this morning we are still finding a need to train users on the new product. How can or should these training methods be coordinated with general informational retrieval training and what does that really imply for CD-ROM products and for online services?

With regard to interface problems, does the CD-ROM really make sense as a primary delivery mechanism for extremely large bibliographic databases or are there technological limitations or alternate technologies which might be more appropriate? Will technological limitations make it a supplementary or a niche application? How would librarians and end-users incorporate the many non-medical non-MEDLINE resources into their informational environment if MEDLINE is the primary resource? Considering cost, local control and wider dissemination, the real issues are a need for alternatives to CD-ROM that better address these issues.

There are some things that you will soon see with CD-ROM. I would like to talk briefly about a product that will soon be marketed which was produced by the publishing group of the Massachusetts Medical Society. It's called Compact Library AIDS. This product includes the AIDS knowledge base, which is an original electronical textbook on AIDS. It includes a subset of AIDS literature from MEDLINE and full text of original articles on AIDS from leading medical and scientific publications. All of these databases are fully integrated. This product was presented at the International Conference on AIDS in Stockholm where it created a great deal of international interest, with orders already coming in from the foreign health organizations as well as from the United States. Now, obviously, this is quite a different approach to MEDLINE searching and we think that it is one that takes advantage of CD-ROM as a publishing medium. I noticed in one of the earlier panel discussions that there was some discussion of the need for non-MEDLINE data to be integrated, backing up bibliographic references. This product is but one such approach. I think you will see different kinds of products coming out very quickly.

JANE KELLY (Compact Cambridge MEDLINE): We have had experience in publishing CD-ROM for about three years now. There are some things that the industry is just now getting under control — one thing is making the medium truly convenient and truly easy to use. If I can speak specifically about our product, we just began sending out a piece of software that is not hardware specific. When you get a piece of software it doesn't matter what reader you are using, and it works after a greatly simplified installation program. That's pretty basic, but it's only happening after three years of experience. We have just gotten our first multi-disc reader; it's a four-disc Hitachi reader. It's the first time we are able to offer the ability to search four years of MEDLINE in one search. It's a pretty basic thing, but we have just begun to offer it.

Currently we are working on networking. One day it seemed that no one cared about it and the next week we received over twenty-five calls on our 800-number wanting to know when we would do networking. So it's a hot issue now and it's something that we are just addressing.

Now to address briefly the evaluation experience. Working closely with our customers during the evaluation period has really shaped our product. With their help we have been able to create a product that we think is really useful and easy for MEDLINE users to use. When we heard from them and realized we had a real consensus, it wasn't difficult to figure out what to do. We were given three suggestions over and over: make it easier to change discs (which we have done), let us search more than one disc, and let us explode and look at the hierarchical MeSH. The evaluation period was a busy time on our 800-number, but it's getting quieter and quieter in terms of technical assistance. We finally got to the point where we can send you a product and you can get it up and running without too much difficulty. That's a big step forward in making the medium acceptable.

WESLEY TAOKA (Dialog OnDisc MEDLINE): Our experience with MEDLINE on CD-ROM was very different from our experience with MEDLINE online. The constraints of CD-ROM limited the amount of data that you could put on disc, and that was a real challenge for us to overcome. We were able to get the entire file on the disc through good compression technology and in addition we were able to integrate a thesaurus which would list cross references. Going from an available online version to a CD-ROM product is not as simple as it may seem.

Another challenge we are working on is multiple access to a CD-ROM workstation. DIALOG is working with a university to establish a LAN for remote access of CD-ROM via personal computers. This is something being established now and we hope to have it working very soon. A future development for LANs could include a cluster of LANs talking to each other. We are very excited about pursuing this.

A very different technology from CD-ROM but related to it is CD-I (compact disc integrated) and DVI (digital video integrated). These technologies not only integrate textual data but video and voice. That is something we feel will definitely enhance textual databases like MEDLINE and other factual databases that are now available. The image capability that optical media allows is something that probably everybody here has an interest in.

I would like to say something about the evaluation as well. We really appreciated all the input that we got from the different Beta test sites as well as other sites where we did place our CD-ROM. The one feature that the University of Nebraska mentioned (save searches in menu mode) is something that we are addressing right now. We do have it in our command mode and realize its utility in the other mode. The ability to upload the search from the CD-ROM into the online system is something that we want to make more seamless. Right now it is more or less doable, but we would like to have it as a one-step process.

RICHARD WERTZ (BiblioMed): When we began marketing CD-ROM products we saw this very clearly as a product for the end-user—physicians, nurses, other medical professionals—and not for medical librarians. I hope this audience is not offended by this, but when we developed our user interface, we knew we had to take into account our customers, your end-users, and not you. We learned this sometime ago. Our company not only sells medical products but we have a successful database in the real estate industry. We have assessors' data of counties and all the properties in counties so that you can view plat maps using graphics that you can zoom up to. We got lots of experience with users, and if you think physicians are klutzes, go out to a few real estate offices and try to put those people on a computer. There aren't any real estate librarians; there are no intermediaries between us and real estate people. With this group we had to go all the way and teach them how to use computers from scratch. With the experience of working with several hundred users at that level we had a fairly good idea about what would work as a user interface for a person who has never touched a computer. What was interesting and somewhat ironic to us when we began working in the field of medicine was that those who had never used a computer before had fewer problems with our CD-ROM product than those who are expecting our system to work like an online system. Those who are experienced users of computer systems are subconsciously expecting certain things to happen on the screen rather than to take things as they happen for granted. This has been a real learning experience for us, working through an intermediary for the end-user. We really can't imagine a busy surgeon being worried about a checklist of features. All he wants to know is what is the latest treatment for a tumor. Our philosophy in product development has been to keep it very clean and simple, perhaps simplistic.

As for where we see things going in this field, I guess one easy way to address this question is to go back to a famous Humphrey Bogart movie. Remember Key Largo, when Boggy is looking Rocko in the eye, and he says, "Rocko what do you want?" Rocko looks back at him, sort of stunned by the question, he hesitates and says, "More." Like Rocko that is the quick answer to where things are going in CD-ROM publishing: more. But I would like to expand on that very briefly. I think we are going to see more graphics. We will see much more interaction, and I personally believe that the days of MEDLINE being a single compact disc will be rapidly gone. We think that single databases are a very temporary thing. We think that there will be various focused markets using portions of MEDLINE. I agree with Lyndon Holmes that we aren't going to see any major jumps, but I disagree about another thing. We are going to see some improvements along this line of storage space. One of the vendors has already added some compression technology. We're doing the same thing. Also, I don't know if many of you knew that when compact disc technology first came out the standard that we got was 550 megabytes, and most of us are over 550 megabytes now. Some of the speakers have been telling us that you can rocket it up to 650 or 700 megabytes—a big jump in capacity. That's really due to improved manufacturing techniques and not to any fundamental change in the compact discs. That together with compression, maybe thirty percent or fifty percent more with compression, will cause us to see some improvement.

I think you are also going to see things get "less," because as we get more and more CD-ROM products out there we can see people affording to put little bits of things on CD-ROM because it will now be economical. I saw an ad in one of the computer magazines (I think PC Magazine) a couple days ago for a $30.00 CD-ROM. Another company has jumped into the business with the complete works of Sherlock Holmes on a CD-ROM, and they are not asking too much for it. I think we are going to see more in terms of size, but we are going to see less in terms of the costs to put out a compact disc, thereby penetrating the large market who will buy them for $30.00 or $50.00.

We have heard lots about networking and jukeboxes. Let me give you my personal bias about such developments. I grew up in the days of the Wurlitzer and there always were jukeboxes around. They never really took off with regular records. Trying to make a CD-ROM become another online system to me does not seem to make a lot of sense either. To us it's been an entity unto itself. We have attempted as much as possible to make the software and product unique unto itself and to find its own characteristics that are different from microfiche and that are different from online. We have not tried to emulate one or the other media. Personally, to me it doesn't make much sense.

Networking, of course, is inevitable in this field, but one of the problems is the intrinsic difficulties with the optical disk technology, particularly when you have a disc that's in a spiral where you have to go to the end of the line to spiral around to find where you are. That's a good design for music because it has a constant linear velocity, not a constant angular velocity. There are some problems with it for text, but the disc drives are getting faster and faster. I hear that Hitachi's newest drive is three times faster than the old one, so the industry is serving us well. Still, there might be some disappointments in that area.

JEANNE SPALA (MEDLINE/EBSCO CD-ROM): As a former hospital librarian I feel very close to this product. First let me talk about the experiences that we have had relative to this technology and the problems of installation. Those of you who have experienced these problems one on one can possibly sympathize with us on the product side who have had to deal with all your questions. We have had to deal with incompatibility of device drives; we have had to learn about the Personal Systems Model 2's and what do they do; we had to deal with the IBM clones that were not compatible with the interface cards available. Fortunately, we now have the infant walking and the infant has moved along to a point where he has got more compatibility and those earlier issues are not issues anymore. We can now place multiple products on CD-ROM workstations and have them work successfully.

Where is the hardware going? We continue to get bombarded with questions about multi-user access and networks and we know that our product will work successfully on a network and that it will not be degraded until you exceed six users. We are now addressing the issues of a pricing policy and licensing agreements relative to selling that to you.

I believe that we may see drives get a little faster. I also believe that you will see the price of drives continue to come down again. As the library marketplace begins to accept this technology and get the funding for it, we will be able to place those products more cheaply than we have in the past. I also think that you are going to see the whole field of optical disc moving forward into the area of electronic publishing.

The evaluation process has been a fascinating one for me. Competition brings excellence and if MEDLINE and the National Library of Medicine has accomplished anything by this evaluation process it has given the library marketplace some excellent CD-ROM interfaces. If you look at other CD-ROM products that are in the marketplace, you notice that people are purchasing them because of the database, because of the contents, not even bothering to evaluate the user interface. They are accepting what they are given. They are accepting Bookshelf, they are accepting Globular, they are accepting McGraw-Hill, but when you come for MEDLINE on CD-ROM they have a choice. All of us, and I know that I speak for the entire panel, had to make a great deal of effort and move perhaps more quickly in product development then what we ever expected to have to do when we first entered this marketplace. You are benefiting from this and I think it's worthy of consideration.

RON RIETDYK (SilverPlatter MEDLINE): What we see happening here is a change, a change from a technology-driven market to a market-driven market, a market driven by users — not technology driven but solution driven. One of the things we keep hearing, especially from the librarians, the people who have to accommodate users by providing a lot of information, is how are we going to make available to all the users the enormous amount of new databases. Today we talk only about MEDLINE. But if we look into catalogs of CD-ROM products we see that there are more than 250 different products available, and next year there will be 2000. The big problem for librarians is how to organize all this. My suggested solution disagrees with one of the previous speakers; I think we need to create a new online system. I think the librarians can afford in the future to make it a meaningful online system. The price of the drive will come down and every library will have in the future large stacks of CD discs being accessed through a network. This week we installed in a Boston college a system with twelve terminals able to access sixty different CD-ROM drives and we believe that that situation will become more common in the future. What it will lead to is a major overhaul of pricing. The MEDLINE database is a very affordable database. If you calculate and compare the amount of dollars per byte, or should I say the amount of cents per byte, for a database like MEDLINE which maintains a high quality of information supply, we have little fear that in the future people will expect to see the same kind of prices for other quality databases. This will only be possible if the volume can be large enough. CD-ROM is a volume-oriented product. Producing extra discs costs maybe $2.00 to $3.00. If there's enough volume, then we are able to maintain a pricing level for a private database somewhere in the area indicated by MEDLINE prices.

MARK NELSON (MED-BASE): I disagree with some of my colleagues here. I feel that CD-ROM is going the way of every other computer technology. It will become much faster and much cheaper, to the point where owning a database on CD-ROM is no more outrageous than buying a word processing program or a piece of software. I think it's inevitable that the prices will drop and that we will see drastic cuts. I was thinking back to the early 1970's as I listened to the evaluation reports today. There must have been a similar forum at that time when they were discussing the whole idea of online searching. If we went back to their taped proceedings would we hear people talking about some of the same issues? Relistening to their tapes might gives us a good perspective on what we are thinking about today. I think that what is happening in CD-ROM right now is great for the users, but for the vendors it means that we are going to have to scramble. We have seen the evolution from the first generation of CD-ROM drives to second generation of CD-ROM drives, but there is more to come. One thing that I haven't heard much talk about today, but what I think will soon be the norm, is the use of a caddy. A caddy makes it absolutely impossible to stick a CD-ROM disk in a floppy disk drive or to put it in the wrong way. This will be a feature of most second-generation CD-ROM readers, and it really will make them ideal for a public access sitting. You would take a CD-ROM disc and put it inside the caddy and it stays there and no one touches it. It slides inside a CD-ROM drive and it is always protected. We will see a substantial price drop when the vendors move from their first generation of CD-ROM drives to a second generation drive. That is notable. CD-ROM designers are making their compact disc drives smaller and faster. So now we have this new generation of half-height CD-ROM drives. They are in production. There are still some glitches in them, but I think once that is in place we are going to see prices drop radically. We are projecting that in two years or so the price of a CD-ROM drive will not be as expensive as the floppy disk drive, about $100 or $150.

Our product was not part of the evaluation reported here. We came out after the end of the experimental period. We have the entire MEDLINE database, including citations and abstracts, back to 1966 on eight CD's, and this week we shipped our first monthly update covering the most recent five years of the database. The database is split up much like an online file would be, into four to five year segments. Our software will work with with one, two, or three CD-ROM drives and we are now announcing at this forum an eight CD-ROM drive box so you can put the entire MEDLINE file online with no disc swapping.

We have learned a great deal in producing MEDLINE on CD-ROM. We have learned from the vendors who preceded us. That's one of the advantages of being last I guess. We reviewed all the issues and we tried to focus on the development of the product, which was an end-user product and also a product that a professional could use. We assumed that there are a lot of people out there who will be using MEDLINE on CD-ROM as a primary search mode, thereby saving money. We know there are some trade offs and I guess it depends on some of the situations, but in designing our product what we're aiming to do is provide a professional level of interface and one an end-user could use. To us the end-user is able to exploit the strength of the NLM vocabulary. Given the quality of the MEDLINE database, you have the opportunity to provide a sophisticated end-user interface that doesn't have to be complex and that can help end-users use MESH headings and subheadings.

I'd like to briefly touch on a couple of other issues. For people who have networks installed, I think networking is a good idea, but for people who don't, I don't think it's a good idea. As a friend of mine said about networking so that you can run CD-ROM drive, "It is sort of like feeling you need a space shuttle when in reality all you need is a wheelbarrow." Space shuttles are a very expensive option. What we need to do is focus on a single user station that will allow multiple access without networking. There are some networking issues that you must be aware of: for one, you must include a budget for a full-time network administrator, rather expensive network cards and things like that. At this point we are taking a sort of wait and see attitude with networking. Our hunch is that the pricing will drop to the point where networking will not be worthwhile.

There are of course other issues, and one of them is performance. A CD-ROM drive of even a new generation has an access time of about 400 milliseconds; that about the best I've heard. That's about twenty times more than a typical network file server. We are very wary of that, and I think there's a lot to be done in that area before networking becomes a real alternative.

PENNIMAN: There are international aspects of this particular technology which are quite intriguing. Also, in certain areas of the United States remote from urban centers, this technology could be applied where information services are currently very thin. I would like to ask the panel to tell us of any plans they may have in these areas.

MARK NELSON (Online Research Systems, Inc.): Outside the U.S. there are many countries where telecommunications is quite expensive. There CD-ROM is an instant solution to the problem of information access. The interesting thing to note about CD-ROM in developing countries is that these systems will be used by professionals. They aren't interested at this point in systems for end users. What they need to do is eliminate those telecommunications costs and get the databases they need on CD-ROM. Problems related to this development have to do with getting the CD-ROM drives. We have seen a case of dumping by a CD-ROM vendor—old drives at very good prices. Obtaining the hardware is an issue for developing countries, much more so than here in the states. Another issue has to do with who will support the CD-ROM technology in their country. When it comes to an international distribution you will have all of the same issues you have here in the United States plus some others related primarily to hardware.

RON RIETDYK (SilverPlatter Information, Inc.): SilverPlatter has a tremendous interest in the overseas market. As a matter of fact, we first received requests to provide MEDLINE on CD-ROM from our overseas customers. They had ordered other SilverPlatter products and they came to us and asked us to put up MEDLINE. At the moment SilverPlatter MEDLINE is being used all over the world—Africa, Australia, China. One of the big problems they face is that once they find the information it's only a bibliographic reference. Trying to get the full text of the article can be very frustrating. For CD-ROM to succeed in the developing world it will have to face the problem of document delivery. The beginning of this year we started a project with the United Nations. In developing countries we hope to find what people are seeking and what they would need on a CD-ROM. It is an ideal medium for forwarding information to developing countries, but we have to solve the issue of document delivery.

JEANNE SPALA (EBSCO Electronic Information, Inc.): We too are seeing a great deal of interest in this non-United States marketplace. It tends to be in places where they speak English, in Europe, Australia, and other places that have money. Getting the appropriate hardware installed and paid for in Third World countries can be extremely difficult. We actually had people tell us that as we are a rich country why don't we give it to them! There are problems in exporting and importing these items. It takes five and half months to obtain authorization to actually export CD-ROM drives from the United States into the People's Republic of China.

Another problem comes from database producers who are concerned about losing the non-US market for their printed indexes. Again, there is the delivery problem. The printed index is getting there slowly and they see the CD-ROM version getting there faster and replacing the printed version.

That brings up an additional issue, which is the misunderstanding of whether they are actually purchasing a product or leasing the right to access a database. The vendors here all understand that we are actually providing access to a database, and that when NLM updates their files we have an obligation to update that database to insure that these people are searching from a current database. That is a very difficult concept to get across when you are speaking through translators.

I think we have to learn from the European marketplace that there is some concern from professional librarians that by providing direct access to their clients we may be restricting what they feel was their professional right as a librarian, namely, to search for literature.

RICHARD WERTZ (Digital Diagnostics, Inc.): We are not a large company, but we do have a number of distributors around the world. Our first approach to a Third World country was with stars in our eyes. We wrote letters to the World Health Organization. We didn't get a answer back for a year, just before a trip I had planned to Switzerland. We prevailed upon WHO to allow us to show our CD-ROM product. The fuse blew, but we got that fixed and went through a demo in Geneva. We have found it rather difficult to work our way through the bureaucracy at WHO, the Pan American Health Organization and so on. Our experience with China has not been much better. In Europe we have a lot more activity going on. Because modems are so expensive there, a CD-ROM drive is much more attractive. We have had a great deal of interest shown by physicians and other health professionals in Europe.

WESLEY TAOKA (DIALOG Information Services, Inc.): DIALOG has been selling online services internationally for a number of years. We have distributors who are used to handling computer-related technology. Our international sales have been very good and we have products in Japan, China, Hong Kong, throughout the whole Pacific region and also throughout Europe. We do see CD-ROM as a complement to online services. Because telecommunications costs internationally can be several times the cost of the database itself, it is cheaper to search the database on CD-ROM than to pay the telephone company. There is a problem of getting the CD-ROM drive into some of the Third World countries. We have been approached by some companies in the Third World who are interested in distributing our product, but just getting the CD-ROM into their country will not be as much of a problem as getting the drive into their country.

JANE KELLY (Cambridge Scientific Abstracts): I don't have the exact statistics, but about four months ago approximately fifty percent of our MEDLINE locations were located outside the US and Canada. We have a large number located all around the world, in the Pacific region, in Australia, and quite a few in the Middle East, Europe and South America. I think that the goal of any database producer is to get the information out to more people. One of the things we are seeing is that CD-ROM allows people to do searching without telecommunications charges. As a result there is more searching of databases like MEDLINE by their original overseas users.

BETTE BRUNELLE (BRS Information Technologies): BRS' experience with foreign sales is not great. Our CD-ROM product is very closely identified with BRS Colleague, which is very much a US-based system. The exception to that is in Japan, where a database distributor has translated the BRS Colleague Disc into Kanji, and they are in the process of marketing this. In Japan they had a CD-ROM fair which was attended by over sixty librarians. They were very excited, and so we are interested to see how that goes.

Another development is that CD library for AIDS, which I mentioned earlier was presented in Stockholm. The fact that it has full text on it minimizes some of the document delivery problems. I don't know if that is the reason, but the health organizations around the world have been very interested and the European Community has also shown great interest in that product.

LYNDON HOLMES (Aries Systems Corp.): I think the international market is probably out of our league, but it may become more significant than the US market is. I think it all will come out in the population count. I think we're all experiencing short-term dislocations in terms of hardware distribution problems. I know we have brought some of the export-import problems on ourselves. Our biggest worry over the long term is the cultural eccentricity of MEDLINE today. It is an English language database, but 25% of the literature is published in a foreign language. That makes me worry about 25% of the population who I fear will have a hard time accessing the MEDLINE database. I am not sure how that problem can be solved.

PUTTING IT ALL IN PERSPECTIVE
A Roundtable Discussion

Moderator: W. DAVID PENNIMAN (AT&T Bell Laboratories)
Panelists: Prudence W. Dalrymple (University of Illinois, Rockford)
Paul B. Kantor (Tantalus, Inc.)
Nancy K. Roderer (Columbia University)
Nancy N. Woelfl (University of Nebraska)

PENNIMAN: In Dr. Lindberg's opening remarks he indicated that he saw trade-offs between CD-ROM and online and for many searchers CD-ROM would be the starting point but hopefully not the end point. I would say that this conference may be a starting point as well and not an end point. One of the things that I hope you will be thinking about tomorrow is where do we go from here. We have reviewed the international challenge for this new medium and I think we have shown what a wonderful opportunity this has been for NLM to work with manufacturers who had these new CD-ROM systems.

Nancy Roderer's panel reported that there was not a stampede of new library users as a result of CD-ROM, but that this new technology did generate new online searchers. Cost factors contributed to the decision to use the systems but once used, most had a very favorable response. Searchers, once initiated, want to retain the CD-ROM system, or at least the simplicity of the CD-ROM system if not the CD-ROM system itself, and that leads to some key points. Don't underestimate the commitment to training that is required when you introduce CD-ROM. I heard that for sure from a number of people today.

One question that came to me after hearing Nancy's panel is, What are the niches that this new technology can successfully fill? A related question is, How will the technology evolve and as it evolves what changes will occur in those niches? The concept of one-stop shopping in a single window was mentioned first in this panel, but it occurred again in later panels. Associated with that idea of one-stop shopping in a single window is the document delivery question.

In the clinical setting panel, we heard that individuals in that particular setting wanted information, not citations. That is the name of the game there. The physical location of the device can be problematic given the nature of a clinical site. The training needs to be focused on the intellectual aspect of searching, and that is more important than the physical aspects. Also, we need to prepare the users psychologically for this.

We heard new ways of classifying users, "the thinkers" versus "the cutters" and "the satisfied" and "dissatisfied" and "ept" and "inept." I didn't know there was such a word as "ept." I guess there must be, and then there's the "not-so ept." That brought a question to my mind about the role of the information professional, not just at a clinical site but in other settings. Is the information professional searcher in those environments with CD-ROM a trainer or more importantly maybe a change agent? Must we train people before we put out the CD-ROM or can we just put them out?

For remote or rural locations, CD-ROM technology is better perhaps than what they have now. What will this mean for the information professionals in terms of serving these locations once CD-ROM is installed? We have heard again about the concept of one-stop shopping, using the same terminal for multiple uses. The question that came to me out of that was, What will constitute one-stop shopping in a clinical setting? Will it include information, illustration and extended document displays as well as the kind of information you see right now? Do clinicians want immediate document delivery right then online?

We heard from Paul Kantor about the cost model that shows numerous factors that have to be considered. He highlighted the problems of the availability of the benchmark and shared usage data. The next question that I would raise is, Where can economic data necessary for informed decisions be acquired? Will this group that is gathered here today be such a source and if so, how?

From Nancy Woelfl's panel we heard again about how hard it will be to send the CD-ROM back once you have installed it. I also heard a repeat of the idea that the most effective searching can be done if we limit the subset of available information, provide training directly to users and thereby improve their search performance. Users were not as ept as they thought, according to the panel's reports. Some searches were ill-conceived, and yet only a few of the CD-ROM users asked librarians for help. They didn't know that they didn't know. CD-ROM may be a choice for ease of use but not for comprehensive searching, and that gave rise to even more questions.

We heard something about the best features of CD-ROM and needed changes. Vendors, I am sure, will be responding to that, but my question is, How are they going to respond to what they have heard today? I, for one, heard something today that really bothered me. Some librarians assume that users are ignorant of their ignorance (which may be true) and that they should not be left alone either in the library or with an information system like a CD-ROM workstation. Can we continue to condone that attitude, and if not, what shall we do about it?

With all of those questions on the table, perhaps we can begin our round-table discussion, putting it all in perspective, by starting with the question: What are the niches that this CD-ROM technology can fill, and how will the evolution of technology change?

RODERER: I think I would like to take the first part of that question. The second part is too puzzling for me. As I think back over my years in the information business, as new technologies have come out I speculated on what the future might be. I haven't always been wrong, at least in the short term. We have never deviated from our objective of providing our library users with access to MED-LINE. This might be provided in many ways—online, CD-ROM, in print, whatever. Not one of these provides everything. So I think that is a very simple way of saying what the role of CD is at this stage; it is to provide an alternative way of accessing MEDLINE and getting new online users.

PENNIMAN: The next question is, What role will the information professional play first in a clinical session and then beyond that.

DALRYMPLE: I think we have seen various responses to the CD-ROM technology in the clinics. I think that MEDLINE is seen as a library product and we may need a different kind of product mix for clinical information needs. My bias is to look at those information needs and the information seeking behaviors of our clinicians and then to design products around that. This evaluation experience has given us an opportunity to see what the response has been to a particular product, and now I think we can go back and think about what/how we would like to begin to approach providing information in a clinical setting. I was very pleased to hear a couple of vendors on the last panel mention some of their electronic publishing products, trying again to provide a mixture of MEDLINE within a module of other kinds of information.

I think that the information professional has a role and perhaps an obligation to provide input of the kind that we have had today, not only acting as an intermediary but, because we understand the needs of clinicians, communicating these needs to the vendors and engaging in the kind of dialogue we have had today, helping them design their products and get into some cyclical testing.

I do believe that one way of looking at the problem of instructions and quality or evaluation of search results is to ask ourselves where the burden for that intellectual conceptualization rests. Do we want the burden to be on our users? Do we want the burden to be on our professionals? As Paul Kantor correctly pointed out, the professional service is not cheap and it's certainly not free. Or do we want to define that intellectual burden as part of the system itself?

PENNIMAN: Thank you. Would any of the other panelists care to comment on Prudence's response or to the question?

RODERER: I would like to expand on that a little bit because it's along the lines of what I have been thinking about. The librarian is the person in between the user and the vendor. How they can best facilitate that process? One of the things that librarians are good at is searching, learning to use a whole variety of systems, and researching. Given that expertise they can be of help to users, helping them to learn the systems, and they can be of help to vendors, telling them what should be built into the systems. I think it's that last aspect, sharing our expertise with vendors, which we sometimes neglect.

PENNIMAN: Now I would like Prudence to respond to the one-stop shopping concept as it might be implemented in the clinical setting, and I would like Nancy Woelfl to comment on the wider environment and what one-stop shopping might mean.

DALRYMPLE: I would like to share with you some perceptions that a couple of the people in the clinic shared with me. It has to do with the role of the abstract. Document delivery is certainly a problem, and I don't see how that is always going to fit together. I can't see the entire universe of published medical literature available on CDs, but a number of people mentioned to me that having the abstract online was very, very helpful. It took care of the immediate need to get some information right there in the clinic. It also served a current awareness role for people who were browsing after hours in a more relaxed fashion. It didn't eliminate entirely the need to go and get the document, but it deferred that need to a later time. I mentioned this morning that Knowledge Finder has a transaction log. In the clinical evaluation we had these transaction logs that I could look at, and in fact I did see that pattern confirmed in the logs that people, once they found a set of citations that they wanted, would press the button for the full display with the abstract. It is my sense that they were in fact reading the abstract. In our current environment that gives you some one-stop shopping, possibly going into a separate file with some kind of electronic book information. I don't have a clear picture of what that would look like, but some combination would appear useful.

WOELFL: In terms of the one-stop shopping concept, it's rather difficult for me to imagine right now how we might expand beyond the phase of looking at abstracts. I would say that in our environment I know that the abstract gives the user a fair amount of what they want, and the abstract feature in any system really is essential. I watch people outside my office in the reference area doing lengthy searches, some as long as an hour. They will walk away with an inch of paper in their hands because they want to take the abstract with them. When they come back, they want to find out what is available of those items they have marked relevant. Now, some of them can decide that by looking at titles on the screen, but the abstract is a valuable feature. At the present time I can't see that much more is to be gained by giving them full text rather than the abstract. I think it would almost complicate matters in that they would have so much material to deal with. I think the idea of one-stop shopping is really a complicated one.

KANTOR: I don't know what the various competing systems can do, but one feature of any baseline system, I should think, would give people the option to say what I see on the screen right now is what I want, and print it right then. If you went to the text of a book, people should be able to find the page and take it home. So it might not make the situation worse, and it might ultimately make it better.

PENNIMAN: What we mean by one-stop shopping in our environment is that we present the user with a single window. They don't need to understand either the organizational environment in which the service resides or how the service is structured. If they go into any physical location, they can get all the service they need through that location. If they are at a terminal, they can access the full range of databases from that terminal. That is what we mean by one-stop shopping.

RODERER: One of the things that we have at Columbia University is a hypertext textbook of internal medicine. Its content was written at various levels, and one of the things we are going to do with that is connect it to MEDLINE so that you can go back and forth between the explanations in that textbook and the references in MEDLINE. I think that is a start on one of the assumptions of a single window.

PENNIMAN: Our next question is where can data, economic or other useful data that is necessary for informed decisions, be acquired? Can this group gathered here be such a source, and if so, how? Paul Kantor, I would like you to be the first to respond.

KANTOR: I think this is a rare opportunity for a community of users of a new technology. With very little investment in the preliminary design of a data collection form, it should be possible for anybody who makes the CD-ROM investment to collect the kind of data that I was talking about. Rates of growth, the fraction of the patrons who need help, and time required to help new patrons and old ones are some of the needed data. If this was contributed, even anonymously, to some kind of shared data bank, those who follow would have more information to go on before they make their decisions. I hope that people will take the opportunity and move forward to do it.

I would like to take this opportunity to mention a new idea. I have been involved in some research on the effectiveness of database searches and database systems, and the key question that comes up is this: when you have an end-user who is working at the terminal, that end-user examines some set of titles or abstracts and eventually decides that some subset of those are worth having. What I regard as a baseline system would then allow the user to indicate by numbers, 1, 2, and 3, etc. which ones are to be examined further. Vendors could easily capture that information. The hard question is, once you've caught the tiger, how do you get him out of the cage and how do you get the information shared? These data will be of value to the vendor because you can see which system performs better. To sum up, I would like to see some kind of evaluation data built into the CD-ROM systems of the future.

WOELFL: I don't think you are ever going to take the problem of precision off the back of either the mediated searcher or the end-user searcher, even if we have an increasingly knowledgeable end-user searcher. As you search more and more, you learn to develop your searches in such a way that you're cutting down on the size of the retrieved set and not getting such a large stack of irrelevant items. I am not sure you are ever going to build that into a system. This idea goes back to some of the original evaluation studies that Wilf Lancaster did when he looked at what very highly trained searchers were retrieving.

KANTOR: I don't want to turn this into an extended debate, but as others have just said we have gotten better systems; eight new interfaces are in the lobby of this auditorium and they are not just cosmetically different. They are different systems, and the door is open for further systems to be introduced. In fact the National Library of Medicine has developed other ways to search things, and I have every reason to believe that some systems are better than others.

PENNIMAN: Let me suggest that not only in that area but in some of the other areas where we heard about needed changes to systems or features that need to be modified, we will hear responses from the vendors but not here today. We will hear it in the marketplace, and that's where the real answer comes anyway. There is one final question concerning the issue I posed that some librarians assume that the users are ignorant of their ignorance, that they cannot be left alone in the library or with an information system. Can we continue to condone that attitude? If we can't condone it, what should be done about it?

KANTOR: There are a lot more end-users out there than there are any other kind of animal. I think that eventually they are going to be their own user whether we would like to keep them from being that or not.

WOELFL: Paul, most of us wouldn't like to keep them from it. You know our efforts are to assist them in finding—helping them to find what they need, whether they find it for themselves or whether they get some help from us. But we see ourselves, at least, as agents in the process of helping them to get to know these systems and to effectively use them.

PENNIMAN: So it's a role of training, rather than as an intermediary doing searches each time.

WOELFL: I see the professionals as having a very large training role. In our library, now that we have two end-user systems available, both the MEDLINE subset and the CD-ROM, our effort goes very much into training people. The training happens on a one-on-one basis. We have not had formal classes because we have found it effective to work with people as they arrive at the point of service and need help. At some point we may change that, but the one-on-one concentrated work with them seems to produce the best results.

DALRYMPLE: I will extend what has been said by saying that besides one-on-one training there may be one-on-machine. I think that the training can happen in the iterative process, as long as you can keep people from not getting turned off. If you can keep the carrot and stick going, I think people will learn. The systems need to be well defined, with enough levels of access. I think Jackie Doyle and Peter Vigil talked about that. If you give people enough levels they will work their way up the hierarchy and can become trained as they access the system.

PART II

Individual Evaluation Study Reports

Editors' Note:

       The individual field trials reported here were independently carried out with minimal supervision by the National Library of Medicine. NLM has served as a coordinator, helped place the CD-ROM workstations, facilitated the use of a "generic" questionnaire as an evaluation instrument if acceptable at the individual sites, and organized a forum for the reporting of results and for the discussion of MEDLINE on CD-ROM by vendors, librarians, and interested health practitioners.

       It was never the intention of NLM to compare systems with each other, but some sites have reported comparative data because of the availability of and interest in systems other than the one used for their part in the NLM evaluation project. The study design for such comparisons was planned and executed independently. The results should be attributed to the authors of the individual reports and not to the National Library of Medicine.

MEDLINE
CD-ROM

AT MEDICAL UNIVERSITY
OF SOUTH CAROLINA LIBRARY

A Comparative Study of Knowledge Finder,
MiniMEDLINE, EBSCO, and MEDLINE

By: *Nancy Smith*
Marcia Anderson
Nancy McKeehan

Medical University of South
Carolina Library
171 Ashley Ave.
Charleston, South Carolina, 29425

MEDLINE CD-ROM
AT MEDICAL UNIVERSITY
OF SOUTH CAROLINA LIBRARY

Setting

The Medical University of South Carolina is comprised of six colleges (Medicine, Dental Medicine, Nursing, Health-Related Professions, Pharmacy, and Graduate Studies) and affiliated teaching hospitals. The oldest medical institution in the South, MUSC is the core of the largest medical complex in the state of South Carolina. At present, approximately 2,050 students are enrolled at the University. The teaching staff consists of 700 core and 1,200 part-time faculty members. The University awards baccalaureate, masters, and doctoral degrees, as well as certificates, in 30 fields of study. In addition, the University coordinates the training of over 700 interns and residents in a variety of medical specialties throughout the state.

The MUSC Library is centrally located on the campus. Access to the entire collection of over 180,000 volumes has been automated since 1986, using MUSCLS, an integrated library system based on the Library Information System (LIS) developed at Georgetown University Medical Center Library. A fully-integrated and fully-functional library system, MUSCLS also includes a MiniMEDLINE module, offering free user-friendly searching of a database of journal literature published since 1985. Over 350 journals are indexed in MiniMEDLINE, giving access to almost 350,000 articles.

In addition to the online system, the library offers a full range of information services, including free MEDLINE searches to MUSC faculty and graduate students (other MUSC students are charged $5.00). Searches on BRS, DIALOG, and other systems are also available for a fee. A total of 2555 searches were conducted during FY 1987/88, 91.3% on NLM databases. 12.9% of all searches were requested for research purposes; 9.2% were requested for patient care.

The University's personal computer environment includes IBM, IBM-compatible, and Macintosh hardware. Approximately 200 of the estimated 600 personal computers used on campus are Macintosh systems and 16% of the Library's dial access patrons use Macintosh hardware. The University has supported a Macintosh-based computer literacy course and microcomputer laboratory for students since 1985. In 1986, a formal Macintosh User Group was established on campus to provide a community-wide forum for Macintosh interests. During FY 1987/88, there was a 50% increase in personal Macintosh purchases at MUSC, the highest growth of any personal use system.

The Library's microcomputer environment includes ten IBM-type and three Macintosh Plus microcomputers. All of these are restricted to staff use. MEDLINE Knowledge Finder was the first Macintosh-based system used in the Library's public access area.

The Knowledge Finder workstation was set up in the main reference area of the Library, within view of the Reference and Circulation desks and convenient to the main entrance to the Library and the stairway to the third floor. Prior to system availability, an article announcing Knowledge Finder and describing the system and CD-ROM technology was placed in the campus newspaper, the Catalyst. Announcements were also mailed to all departments on campus and to dial access users of the library system.

Reference and Systems staff conferred to decide policy and organize the evaluation project. A member of the Systems staff was responsible for setting up the hardware and configuring the system, while a Reference librarian was selected as "resident expert" from the user perspective. These librarians worked together to ensure that the system worked smoothly, appropriate user aids were designed and available, and that other reference staff were trained to help patrons.

Knowledge Finder was initially available for use during all hours that a reference librarian was on duty (60 to 76 hours per week). User interest, and the philosophical position that an "cnd-user" system should be able to support itself, soon prevailed and the hours of availability were extended to all hours of library operation. The CD-ROM disks were kept at the Circulation Desk where patrons could check them out for use at the workstation. The Knowledge Finder documentation was kept in the Reference Office, but was available for consultation by patrons if requested.

Evaluation

HARDWARE

Installation and Documentation

Aries supplied all hardware components including cables and an extra box of Imagewriter printer ribbons. Equipment manuals were included with each component and Aries included a special CD-ROM drive installation chapter in its Knowledge Finder manual.

Because installing the Macintosh SE and the Toshiba CD-ROM drive were new experiences for the Systems Office staff, all manuals required some level of consultation. For the purpose of this testing and evaluation situation, more written guidance from Aries, perhaps in the form of a simple check-list (e.g., "1. The set-up should contain. . .; 2. Begin by connecting . . . "), would have been welcome. The equipment instructions that were supplied by Aries (i.e, for the Toshiba CD-ROM drive) were especially clear and helpful. Considering that Aries markets both MEDLINE Knowledge Finder and CD-ROM drives, but not Macintosh microcomputers and printers, the documentation supplied by Aries was appropriate.

Security

Macintoshes and their peripherals (except the Imagewriter) are fairly portable machines. A decision was made to detach the mouse and the keyboard during the hours that Knowledge Finder was unavailable for use (i.e., when the reference staff was not on duty). Because of user interest and the belief that an end-user access tool should be self-supporting, Knowledge Finder was made available for use during all hours of Library operation. The mouse and keyboard are still removed as part of the Library closing procedure to ensure (1) that they are still attached to the Mac, and (2) that the workstation is properly shut down each night. Because the workstation is located in a very busy public area and in full view of both the Circulation and Reference desks, no other security measures have been instituted.

Vendor Support

Aries support is of the highest possible quality: consistently accessible and always helpful. Questions concerning hardware configuration and performance have been met with quick solutions or reliable suggestions. The company president, Lyndon Holmes, is readily available and has proven to be an excellent long-distance educator in the use of the Macintosh hardware as well as in the use of Knowledge Finder.

Performance

The Macintosh SE microcomputer, Imagewriter II printer, and Toshiba XM-2100A CD-ROM disk drive performed well and required little daily maintenance attention.

The SE experienced six "lock-ups" that were probably due to software/user interface problems and one hardware harddisk failure. The "lock-ups" only momentarily interrupted use while simple system restarts were performed; the harddisk failure required removal of the workstation for ten days and replacement of the harddisk by a local Apple dealer ($280). Considering the reported survival rate of SE harddisks in general, an annual service contract with a local dealer ($378) would be a good investment.

The Imagewriter II printer was the least popular component of the workstation. It seemed extremely loud and annoyingly "whiny" compared to the public area's other printers (ink jets used with MUSCLS). An acoustic cover is recommended for environments that are accustomed to or require a low-noise level.

Because the Knowledge Finder default printing format includes bolding and underlining, the Imagewriter prints references somewhat slowly even in draft mode. Knowledge Finder software does offer the user custom-print formatting options that can increase overall printing speed, but these options are not readily apparent to the casual user.

Both the noise and the speed of the printer seemed to encourage more judicious printing on the part of users. Considering paper and ribbon costs, these seeming disadvantages of the Imagewriter may actually be advantageous to the Library's supply budget.

The Toshiba CD-ROM drive performed well. Because the opening and closing mechanism for the disk caddy had to be depressed and held, users experienced some difficulty inserting and removing disks. Prominent instructions (i.e., to press and hold the blue button) helped to alleviate most of these problems.

SOFTWARE

Installation

Installing the Macintosh operating system was a new experience for the Systems Office staff. Using the step-by-step instructions in the Macintosh manuals, system and utility folders were easily created. The Macintosh software included a "Guided Tour of the Macintosh" which was used to further acquaint staff with mouse manipulation and opening, closing, and copying files. Aries included easy-to-follow Knowledge Finder software installation instructions in its manual. Both the Macintosh operating system and Knowledge Finder were installed quickly and without difficulty.

Documentation

Aries documentation is excellent! The manual includes a detailed table of contents and an index. Page numbers cited actually refer to the correct pages! A "Messages" glossary and five appendices that list binding prefixes, stop words, word variants, citation fields, and Core database journal titles are included. A tutorial that emphasizes the basic application of a free-form search and a subject heading search is included to provide an organized introduction to using the software. All text is clearly stated and numerous examples and screen displays are presented to illustrate specific search features.

Only one documentation short-coming was noted: there is no comprehensive explanation of the algorithm used to determine citation relevancy. Because Knowledge Finder's thesis is to gather references that it judges to be most relevant to the search terms entered, it is incumbent upon Aries to provide a definition of "relevancy." It was especially difficult for experienced online searchers accustomed to strict Boolean operants to determine why some references were retrieved and others were not. "Probabilistic retrieval" is what sets Knowledge Finder apart from the other MEDLINE system vendors; it needs fuller explanation in the documentation.

Security

Part of the attraction of the Macintosh operating system is its ease-of-use and ease-of-system exploration. While this may be ideal for personal computer use, it presents a problem for public use workstations. Using the Macintosh's "Finder" capability, the Knowledge Finder workstation was set to "start-up" with Knowledge Finder. A simple "QUIT" and "SHUTDOWN" or "RESTART" were all that was necessary to leave the program and prepare it for the next user. Some user's, however, took full advantage of the Macintosh's ease-of-maneuverability and would explore other files on the workstation, reset the start-up, or change the names of files. Whether it was intentional misuse of the system or inexperienced user errors does not really matter. What does matter is finding a way to secure software access. Utility programs that limit access to certain files either by a password or by a "Guard Dog" approach will be investigated to ensure that files other than Knowledge Finder and other public use programs are protected.

Vendor Support

Software support from Aries was exceptional! Lyndon Holmes, the company president, is readily available to explain the intricacies of the Knowledge Finder search system. The intellectual shift from an environment that previously only used "hard" Boolean operators, to Knowledge Finder's "soft" Boolean has required a great deal of explanation and interpretation. Dr. Holmes has patiently listened to our questions and provided the answers that, in turn, have enabled us to interpret search results for patrons. Aries believes in the product and freely offers its full support toward effective use of Knowledge Finder.

Performance

During four months of constant use, only six system software "lock-ups" were recorded. Turning the system off and then on again resolved the lock-ups. Users did "lose" their searches and have to begin again, but all took the inconvenience without complaint and were relieved that they had not "broken" anything.

In order to examine the performance of Knowledge Finder software features, three comparative studies were conducted. The first compared retrievals obtained by NLM's MEDLINE, MUSC's MiniMEDLINE, EBSCO's Core MEDLINE, and Knowledge Finder's Core MEDLINE. The second compared retrievals obtained by NLM's MEDLINE with Knowledge Finder Unabridged MEDLINE, and the third compared retrievals resulting from variations in Knowledge Finder search control settings.

Comparison #1

Methodology: Seven simple searches were conducted on each system by the same person. To eliminate date coverage variability between subsets, search results were manually filtered to limit the retrieval to a year of common coverage, 1986. Results were compared, discrepancies noted, and discrepancy-producing features identified. Additional software capabilities and an overall time for searching each system were recorded. The searches included:

1) an author search = RIGOTTI, NA
2) a text-word or free-form search = EATING DISORDERS

3) a MeSH vocabulary search = ANOREXIA NERVOSA
4) a Boolean OR search = ANOREXIA NERVOSA OR BULIMIA
   OR HYPERPHAGIA
5) a Boolean AND search = <above results> AND OSTEOPOROSIS
6) an exploded MeSH search = APPETITE DISORDERS
7) a limiting search = <above results> limited to ENGLISH
   LANGUAGE and 1986

Results: A comparison of the contents of each system as a whole is shown in Table 1. Overall "online time" spent conducting the seven searches and printing selected references is shown in Table 2. An average-per-search time has been calculated for each system based on this same small sample. Table 3 compares the numeric results from the author search, the Boolean search that combined (ANOREXIA NERVOSA OR BULIMIA OR HYPERPHAGIA) AND OSTEOPOROSIS, and the text-word search.

Using NLM MEDLINE results as the basis for judging total retrieval, the author search resulted in the possible retrieval of three references. All of the subsets found 2 of the 3, losing one reference because of subset composition: *The Journal of Psychiatric Research* is not included in any of the subsets, but is included in MEDLINE.

NLM requires the use of last name and initials (or last name and a colon, or an (AU) designator) to limit a search to an author field. MiniMEDLINE, EBSCO, and Knowledge Finder require that an author search option be selected. Using MiniMEDLINE, a menu option for AUTHOR is chosen, then the name being searched is keyed; all possible

Table 1

COMPARISON OF TITLE COVERAGE

	# of Titles	% of MEDLINE	% of Titles in Common
NLM	3100+	100%	4%
miniMEDLINE	319	10%	42%
EBSCO	550	18%	24.5%
KF	220	7%	61%

Table 2

COMPARISON OF "ONLINE TIME"
(Includes 7 Searches and Printing)

	Total	Average/Search
NLM	13 minutes	1.85 minutes
miniMEDLINE	20 minutes	2.85 minutes
EBSCO	31 minutes	4.43 minutes
KF	32 minutes	4.57 minutes

matches are retrieved. Using EBSCO, the author field of the EBSCO search template is filled in with the name being searched; all possible matches are retrieved. If an author's initials are included in an EBSCO search, the entire name must be enclosed in quotation marks. There are multiple steps to conducting an author search in Knowledge Finder: the mouse is used to select the Author Name(s) dictionary, the keyboard is used to enter a specific name, the dictionary is opened to the appropriate alphabetic "page," the mouse is used to select the name from the page and a

Table 3

COMPARISON OF RETRIEVAL RESULTS

	Author Search	Boolean/MeSH Search	Text-Word Search
NLM	3	3	110
miniMEDLINE	2	1	16
EBSCO	2	1	23
KF	2	1	18

Boolean-type search option (i.e., "USE ONLY", "TRY TO USE", "DON'T USE") from the right side of the screen. These minute steps can become tedious, but proceed so quickly and logically that user tolerance-level is generally not exceeded. MiniMEDLINE and EBSCO do not prefilter author searches through a name authority file or dictionary as Knowledge Finder does; the user must "manually" filter each reference after retrieval.

Again, using NLM MEDLINE results as the basis for judging total retrieval, the MeSH searches resulted in matching retrieval except for references to journal titles unique to each system.

NLM MEDLINE assumes that search terms entered at the USER: prompt are MeSH headings unless a special format (e.g., author name, initials, colon, "all", etc.) is used. MiniMEDLINE, EBSCO, and Knowledge Finder require that a MeSH search option be selected.

Using MiniMEDLINE, a menu option for SUBJECT is chosen, then the heading being searched is keyed. MiniMEDLINE applies truncation automatically, allowing a user to type in part of the term (e.g., "APPETITE") to retrieve a listing of all MeSH entries containing the word "APPETITE." MiniMEDLINE also automatically maps MeSH cross-referenced (i.e., "X") headings to the valid MeSH heading, saving the user an extra search entry step. When a subject term is entered, all matching MeSH vocabulary is displayed for selection. When a MeSH heading is selected, it is redisplayed with its retrievable subheadings. A user can select one or all of the subheadings for further retrieval. As MeSH terms are selected, citation sets are built which can be displayed individually or combined with other sets using Boolean OR and AND operators. MiniMEDLINE does not support MeSH EXPLOSIONS.

EBSCO allows MeSH headings to be entered on the "Any field" lines of the search template, but to limit a search to the MeSH vocabulary, the terms should be entered on the template's "MeSH" line. Quotation marks must be used to identify multiple-word MeSH headings. Boolean OR, AND, and NOT operators are supported, as is EXPLODING.

Medical Subject Heading searches using Knowledge Finder begin with the selection of the "Subject Heading Thesaurus." As in the author search, there are several steps involved in selecting a term: the thesaurus is opened, a subject entry is keyed in, the alphabetic "page" containing the term is displayed along with its cross-referencing notes. A user can "double click" on a heading to see the MeSH detail (i.e., *Annotated MeSH*) for further information about the term's usage. A user can also "click" on "Context" to see the MeSH tree and to EXPLODE the term using the "Command" key in combination with the mouse. Knowledge Finder politely refers to EXPLODING terms as "creating CONTEXT GROUPS." This is a very simple and straight-forward process once the user discovers its location. Knowledge Finder also offers selection of topical subheadings, "floating" subheadings, and subject check tags - all at the click (or several clicks) of the mouse.

Knowledge Finder supports Boolean OR, AND, and NOT operators, but calls them "USE ONLY," "TRY TO USE," and "DON'T USE." This departure from the experienced online searcher's vocabulary created a controversy at the test site! Both librarians and experienced non-librarian searchers had difficulty making the transition from what they expressed as "precise language" to terms that they thought obfuscated an otherwise straight-forward process. Inexperienced searchers were less indignant.

While all the systems studied retrieved similar results for MeSH searches, Knowledge Finder, in terms of ease-of-use and variety of features, presented the most comprehensive approach to MeSH.

The "limiting" searches conducted on the systems were not particularly useful. All subsets included English only titles, so limiting to English was unnecessary except on NLM. (Note: the Knowledge Finder *UN-ABRIDGED* includes both English and foreign titles, but defaults to English.) MiniMEDLINE does not support date limitations and Knowledge Finder's date selections are based on MEDLINE entry *months* (i.e., tape-by-tape) rather than years. It's a tedious process to select a specific year on Knowledge Finder CORE, but it is a very handy SDI tool for saved searches. EBSCO supports both year and "year month" entries for retrieving dates of publication. NLM's simple "AND 86" seemed the most direct and best approach.

Text-word or free-form retrieval differed most among the systems. Subset "performance" was compared to the full NLM MEDLINE retrieval of 110 references (Table 4) and to the possible retrieval of 26 references to journals that are included in the title coverage of all subsets (Table 5).

Table 4

COMPARISON OF SUBSET RETRIEVAL
(Using NLM as the Percentage Base)

	System Retrieval	% Retrieved
NLM	110	100%
miniMEDLINE	16	14.5%
EBSCO	23	20.9%
KF	15*	13.6%

* KF actually retrieved 18 references, 3 of which were not included in the NLM retrieval.

Table 5

COMPARISON OF SUBSET RETRIEVAL
(Using Common Titles as the Percentage Base)

	System Retrieval	% Retrieved
NLM	26	100%
miniMEDLINE	10	38.5%
EBSCO	19	73%
KF	14	53.8%

While it may appear that Knowledge Finder is the least productive of the subsets when using NLM as a base, it should be emphasized that it is the smallest of the subsets (220 titles). MiniMEDLINE, containing 319 titles, retrieved only 14.5% of the base NLM set, and only 38.5% of the common title retrieval. Because MiniMEDLINE's text-word search capability is limited only to the title field, 15 references that included "EATING" and "DISORDERS" in the abstract were not retrieved from the common title group of references.

EBSCO's free-form search is applied to the title and abstract fields and supports phrases (by enclosing terms in quotation marks) and proximity (by enclosing terms in square brackets). For the purposes of this study, quotation marks were used to indicate "EATING DISORDER*" as a phrase. As a result, EBSCO's retrieval omitted references that contained "EATING" and "DISORDER*" as isolated words in the record. It is assumed that entering the search using proximity [EATING DISORDER*] would increase the number of references retrieved. EBSCO's proximity default of "within 50 words" is user-controlled; proximity can be set closer or farther apart.

Knowledge Finder's "free-form" (i.e., text-word) search is applied to all text fields within the record: title, MeSH descriptors, abstract. MeSH descriptors are unbound and treated as separate words when matched against the search terms. The search software's default settings include "Word Variants ON." This setting results in the automatic retrieval of search words plus suffixes such as -ability, -ally, -ancies, -ancy, -ed, -es, -ing, -s, -y, etc. (Note: over 135 suffixes are automatically applied.) Use of Word Variants relieves the searcher of having to use truncation or having to think of suffix possibilities. In the example EATING DISORDERS, three references were retrieved by Knowledge Finder and not by NLM because the word DISORDERS or EATING was used in a MeSH heading, or because a record containing a word variant (EAT) was retrieved. It should be noted that the search strategy used on NLM MEDLINE was "all eating (tw) and all disorder# (tw)" which excluded the possibility of retrieving MeSH heading matches. Knowledge Finder applies these search capabilities automatically; a user does not have to be trained in the idiosyncracies of command-mode MEDLINE to formulate and reformulate searches.

It is Knowledge Finder's automatic search capabilities that at once make it an easy retrieval system for novice searchers and an enigma to experienced searchers. Considering that the product is marketed as an end-user MEDLINE tool, the approach that Knowledge Finder has taken seems appropriate. While the Knowledge Finder search environment is loaded with automatic features, most of them are under the user's control. This control is not readily apparent to the casual user. The "Search Control Options" setting is found in the Search Window. When these options are revealed by a quick mouse click, the soul of Knowledge Finder is revealed: the "RELEVANCE FILTER."

Knowledge Finder uses a "probabilistic search mechanism" (or algorithm) to examine the occurrence of the search words in the database and to retrieve only those references judged to be *most relevant*. Relevancy is based on the frequency of word occurrence in the record, the fields the word appears in (more value is placed on the title than the abstract; more value is placed on major descriptors than minor descriptors), and frequency of occurrence in the database as a whole. A very frequently used word, such as "disease" is given less value than a less frequently occurring word. A value is also assigned based upon the length of citation. While Knowledge Finder defaults to a "middle-of-the-relevancy-filter" setting, a knowing user can adjust that setting to meet the needs of any particular search or group of searches. There are eleven shades-of-relevancy; each can retrieve a different result depending upon the search, but the references judged by Knowledge Finder to be "most relevant" will always be displayed first.

Other search options under the user's control include WORD VARI-ANTS and ARTICLE COUNT LIMIT. The Word Variants option is set ON, but can easily be clicked off. When ON, over 135 suffixes are automatically considered as retrieval possibilities for the search terms entered; when OFF, only matches for the term entered will be retrieved. The Article Count Limit is initially set to 100. Knowledge Finder assumes that a few highly relevant articles are better than a comprehensive retrieval of all search term matches. The default setting of 100 is a logical starting point. The setting can be changed to retrieve as few as 1 or as many as 1000 articles by simply clicking on the box and keying in the new value.

In addition to these automatic features, Knowledge Finder, like NLM MEDLINE and EBSCO, does support user-defined truncation and character substitution (using #, ?, or $) for more user control. MiniMEDLINE automatically applies truncation, but does not support character substitution.

Knowledge Finder offers a wide variety of personalized user features that are unavailable on the other systems. Personal annotations can be added to references as reminders. The length, field composition, and field order of display and print formats can be completely customized and the formatting saved for future use. Like NLM MEDLINE and EBSCO, search strategies can be saved for reuse. Again, like EBSCO (and NLM MEDLINE and MiniMEDLINE online), retrieval can be saved to either paper or disk. Knowledge Finder disk output is compatible with other standard Macintosh applications (e.g., MacWrite, Word, etc.), and with Personal Bibliographic Software, Inc.'s NLM Biblio-Link and Pro-Cite bibliography management software. This, coupled with the personal annotation feature, is an especially useful feature for researchers who maintain personal reference databases.

Comparison #2

While Knowledge Finder's automatic retrieval of references it judges to be relevant is very attractive and easy-to-use, a closer comparison of the retrieval results produced by Knowledge Finder and those obtained using by NLM MEDLINE was needed to determine whether relevant articles were missed by Knowledge Finder.

Methodology: Knowledge Finder documentation contains a clear statement of the subjectiveness of relevancy: "whether or not the citation is relevant is ultimately a decision that only you can make" (MEDLINE Knowledge Finder [Manual], January 1988, p.3-25). With this in mind, the retrieval from the EATING DISORDER# text-word search on NLM MEDLINE was compared to the retrieval obtained from Knowledge Finder UNABRIDGED. "Relevancy" was determined by the searcher. All articles addressing "eating disorders" as an appetite disorder, such as anorexia nervosa or bulimia were considered relevant to the information need. Note that this was a test of one search by one searcher. As quantitative analysis goes, an extremely small sample, but as a judgement of satisfaction by a system user, perhaps the only data necessary. The search statements used on NLM MEDLINE were: "all eating: and all disorder:", followed by limitations to English language and 1986. Using Knowledge Finder, the free-form search "eating disorders" was entered.

Results: Tables 6, 7, and 8 show the results of the searches and the relevancy judgements. The precision ratio (as defined by F.W. Lancaster in *Vocabulary Control for Information Retrieval*, Washington, D.C.: Information Resources Press, 1972, p.108-110) was calculated by dividing the total relevant retrieval by the total retrieval and multiplying by 100.

While Knowledge Finder's overall precision was slightly better than NLM MEDLINE's for this search, Knowledge Finder's unique retrieval precision was much lower than NLM MEDLINE's. Of the five unique articles that Knowledge Finder retrieved, four were judged to be not relevant to the

Table 6

COMPARISON OF NLM MEDLINE and KNOWLEDGE FINDER UNABRIDGED			
	Total Retrieval	Total Relevant	Precision Ratio
NLM MEDLINE	119	100	84.0
KF UNABRIDGED	63	55	87.3

Table 7

COMPARISON OF NLM MEDLINE and KNOWLEDGE FINDER UNABRIDGED		
Common Retrieval	Total Relevant	Precision Ratio
58	54	93

Table 8

COMPARISON OF NLM MEDLINE and KNOWLEDGE FINDER UNABRIDGED			
	Unique Retrieval	Total Relevant	Precision Ratio
NLM MEDLINE	61	46	75.4
KF UNABRIDGED	5	1	20.0

searcher's need. Matches with the unbound MeSH descriptor "Disorders" was a factor in all four records. "Disorders" was weighted as a major descriptor in two articles which also included "eating" as either a major descriptor or word in the abstract. One of these two articles also counted "eat" in the title when determining relevancy for retrieval. The other two records contained "Disorders" as a minor descriptor and "eat" or "eating" in the title or multiple times in the abstract. In this one particular search, Knowledge Finder's relevancy algorithm appears to have created more "noise" than precision.

To further compare retrieval using Knowledge Finder and NLM MEDLINE, a small sample of "real searches," i.e., searches conducted by users of Knowledge Finder was analyzed. Knowledge Finder users were approached and asked to make a second copy of the references they printed. A reference librarian then ran the search on NLM's MEDLINE without conducting a reference interview and basing the strategy on the words input by the Knowledge Finder searcher. In all cases, some articles printed by the Knowledge Finder searcher, and therefore assumed to be relevant, were not retrieved by the NLM search. HOWEVER, when these references were analyzed, it was discovered that they did not actually contain all the concepts stated by the user.

For example, one search was "sickle cell membrane permeability". Many of the references retrieved with Knowledge Finder were about cell membrane permeability but not sickle cells. Such articles would rarely be retrieved in a "first pass" search by a trained searcher. The Knowledge Finder software makes various permutations and combinations of the words input by a searcher often netting a larger retrieval with lower precision. The question of course is: "Do end-users want to plow through less precise references?" This is, of course, a matter of individual preference, but most people do not seem to mind looking at large numbers of references. Indeed, one of the Knowledge Finder search participants spent three hours looking at 163 citations! This type of browsing also often nets articles which are not precisely pertinent to the question at hand but are related to an individual's overall work. To fully determine the effectiveness of the relevancy factor, more searches would need to be compared between Knowledge Finder and NLM MEDLINE.

Comparison #3

The question arose: what effect do changes in the search control options have on Knowledge Finder's retrieval? The answer to this question was only addressed quantitatively; there was no attempt to identify relevant articles or determine a precision ratio as in Comparison #2.

Methodology: All six disks of Knowledge Finder Unabridged MEDLINE were searched three times, again using "Eating Disorders" as a free-form search. The first time the search was conducted, the default Knowledge Finder settings were used: RELEVANCE FILTER at the mid-range setting, ARTICLE COUNT LIMIT = 100, WORD VARIANTS = ON). The second time the search was conducted, the RELEVANCE FILTER was adjusted to "emphasize relevancy"; the other settings remained at their defaults. The third time the search was conducted, the RELEVANCE FILTER was adjusted to "emphasize quantity" and the ARTICLE COUNT LIMIT was changed to its highest setting (1000); the WORD VARIANTS remained at "ON." Table 9 lists the results of these searches. In a separate process, the WORD VARIANTS setting was compared throughout the RELEVANCY scale at the ARTICLE COUNT LIMIT of 100 and 1000 (Table 10).

Table 9

COMPARISON OF KNOWLEDGE FINDER SEARCH CONTROL SETTINGS

	Year	KF Retrieved as "Relevant"	Total Articles Considered for Relevancy	Disk Access Time (Sec.)
Default	1988	39	2980	10.8
Settings	1987	49	3917	13.2
	1986	63	4316	14.2
	1985	41	4239	15.4
	1984	43	4236	13.9
	1983	39	3471	12.4
		274	23069	79.9
Emphasize	1988	1	1790	8.7
Relevancy	1987	1	2379	11.6
	1986	1	2647	12.7
	1985	1	2645	12.7
	1984	1	2641	11.7
	1983	1	2114	11.2
		6	14216	68.6
Emphasize	1988	1000	6850	27.8
Quantity	1987	1000	12796	28.8
	1986	1000	13346	29.9
	1985	1000	12300	30.9
	1984	1000	12028	30.0
	1984	1000	11388	33.0
		6000	68708	179.6

Table 10

COMPARISON OF KNOWLEDGE FINDER SEARCH CONTROL SETTINGS
(Using KF Unabridged MEDLINE, 1986 disk)

EMPHASIZE RELEVANCY <<<<< RELEVANCY FILTER >>>>> EMPHASIZE QUANTITY

	000	010	020	030	040	050	060	070	080	090	100
WV ON/ACL = 100											
Retrieved	1	2	13	13	20	63	94	100	100	100	100
Total Considered	2647	2918	3142	3423	3814	4316	5069	6302	8471	11745	10843
WV OFF/ACL = 100											
Retrieved	1	4	17	21	23	33	84	100	100	100	100
Total Considered	386	426	480	546	636	763	947	1257	1858	2758	13346
WV ON/ACL = 1000											
Retrieved	1	11	36	158	177	590	590	590	1000	1000	1000
Total Considered	12383	13252	13346	13346	13346	13346	13346	13346	13346	13346	13346
WV OFF/ACL = 1000											
Retrieved	1	12	53	144	165	991	991	991	991	991	1000
Total Considered	2917	3134	3402	3747	4206	4837	5775	7333	10374	10843	10843

KNOWLEDGE FINDER DEFAULT SETTINGS
RELEVANCY FILTER 050
WORD VARIANTS ON
ARTICLE COUNT 100

WV: WORD VARIANTS
ACL: ARTICLE COUNT LIMIT

Results: Knowledge Finder looks at fewer articles when relevancy is emphasized than it does at the default setting or when quantity is emphasized. This is due to Knowledge Finder's method of sorting, or ordering, entries in its index structure. Unlike traditional database indexes that list document accession numbers as matches for a particular search term, Knowledge Finder indexes are sorted by the search term's valued "weight" in a given document. Those documents having the highest relevancy value or "weight" are listed first in the indexes. Taking both the RELEVANCY FILTER setting and the the ARTICLE COUNT LIMIT into account, Knowledge Finder determines how many documents to consider as retrieval possibilities. The WORD VARIANTS setting also affects the number of documents Knowledge Finder considers for retrieval. If WORD VARIANTS is set "ON," more documents are "looked at" than when WORD VARIANTS is "OFF."

How does this help the user? The most relevant articles can be identified quickly, without having to sift through a long retrieval list. If more articles are needed, adjustments can be made in the SEARCH CONTROL OPTIONS to modify the retrieval without keying in additional search terms. With experience, users can customize the size and relevancy expectations of the retrieval results to meet their specific information needs. Because both individual searchers and individual search needs are so varied, Knowledge Finder's adjustable SEARCH CONTROL OPTIONS are a distinct benefit.

User Survey

PLANNING AND IMPLEMENTATION

Getting Ready

Reference Staff developed a questionnaire to be completed each time a patron used Knowledge Finder (it was difficult to persuade users to fill out more than one). One reference librarian was designated the system "expert" and developed the patron instructions. She also served as staff instructor and troubleshooter. Systems Staff provided hardware information and maintenance.

The "expert" read the user manual and performed sample searches on Knowledge Finder to become familiar with the system features. These initial searches netted results which were inconsistent with the expectations of a very experienced searcher. Dr. Lyndon Holmes, president of Aries, was contacted and he explained the concept of "soft" Boolean (artificial intelligence-based logic) which is used in Knowledge Finder. This conversation explained the mysterious results. It would be very useful to have this explanation in the user manual.

Patron Instruction

Reference Staff decided that an end-user system should be self-instructional. Therefore, no "Introduction to Knowledge Finder" classes were held and only minimal individual instruction was given to patrons during their use of Knowledge Finder. To supplement the online help screens, one sheet of written instructions was placed next to the workstation (Appendix A). Library staff loaded the disks for CORE users; first time UNABRIDGED users were given instruction on loading and changing disks. Library staff relaxed considerably as patrons proved capable of loading the disks with no trouble. Once disks were loaded, patrons were very much on their own. However, if problems or questions arose during the course of the search, a reference librarian was available for consultation. Most patrons were able to execute a search, view citations, and print them with the single sheet of instructions available.

EVALUATION

Internal Log Information

Aries Knowledge Finder offers an internal logging process to record searches. The log records a wealth of significant information about searches including the actual search formulation. The log file must be emptied frequently or information can become inaccessible due to the size of the file.

Logs covering two week periods for each of the versions of KNOWLEDGE FINDER were analyzed. During those two week periods logins and searches were counted. A login was defined as a search session followed by a system shutdown. A search was defined as system interaction which ended in the viewing of citations. This means an intellectual search was counted more than once if performed across multiple years in the UNABRIDGED version. There were 27 logins on the CORE version and 58 logins on the UNABRIDGED version. Table 11 outlines the types of searches performed on each version.

The free-form search was the most popular of the search options for the Knowledge Finder CORE. This may have been a reflection of the decision not to provide formal instruction; it might also indicate that this particular search option is the most obvious choice and the easiest to use. The free-form search option was used to much lesser degree in the UNABRIDGED version; the use of each of the other options was increased significantly. This change clearly reflects an increase in the numbers of experienced users. Repeat users were far more likely to question the reference staff about alternative ways to perform a search and to begin to experiment with the various options available on the KNOWLEDGE FINDER screen.

Table 11

	CORE	UNABRIDGED

COMPARISON OF PATRON USE OF
KNOWLEDGE FINDER CORE AND UNABRIDGED

	CORE	UNABRIDGED
<u>Free-form</u>	<u>74.0%</u>	<u>48.3%</u>
1 word	52.7%	36.0%
2 word	24.0%	25.0%
3 words or more	23.3%	38.0%
<u>Dictionary/</u> <u>Thesaurus</u>	<u>19.3%</u>	<u>36.0%</u>
author	23.7%	38.2%
subject	68.4%	56.2%
journal	7.9%	5.6%
<u>Combination*</u>	<u>6.1%</u>	<u>15.7%</u>

*This includes various combinations: dictionary/thesaurus with free-form, free-form with author or journal, journal with subject or author

The log records were also used to see how many of the six years (disks) were searched. For this purpose, a search was defined as an intellectual one rather than the more arbitrary definition of a search described above; the January June, 1988 disk was considered a year. Fifty percent of the searches covered 1 year; 23 %, 2 years; 11%, 3 years; 6%, 4 years; 2%, 5 years and 8%, 6 years. These percentages do not necessarily indicate that 50% of the searches were on the Jan-June, 1988 disk; many people chose a single disk seemingly at random and did not continue searching any further. Many people searched one or two years in one session and returned hours or days later to run the same search on additional years.

User Survey

To accommodate patron evaluation, the reference staff developed a 25-item questionnaire (Appendix B). Questions 1-17 were designed to elicit opinions about the system and its features. Questions 18-25 were designed to obtain demographic information about the people using the system. The questionnaires with percentage responses are reproduced as Appendix B and C.

The user survey produced no great surprises. Patrons were generally positive about all aspects of the system. Studies of the Knowledge Finder CORE correlating demographics and the general opinions about the system revealed no significant differences in the responses of physicians versus non-physicians or the responses of experienced Macintosh users versus non-Mac users. Of the correlations done, only one produced a statistically significant difference, and that was on only one item. Item 9 stated that MiniMEDLINE had more information than Knowledge Finder CORE. Faculty agreed with the statement more than non-faculty did. This is probably explained by two factors: (1) basic sciences faculty are more likely to identify themselves as faculty (though physicians could have chosen both physician and faculty), and (2) Knowledge Finder CORE provides a very limited database for basic scientists.

The survey also requested comments. The comments for Knowledge Finder CORE fell into three categories: dissatisfaction with the database, with the printer or general positive comments. Basic scientists felt the database was too clinically oriented and others felt the database was too small or did not cover enough years. Everyone who commented on the printer found it to be too noisy and too slow. Users also wanted to continue searching while printing. However, a number of people who made these comments added that they were very pleased with the system anyway. The third category included general positive comments about the system, with no specifics. Less than half of the questionnaires had comments of any kind.

Analysis of the survey response to Knowledge Finder UNABRIDGED again produced no great surprises. The most significant difference in response was to item 6: "I found all the information I needed." 38.1% of Knowledge Finder CORE users responded positively to the question; 68.6% of the UNABRIDGED users responded positively to this item. No significant differences appeared in the groups of people using the CORE version versus the UNABRIDGED version. Percentages of positive responses increased for the UNABRIDGED version on the questions dealing with the size and scope of the database. Very few comments appeared on the UNABRIDGED version surveys: none complained about the size and scope of the database; only one or two complained about the printer.

General Comments

Some members of the reference staff had difficulty adjusting to the "soft" Boolean and wanted an option for hard **ands** and **ors.** A number of people who had taken "The Basics of Searching Medline" class had similar difficulties. MiniMEDLINE, the Medical University's MEDLINE subset, uses strict Boolean logic and the reference staff has worked very hard to teach that concept to system users. This desire for "hard" Boolean might not be a problem elsewhere.

While people with some knowledge of Boolean logic had difficulties with the system, the "soft" Boolean concept is a major step in the right direction as far as end-user searching goes. Knowledge Finder enables people with no searching experience to quickly search and print references with little or no instruction from a reference librarian. To take full advantage of the system, individuals need instruction or a manual but does everyone want to take full advantage of searching capabilities? Knowledge Finder delays the necessity of teaching such thorny issues as Boolean logic and truncation until a time when a patron is willing to invest the time in learning more sophisticated techniques and has done enough searching to realize that there are ways to improve his search results.

Conclusion

Knowledge Finder offers unique.and extensive features in a highly reliable package designed especially for the end-user. The evaluation at the Medical University of South Carolina revealed the system's strengths to be (1) search software designed to give novice users the capability of searching successfully with little or no instruction, (2) adjustable search control options, (3) excellent documentation, and (4) strong vendor support. Knowledge Finder has become a popular resource at the Medical University Library. It is steadily used and enthusiastically accepted by library patrons—the ultimate evaluators of any "end-user service."

GETTING STARTED ON MEDLINE
CD-ROM KNOWLEDGE FINDER

Read the screen. Move the arrow to the COPYRIGHTS ACKNOWLEDGED bar and click on the MOUSE

SCREEN CONTROLS

MOUSE Controls arrow on screen
Move the arrow using the MOUSE to the menu option or terms you want to select; click on the MOUSE to select the desired menu option or term

 Click on this option to look at citations

 Click on this option to initiate a search

 Click on this option to erase all search input

 Search or operation in progress; no other operations possible

CURSOR Blinking vertical line
Shows where you can type terms such as subject headings, authors' names etc.

  Search in progress; no other operations possible

 Search or operation in progress; no other operations possible

SEARCHING

FREE-FORM TOPIC SEARCH Type keywords for your topic

SUBJECT, AUTHOR, ETC. Click on desired search type with MOUSE; click on selected terms; choose one of three options:
USE ONLY... if you want a precise search retrieving only the terms you've indicated
TRY TO USE... if you want a less precise search
DON'T USE if you do not want a term included

ORing TERMS TOGETHER Hold down COMMAND key; click MOUSE on desired terms to form a synonym group

EXPLODING SUBJECT HEADINGS Select subject heading; double-click MOUSE for context; hold down COMMAND key, click MOUSE on desired broad heading, all subordinate headings will be included in a synonym group

VIEWING AND PRINTING

Click on to look at citations

Select items for printing by clicking MOUSE on

To **PRINT**, select the FILE command from the top of the screen; choose the PRINT SELECTED ARTICLES option; check print parameters screen; click on the OK box to initiate printing

LEAVING THE SYSTEM

Select the FILE command from the top of the screen; choose the QUIT option; after processing has stopped choose the SPECIAL option from the top of the screen; select the SHUTDOWN option; remove the disk and return it to the Circulation desk

Appendix B-1

KNOWLEDGE FINDER <u>CORE</u> CD-ROM EVALUATION

Please answer the following questions using the scale below:

5=STRONGLY AGREE 4=AGREE 3=NEUTRAL 2=DISAGREE 1=STRONGLY DISAGREE

1. I was able to turn on the computer and the CD-ROM player with ease.

5	4	3	2	1
68.4%	20.3%	3.8%	7.6%	-

2. The printed instructions located at the computer gave me the information I needed to search the system.

5	4	3	2	1
44.7%	37.6%	10.6%	3.5%	3.5%

3. KNOWLEDGE FINDER did not go far enough back in time for my purpose.

5	4	3	2	1
17.9%	17.9%	37.2%	19.2%	7.7%

4. I thought the system response time was fast.

5	4	3	2	1
43.5%	41.2%	14.1%	1.2%	-

5. The screen/help instructions on KNOWLEDGE FINDER were not helpful.

5	4	3	2	1
12.0%	10.8%	13.3%	32.5%	31.3%

6. I found all the information I needed.

5	4	3	2	1
11.9%	26.2%	19.0%	33.3%	9.5%

7. I expected to find more information than I did.

5	4	3	2	1
9.9%	34.6%	14.8%	32.1%	8.6%

8. This system is easier to use than MiniMEDLINE.

5	4	3	2	1
32.1%	21.0%	24.7%	12.3%	9.9%

9. MiniMEDLINE has more information than KNOWLEDGE FINDER.

5	4	3	2	1
9.1%	16.9%	40.3%	15.6%	18.2%

THE FOLLOWING QUESTIONS PERTAIN TO THE TYPES OF SEARCHES YOU PERFORMED. PLEASE CIRCLE THE TYPES OF SEARCHES YOU DID AT EACH SESSION; YOU MAY HAVE MORE THAN ONE TYPE IN A GIVEN SESSION. THE SCALE IS THE SAME AS THE SCALE FOR THE PREVIOUS QUESTIONS.

10. 1. Author-**18.6%**　　2. topic (includes keywords, subjects, title words)-**81.4%**　　3. journal title-**1.2%**　　4. year-**2.3%**　　5. combination of two or more above using Boolean _and_ or _or_-**14.0%**　　6. other (please specify)-**1.2%**

11. I was able to broaden my search to retrieve more articles when necessary

5	4	3	2	1
12.9%	42.9%	34.3%	4.3%	5.7%

12. I was able to narrow my search to retrieve fewer articles when necessary.

5	4	3	2	1
17.8%	35.6%	32.9%	8.2%	5.5%

13. Searching by topic was easy.

5	4	3	2	1
47.6%	40.2%	8.5%	1.2%	2.4%

14. Limiting my search to a specific journal title was easy.

5	4	3	2	1
28.9%	13.3%	44.4%	8.9%	4.4%

15. Searching by author was easy.

5	4	3	2	1
41.5%	17.1%	39.0%	-	2.4%

16. Limiting my search to a specific year was easy.

5	4	3	2	1
20.5%	15.4%	59.0%	-	5.1%

17. Combining sets with boolean logic was a successful technique when using KNOWLEDGE FINDER

5	4	3	2	1
17.3%	25.0%	42.3%	1.9%	13.5%

FOR EACH QUESTION, PLEASE CIRCLE **ALL** THE FOLLOWING ANSWERS THAT APPLY

18. I am affiliated with:
    1. Medicine-**50.0%** 2. Dental Medicine-**2.3%** 3. Nursing-**3.5%** 4. Pharmacy-**4.7%**
    5. Hospital-**1.2%** 6. Health related professions-**7.0%** 7. Basic Sciences-**19.8%**
    8. Other-**11.6%**

19. I am a :
    1. Physician-**32.6%** 2. Nurse-**4.7%** 3. Dentist-**1.2%**   4. Other Health Professional-**3.5%** 5. Faculty-**16.3%** 6.Researcher-**14.0%** 7. Support Staff-**1.2%** 8. Student-**37.2%**
    9. Other-**4.7%**

20. I need information for:
    1. Patient care-**24.4%** 2. Lecture/speech-**17.4%** 3. Paper/publication-**43.0%**
    4. Grant/research-**41.9%** 5. Current awareness-**11.6%** 6. Didn't need anything, just curious-**14.7%** 7. Other-**2.3%**

21. I have previously used:
    1. Index Medicus etc. **79.1%**
    2. Other printed indexes... **52.3%**
    3. MiniMEDLINE **84.9%**
    4. Database searches performed by a librarian **62.8%**
    5. Computerized databases other than MiniMEDLINE to perform my own searches **19.8%**

22. I have used Knowledge Finder _____ times.

0	1-2	3-5	6-9	10 or more
80.5%	12.2%	6.1%	1.2%	-

23. I retrieved _____ references.

1-10	11-20	21-50	51-100	100+
46.8%	16.9%	20.8%	7.8%	7.8%

24. I printed _____ references.

1-10	11-20	21-50	51-100	100+
57.7%	25.4%	15.5%	-	-

25. I have used a Macintosh microcomputer

never	occasionally	frequently
17.1%	30.5%	52.4%

KNOWLEDGE FINDER <u>UNABRIDGED</u> CD-ROM EVALUATION

Please answer the following questions using the scale below:

5=STRONGLY AGREE 4=AGREE 3=NEUTRAL 2=DISAGREE 1=STRONGLY DISAGREE

1. I was able to turn on the computer and the CD-ROM player with ease.

5	4	3	2	1
80.5%	13.4%	4.9%	1.2%	-

2. The printed instructions located at the computer gave me the information I needed to search the system.

5	4	3	2	1
45.2%	36.9%	9.5%	4.8%	3.6%

3. KNOWLEDGE FINDER did not go far enough back in time for my purpose.

5	4	3	2	1
10.8%	14.5%	10.8%	33.7%	30.1%

4. I thought the system response time was fast.

5	4	3	2	1
51.1%	35.7%	4.8%	2.4%	-

5. The screen/help instructions on KNOWLEDGE FINDER were not helpful.

5	4	3	2	1
2.4%	7.3%	22.0%	24.4%	43.9%

6. I found all the information I needed.

5	4	3	2	1
31.3%	37.3%	19.3%	8.4%	3.6%

7. I expected to find more information than I did.

5	4	3	2	1
10.8%	10.8%	31.3%	22.9%	24.1%

8. This system is easier to use than MiniMEDLINE.

5	4	3	2	1
29.1%	32.9%	27.8%	6.3%	3.8%

9. MiniMEDLINE has more information than KNOWLEDGE FINDER.

5	4	3	2	1
3.8%	2.5%	22.5%	20.0%	51.3%

THE FOLLOWING QUESTIONS PERTAIN TO THE TYPES OF SEARCHES YOU
PERFORMED. PLEASE CIRCLE THE TYPES OF SEARCHES YOU DID AT EACH
SESSION; YOU MAY HAVE MORE THAN ONE TYPE IN A GIVEN SESSION. THE
SCALE IS THE SAME AS THE SCALE FOR THE PREVIOUS QUESTIONS.

10. 1. Author-**29.4%**   2. topic (includes keywords, subjects, title words)-**80.0%**   3. journal
title-**4.7%**   4. year-**3.5%**   5. combination of two or more above using Boolean
<u>and</u> or <u>or</u>-**14.1%**   6. other (please specify)-**1.2%**

11. I was able to broaden my search to retrieve more articles when necessary

5	4	3	2	1
29.7%	41.9%	24.3%	2.7%	1.4%

12. I was able to narrow my search to retrieve fewer articles when necessary.

5	4	3	2	1
55.0%	35.0%	6.3%	3.8%	-

13. Searching by topic was easy.

5	4	3	2	1
27.3 %	12.7%	54.5%	3.6%	1.8%

14. Limiting my search to a specific journal title was easy.

5	4	3	2	1
27.3%	12.7%	54.5%	3.6%	1.8%

15. Searching by author was easy.

5	4	3	2	1
50.0%	3.1%	45.3%	1.6%	-

16. Limiting my search to a specific year was easy.

5	4	3	2	1
51.5%	8.8%	35.3%	2.9%	1.5%

17. Combining sets with boolean logic was a successful technique when using
KNOWLEDGE FINDER.

5	4	3	2	1
22.8%	19.3%	52.6%	5.3%	-

FOR EACH QUESTION, PLEASE CIRCLE **ALL** THE FOLLOWING ANSWERS THAT APPLY

18. I am affiliated with:
    1. Medicine-**37.6%** 2. Dental Medicine-**5.9%** 3. Nursing-**1.2%** 4. Pharmacy-**11.8%**
    5. Hospital-**3.5%** 6. Health related professions-**5.9%** 7. Basic Sciences-**20.0%**
    8. Other-**7.1%**

19. I am a :
    1. Physician-**28.2%** 2. Nurse-**1.2%** 3. Dentist-**2.4%** 4. Other Health Professional-**4.7%** 5. Faculty-**12.9%** 6. Researcher-**8.2%** 7. Support Staff-**0.0%** 8. Student-**31.8%** 9. Other-**14.1%**

20. I need information for:
    1. Patient care-**24.7%** 2. Lecture/speech-**28.2%** 3.Paper/publication-**35.3%**
    4. Grant/research-**41.2%** 5. Current awareness-**14.1%** 6. Didn't need anything,just curious-**0.0%** 7. Other-**2.4%**

21. I have previously used:
    1. Index Medicus etc. **75.3%**
    2. Other printed indexes... **50.6%**
    3. MiniMEDLINE **78.8%**
    4. Database searches performed by a librarian **61.2%**
    5. Computerized databases other than MiniMEDLINE to perform my own searches **18.8%**

22. I have used Knowledge Finder _____ times:

0	1-2	3-5	6-9	10 or more
51.9%	18.2%	22.1%	5.2%	2.6%

23. I retrieved _____ references:

1-10	11-20	21-50	51-100	100+
24.0%	22.7%	24.0%	10.7%	18.7%

24. I printed _____ references:

0	1-10	11-20	21-50	51-100	100+
1.3%	30.7%	34.7%	25.3%	5.3%	2.7%

25. I have used a Macintosh microcomputer

never	occasionally	frequently
28.6%	29.9%	41.6%

KNOWLEDGE FINDER
AT ROCKFORD

EVALUATION OF A CD-ROM MEDLINE SYSTEM IN A COMMUNITY-BASED MEDICAL SCHOOL LIBRARY AND AN OUTPATIENT CLINIC

By *Prudence Ward Dalrymple,*

Library of the Health Sciences
University of Illinois College of
Medicine at Rockford
1601 Parkview Ave.
Rockford, IL 61107.

Knowledge Finder At Rockford
Evaluation Of A CD-ROM MEDLINE System In A Community-Based Medical School Library And An Outpatient Clinic

I. Introduction

The following report describes an evaluation conducted at the Library of the Health Sciences, University of Illinois College of Medicine at Rockford, of Knowledge Finder, a CD-ROM MEDLINE product developed by Aries Systems. The evaluation was conducted in two stages. The first stage was designed primarily to determine who used Knowledge Finder and how it was used. A secondary objective was to explore certain aspects of the user interface that are unique to Knowledge Finder. In the second stage, the Knowledge Finder was installed in a clinical setting, a primary care clinic operated by the University of Illinois College of Medicine at Rockford.

The data collected in the first stage was conducted in the library using a questionnaire developed by the National Library of Medicine Office of Planning and Evaluation and modified to reflect conditions in the evaluation site. The questionnaire consisted of 24 items examining attribute variables used to describe the user population, as well as variables used to characterize the search session such as purpose of search, session length, sources of help, frequency of re-running a search (search reformulation) and satisfaction with search system and results. One of the items used a semantic differential to determine attitudes toward the search experience; results of the analysis of the semantic differential will be presented in a separate article at a later date. In the clinical evaluation, the CD-ROM was unattended and data were collected by means of transaction logs. The results of both the library-based and the clinic- based evaluations are included in this report.

II. The Medical Information Environment at Rockford

The University of Illinois College of Medicine at Rockford is a community-based medical school with a population of approximately 150 medical students and 30 Family Practice residents. Medical students arrive on campus in the second of their four years of medical school, having obtained their basic science education at the University of Illinois at Urbana-Champaign. The faculty is drawn primarily from clinicians practicing in the community; most appointments are part-time.

The campus consists of the main facility housing the library, administrative offices, and classrooms. The Office for Family Practice (OFP), staffed by the residents, is located in one wing of the building. Three rural community health centers are located 20-30 miles outside of Rockford. The College also supports a small biomedical research department with labs located in the same building as the library.

The Library of the Health Sciences in Rockford is one of the libraries of the University of Illinois at Chicago. Its collection is composed of approximately 52,000 volumes. Reference service is available 8:00-5:00 weekdays. Last year, about 1200 online searches (primarily MEDLINE on BRS) were conducted by librarians. The cost of these searches is subsidized by the academic departments, grants, or a special fund made available by the school's director.

The three teaching hospitals affiliated with the College maintain libraries with online search services available to faculty and staff, and therefore most faculty, medical students, and residents have been exposed to mediated online searches.[1] Although provision of end-user searching facilities has been explored by all the Rockford area health science libraries, none has instituted a program of end-user access such as Grateful Med or PaperChase. There are no CD-ROM database products located in any of the libraries in Rockford. Thus, the presence of Knowledge Finder was unique within the community.

Most students arrive in Rockford with a basic familiarity with microcomputing.[2] A microcomputer lab equipped with an IBM PC and an Apple computer was established in the library in 1985 and has shown steadily increasing use. No Macintosh computers are available at the College of Medicine, although many faculty and students have used them elsewhere.

Because most students and faculty are based in hospitals and clinics away from the library, a flyer announcing the evaluation was sent to all 400 faculty. Two announcements appeared in the library newsletter *Offshoots*. In addition, a series of three flyers was stuffed in student, staff, and in- house faculty mailboxes during the evaluation period.

III. Description of the Knowledge Finder

Knowledge Finder exploits many of the unique features of the Macintosh interface in order to present in graphic format a simple and attractive approach to bibliographic searching that is accessible to the casual user, while at the same time offering a number of highly sophisticated searching options to more advanced users. The interface is designed to be highly interactive and iterative; it encourages users to "run" their searches several times using new terminology or different search parameters. While offering full Boolean and keyword searching capabilities as well as MeSH authority files, the system differs from traditional database searching by employing a probabilistic searching algorithm that ranks retrieval according to the likelihood of its relevance to a given query.[3] Furthermore, it displays this ranking on a "relevancy graph" that can be adjusted to emphasize precision over recall, or vice versa; this is known as the "relevancy filter." Because the software release containing the transaction logging capability was not available at the outset of the library evaluation, it was not possible to observe directly users' understanding and utility to manipulate Knowledge Finder's interface. During the clinical evaluation, the transaction log was the primary method of data collection and provides an indication of the extent to which users tried the various features. Further exploration of this approach to information retrieval may yield greater insights into the ways in which users change and develop their searching patterns over time, and which features are used most frequently.

IV. Description of the Evaluations

Prior to the evaluation, the Knowledge Finder software was loaded onto the Macintosh hard disk. Since the one-disk MEDLINE subset consisting of 225 core medical and nursing journals was used during the evaluation, it was placed in the CD ROM player and no further access to the player was required. A sign requesting that users sign up before using the system was posted at the workstation.

A photocopy of the Knowledge Finder tutorial was placed beside the Macintosh. The Knowledge Finder user manual was available on request. A brief handout (two pages) explaining the evaluation program and giving some helpful hints on getting started with the Macintosh was given to each user along with the questionnaire.

Library staff were instructed to request that users complete a questionnaire each time they used the Knowledge Finder (see Appendix A). This was done for two reasons. First, it was hypothesized that there would be differences in response between users searching Knowledge Finder for the first time and those who had had experience with the system. Second, there was concern that too few responses would be generated, since the evaluation coincided in part with the National Board Exam period, usually a time period associated with fewer information search requests.

Staff noted the beginning and ending times for each session. The session log was numbered to coincide with the pre-numbered questionnaires to facilitate matching the response with the session so as to assist in reviewing any outliers. The session log also made it possible to determine the proportion of repeat users versus new users and thus to observe the ways in which search sessions differed over time. Data collection began April 1 and ended June 21, 1988. One hundred and one (101) sessions were logged.

On June 24, 1988, the Knowledge Finder was relocated to the Office for Family Practice for the clinical evaluation. One week prior to the relocation, the author met with second and third year residents to describe the evaluation and to demonstrate the Knowledge Finder. Copies of an abbreviated version of the questionnaire (13 items) (Appendix B) were placed by the Knowledge Finder, and the telephone number of the library was posted nearby. The abbreviated questionnaire omitted questions regarding the user interface. Early in the evaluation period, the Knowledge Finder was unavailable to users for about a week because of interior re-painting. The author visited the clinic weekly to insure that the system was working properly. Otherwise no other assistance was available to clinicians. The Knowledge Finder was returned to the library on August 17, 1988.

An automatic logging device developed by Aries Systems was installed during the clinical evaluation in order to capture basic information about the searches being conducted on the system. The log provides data such as date and time, search type (author, subject, title), database searched (MEDLINE core, MEDLINE by years covered, MeSH, and others), number of items retrieved, number of items considered by the system to be "relevant," number of citations reviewed by the searcher, and the search formulation. The elapsed time is the number of seconds taken by the processing unit, useful data in terms of system capability but not helpful in understanding the length of the search session from the users' perspective. The log also indicates which of the available search controls was adjusted by the searcher, and which remained in the default mode.

V. The Sample Populations

Ninety-five questionnaires were returned; six users did not complete a questionnaire. Of the questionnaires returned, ten were completed by librarians or library staff and were removed from consideration. The sample therefore consists of 85 questionnaires, and results are reported for this group only. Of these, the majority (66) were affiliated with medicine, 6 with nursing, 6 with allied health or public health, and 4 were other (math, biophysics, etc.). The largest group of questionnaires was from students (39 or 46%) with the next largest from physicians (22 or 26%). Scientists/researchers were 9 (11%) and nurses 6 (7%). Other professions made up the remainder.

The clinical evaluation was restricted to family practice residents. As was expected, users in the clinical setting were not motivated to complete the questionnaire. Four residents completed them in response to a general request at a staff meeting. Two residents and the clinic director agreed to be interviewed regarding their use of Knowledge Finder. Given the non-representative nature of the respondents, the data were not analyzed systematically, but were reviewed to identify any important differences among the groups. The results of the library evaluation are presented below, followed by the findings that results from the clinical evaluation.

VI. Results of the Library Evaluation

A. Library and Computer Experience

In order to identify whether Knowledge Finder users represent a new class of library users, two questions were asked regarding frequency of library materials use and frequency of requesting a computer search. Most of the questionnaires were completed by frequent library users—people who used the library at least once a month, and often more than once a week. Of the few respondents who had never been to the library before, one was an administrator, one a medical student, and two were nurses. The computer search data were collapsed into frequent, moderate, and infrequent users.[4] Most respondents were moderate users of the computer search service, having requested a computer search at least once a year.

Because Knowledge Finder runs on a Macintosh computer, two questions were included to determine previous microcomputer use and previous Macintosh use. Almost every respondent had used a computer—only 15% had not. Thirty-one respondents (36%) had never used a Macintosh before.

Fifteen respondents reported having searched MEDLINE by themselves, whereas 45 reported having had a librarian process a search. When asked to select one of four access mechanisms to MEDLINE (search on their own, gateway search, mediated search or Knowledge Finder), the various forms of end-user access were favored over mediated searches (40 to 9). Since this question was designed to eliminate respondents who had never used MEDLINE in any form, not all respondents stated a preference. It appears, however, that those who have tried end-user searching, prefer it. The frequency of preferences is displayed below:

Preferred Mode of MEDLINE Access

Knowledge Finder 25
End-user search 15
Mediated search 9
Gateway search 2

From the preceding analysis, it was concluded that the response captured in this evaluation described a sample of individuals who were experienced library users possessing a better-than-average familiarity with computers and computerized information retrieval. A substantial number of users had tried end-user searching of MEDLINE, and preferred it over mediated searches.

B. First-time Users vs. Repeat Users

Because respondents logged their sessions, it was possible to determine whether some of the questionnaires were filled out by users who had searched Knowledge Finder one or more times previously. It was also possible to determine which sessions were not represented by a questionnaire. The session log was analyzed to determine how many different individuals comprised the user group. Of the 101 sessions logged, just over half of the sessions reflected repeat users (54), most of whom returned questionnaires. The frequency distribution of repeat use across the sample is displayed here:

No. of uses	Frequency.
1	57
2	19
3	8
4	3
5	2
6	1

Total   90*

(*Logged sessions excluding library staff/libraries—not all returned questionnaires)

When the questionnaires themselves were matched against the log, it was determined that 45 questionnaires were returned from first time users, while the remaining 40 questionnaires represent responses from repeat users. For this reason, the data were broken into two sections: those reflecting first-time users, and those reflecting second or more uses. In the following sections, the data are re-grouped and analyzed in two ways: in the aggregate across all reported sessions, and divided into two groups, first- time users, each of whom is unique, and repeat users who filled out two or more questionnaires.

VII. Description of Search Sessions

The nature of the sessions themselves were analyzed on the following dimensions: length of session, purpose of search, sources of help, and frequency of re-running a search. It was expected that the use of the system would differ depending upon whether the user was a first-time or repeat user. Where relevant, analysis of the questionnaires as a whole is presented.

A. Session Length

The length of the session was determined by examining the log. Sessions ranged in length from 10 minutes to two hours. Only one session lasted longer than 75 minutes, however, so the data were collapsed into five categories, and the outlier removed. A comparison of session length among first time and repeat users revealed that first-time users' sessions lasted 31-45 minutes, while a typical session for a repeat user lasted 16-30 minutes.

From this analysis it cannot be determined whether searchers were becoming more efficient or whether those who took longer among the first time users were so frustrated they did not choose to return. Further analysis on a case-by-case basis may yield greater insight.

B. Purpose of Search

Virtually all users reported that they were searching for articles on subject. Searches were conducted primarily for patient care (31) or for papers and reports (34). Some respondents selected research as the reason for the search (21), although it is likely that the "research" was related to a paper or personal use, rather than to basic research. Current awareness (11) and curiosity (9) were the next most frequent purposes selected. Categories were not mutually exclusive.

C. Sources of Help

The most popular forms of help during a session were asking a librarian (33), working with the tutorial (24), and calling for the HELP screens (23). While some users reported consulting friends (14), virtually no one used the brief reference sheet that was provided with the questionnaire, the user manual, or the Apple Tour of Macintosh. It is possible that respondents did not see the reference sheet since it was attached to the description of the evaluation. Since both the user manual and the Apple Tour were obtainable only by request at the desk, most users preferred to ask their questions of staff directly.

When first time users were compared with repeat users, it was found, not surprisingly, that first time users favored the tutorial (17) and asking library staff (22), while repeat users still favored asking library staff (8) and rarely used the tutorial (3).

D. Re-running a Search (Search Re-formulation)

In Knowledge Finder, search statements are run against the MEDLINE file when the user clicks on the "run" icon. After viewing the results of the search, the parameters of the search can be adjusted in a variety of ways to increase or decrease retrieval, or to emphasize or de-emphasize various aspects of the topic. The evaluation questionnaire was edited in order to determine how searchers used these features (items 15, 16, and 17). Because it was expected that utilization of these features would change over time, the group of first time users was compared to the group of repeat users.

Among first time users, only sixteen reported running their search only once, while 29 reported running their search two or more times. Among repeat users, the pattern was much less distinct. Eleven reported running their search only once, while twelve reported running them two or more times.

Item 16 on the questionnaire presented seven choices plus "other" as reasons for running the search more than once. The choices were: "articles weren't useful", "found too little," "found too much," "adjusted search controls," abandoned search and started over again," "got help from another person," or "chose different search terms." Respondents could select all that applied. The most commonly selected reason for re-running a search was "chose different search terms." Among first time users, eighteen of the 29 respondents who ran their search more than once indicated they chose new terms. Among repeat users, seven of the twelve who ran their search more than once chose new terms.

In both groups, then, changes in search terms were associated with repeated running of the search.

It is worth noting that among the group of first time users, eight respondents selected "found too little" and "articles weren't useful" reasons for running the search. In a case-by-case analysis, four of the eight were discovered to be the same respondent, but the remaining four represented different respondents. In other words, twelve of the first time users re-ran their search because the results of the first search either were not useful or were too sparse. Among repeat users, only two sessions yielded too few articles. From these results, it may be hypothesized that experienced users may have been more proficient at searching and were interested in refining their searches, while first-timers expended more effort in achieving even minimal results. On the other hand, it may be that first-timers did not return for repeat sessions because they perceived the effort as being too great.

Based on previous research into search reformulations[5] item 17 was added to the questionnaire to determine the frequency and nature of the reformulations that occurred during search sessions. The available responses were: I changed the free-form topic search statement, I changed the term selection criteria, I generated new terms using the subject heading thesaurus, I generated new terms using the word dictionary, I got ideas from looking at articles, I thought up new terms on my own, I did not change my search statement, but I used other features to affect the outcome of my search. Respondents could select all that applied. The most frequently selected responses across all sessions were changing the topic search statement (20), following by thinking up new terms on my own (16). Only one person reported consulting the word dictionary, and five reported getting ideas for terms from looking at articles. Of the features provided by the Knowledge Finder software, the subject heading thesaurus (MeSH) and the term selection criteria were selected by twelve and ten respondents respectively.

When the group of first time users was compared with repeat users, the patterns of use appeared to be similar. That is, both groups were more likely to change the search statement and to think up new terms on their own. Changing the term selection criteria and consulting the subject heading thesaurus were selected proportionately in both groups.

VIII. Satisfaction with System and Results

User satisfaction was examined both in terms of the Knowledge Finder itself and the results generated by the search session. Across all sessions, about half of the respondents indicated that the results obtained through Knowledge Finder were sufficient for their needs (42). It is significant, however, that about a third indicated that the results were helpful but incomplete. (The MEDLINE file available in this evaluation was the core subset only.) These findings were consistent when the data were analyzed by first-time users and repeat users as well. It seems that in a library where users are familiar with online mediated searches, the core subset enhances but does not substitute for traditional online searching.

The data indicated that users liked Knowledge Finder, however. When asked what form of access to MEDLINE they would consult the next time they needed information (Knowledge Finder, online, printed, or other) virtually all of the respondents chose the Knowledge Finder (75). Twenty-one indicated they would also consult an online source and a few indicated they would consult a printed source, probably for cost reasons. As pointed out above, Knowledge Finder in the form evaluated here does not replace other methods of access, but clearly is a popular supplement. In the unabridged form, Knowledge Finder might be much more likely to substitute for traditional online access.

IX. Knowledge Finder vs. Online Information Systems

Despite the fact that most online searches for faculty are subsidized in one form or another, cost was considered to be very important or somewhat important on nearly three-quarters of the questionnaires (71%). Five respondents indicated specifically that they would not have requested a computer search of MEDLINE. Since users are not directly charged for online searches, the awareness of cost may seem surprising. On the other hand, in the current fiscal climate in universities generally, awareness of cost has become increasingly apparent. It is not clear, though, whether the online searches are simply perceived to be more expensive than CD-ROM.

Users were also asked to indicate what alternate information sources they might consult if Knowledge Finder were not available. About a third of respondents (30) indicated that they would consult a printed version, while about one fourth of respondents indicated they would request a MEDLINE search (24). Thirteen indicated that had Knowledge Finder not been available to them, they would have done nothing. Most of these responses were from medical students.

As indicated above, the version of Knowledge Finder that was available for evaluation was limited to a core subset of journals. One of the items on the questionnaire asked respondents to indicate which enhancement would be MOST important to them: more journals or more backfiles. Across all the questionnaires, responses were almost evenly split. Thirty-seven respondents selected more journals, while 34 selected more backfiles. Because this choice might affect future purchase decisions, the data were further analyzed by groups. Among first time users, the split was also almost even; 21 selected more journals, while 19 chose more backfiles. Only among repeat users was there any noticeable difference; eight chose more journals, while twelve chose more backfiles. Since there were only a few missing cases, the data are probably an accurate reflection of users' responses. While it appears that many users would like enhancements to the file, it is not clear how best to structure the database. Furthermore, it is not clear whether an unabridged MEDLINE with 5-10 years of backfiles would actually turn out to be desirable since satisfaction with retrieval (and avoiding large sets) is frequently related to searching skill.

X. Results of the Clinical Evaluation

Data collected in the clinical evaluation (Appendix B) consisted of transaction logs, interviews and four questionnaires; it is descriptive and, while it may stimulate thinking on clinicians' use (or non-use) of CD-ROM MEDLINE, it is preliminary and anecdotal.

Use of the Knowledge Finder at the Office for Family Practice was prompted by patient care situations and physicians' wishes to keep up with literature in their areas of interest. The clinical subset was regarded as sufficient for their needs, even desirable, since it automatically limited retrieval by eliminating non-clinical titles. The presence of the abstracts was a boon, making it possible to defer obtaining the article itself, and often making it unnecessary to obtain the document at all. Knowledge Finder was perceived as easy and enjoyable to use, even by someone who had never used a computer before. The only reported problems were with a jammed printer.

While those interviewed expressed an interest in having the Knowledge Finder located at at the clinic, they indicated that their greatest challenge was finding specific information. One difficulty identified was the bibliographic format itself; that is, specific information is more suited to reference materials rather than the journal article format. Another difficulty was problems expressing that need to library personnel who may not have (or may not be perceived to have) the subject expertise required to ferret out the specific item of information. For these reasons, clinicians at this site stated that they would continue to consult with colleagues and refer to textbooks to meet many of their information needs, while continuing to delegate more general and document-based searches to librarians. Direct searching of databases, either bibliographic files such as MEDLINE, or textual files such as Micromedex, was appealing to the clinicians interviewed; however, there is no indication of the prevalence of such attitudes.

The transaction logs indicated that twenty-six searches had been conducted; five of these could be identified as demonstration or tutorial searches and were disregarded, leaving a total of 21 search sessions that were initiated by clinicians at the OFP. Since transaction log analysis can act as a "reality check" on users' reported searching experience, the logs generated at OFP were examined to compare them with the experiences described in the interviews. The transaction logs corroborated clinicians' reports that for most searches, the abstracts were reviewed. Similarly, the clinicians' suspicion that the system had more power and flexibility than they knew how to exploit was reflected in the logs; most of the search controls remained in the default mode.

Some searches were "run" as many as three or four times, each time with terminology variations, indicating at least an intuitive ability to exploit the iterative aspect of the user interface; others were run several times with large retrieval and no refinements, almost surely an indication that the user was "stuck."

The technique most frequently used to refine retrieval was re-running the search with different terminology or more terms added to the search string. For example, "hemorrhage, post partum" became "hemorrhage, post partum, [and] review" reducing the retrieval from 75 items to 30. In another instance, "dyspraxia and hyperactivity or attention deficit disorder" yielding over 100 relevant citations was refined to be "dyspraxia." In still another, "cyst" yielded 33 relevant items. Once a few were viewed, however, the search was re-run with the terms "cyst arachnoid," yielding 33 items, but a different 33, presumably ones that were more useful to the searcher, since 15 were reviewed with abstracts.

XI. Summary and Conclusions

The results reported here hold few surprises, yet some of the findings are provocative and may lead to further research. In the short period of time during which the evaluation was conducted, it appears that few new users were attracted to the library. Time of year, duration of the evaluation period, and deep-seated patterns of information-seeking among Rockford medical personnel may account for these findings. On the other hand, the alternatives to Knowledge Finder suggest that at least some library users discovered new ways to access the medical literature.

Most people liked the Knowledge Finder, and a few *really* liked it. Repeat users probably conducted many more searches using the Knowledge Finder than they would have otherwise. When the Knowledge Finder was relocated to the clinic, those who had come to rely on it requested that it be returned to the library as quickly as possible.

Knowledge Finder exploits the Macintosh interface, and those who had used the Macintosh previously took to Knowledge Finder most quickly. About half-way through the evaluation, it was discovered that word-processing and spreadsheet applications were being loaded into the Mac. In order to keep the machine available for MEDLINE searches, a guardian program was installed that prevented additional applications. During the busy times, a single workstation, particularly if additional applications were tolerated, would probably be insufficient for a library of this size.

The relationship of CD-ROM to other medical information resources is complex. Issues of cost—particularly who pays and how the cost is calculated—are important not only to libraries but also to users. The ability to provide free access to MEDLINE to all library users was particularly attractive to nurses, allied health personnel, and the occasional public library patron for whom requesting a mediated search would be prohibitively expensive.

Most users wanted to begin searching right away. The tutorial with its printed representation of an "online" interactive session seemed more attractive to users than either print or "online" tutorial alone. While users consulted librarians rather frequently, they were also able to search successfully after hours when the library was staffed by a single student.

Knowledge Finder represents an important innovation in information access in medicine. It is not a replacement for mediated searches, but it may offer satisfactory access to the medical literature to users who would not otherwise conduct a systematic search.

This evaluation, like many studies, revealed the difficulty users have with terminology. Knowledge Finder is a highly interactive system in which a trial and error process of searching is tolerated, even encouraged. The interface is particularly rich, yet the methods of data collection available for this study precluded any more than a cursory observation of users' exploration of the many options afforded them. More detailed analysis, particularly of transaction logs in conjunction with other data, may provide greater insight into users' searching behavior. Of particular interest is the relationship between use of the online MeSH and self-generated terms, and the ways in which interface design may affect searching behaviors among new and experienced users.

References

1. All students currently enrolled are required to have demonstrated competency in basic library skills which is determined by their performance in the Medical Information Management curriculum, reported in Kolner, Stuart, Prudence Dalrymple, and Richard Christiansen, "Teaching Skills in Medical Information Management to Medical Students," *Journal of Medical Education* 61 (November 1986): 906-910.

2. Unpublished data collected in conjunction with the Medical Information Management Course, 1985-1987.

3. Bernstein, Lionel M. and Robert E. Williamson, "Testing of a Natural Language Retrieval System for a Full Text Knowledge Base," *Journal of the American Society for Information Science* 35 (1984): 235-247.

4. Frequent library users were defined as those requesting a search more than once a month (13), moderate users were defined as requesting a computer search at least once a year (56), and infrequent users were defined as those requesting a computer search less than once a year (14).

5. Dalrymple, Prudence W. "Retrieval by Reformulation in Two Library Catalogs: Toward a Cognitive Model of Searching Behavior." *Journal of the American Society for Information Science,* in press.

KNOWLEDGE FINDER EVALUATION
FORM FOR THE LIBRARY

The Knowledge Finder CD-ROM MEDLINE is being tested by the Library of the Health Sciences-Rockford. We would like you to fill out this questionnaire in order to help us find out who is using the system, and how useful it is to you. Please answer all the questions and return the questionnaire to the Circulation Desk.

1. My primary affiliation is (Circle one):
   a. medicine
   b. nursing
   c. public health
   d. allied health
   e. other (please specify):_____

2. My profession is (Circle ALL that apply):
   a. physician
   b. scientist/researcher
   c. medical student
   d. resident (medicine)
   e. nurse
   f. librarian
   g. educator
   h. other health care professional
   i. other (please specify)_____

3. I was looking for articles (Circle ALL that apply):
   a. by an author
   b. under a title
   c. on a subject
   d. in a specific journal
   e. other (please specify):_____

4. I needed the information for (circle ALL that apply):
   a. patient care
   b. a paper or report
   c. a research project
   d. keeping current
   e. to check a reference
   f. teaching/planning a course
   g. not needed, just curious
   h. other (please specify):_____

5. The information I found was (circle ONE):
   a. what I needed
   b. more than I needed
   c. some of what I needed
   d. not useful
   e. other (please specify)

6. Have you ever used any of the printed publications produced from the MEDLINE system (e.g., INDEX MEDICUS, INTERNATIONAL NURSING INDEX, INDEX TO DENTAL LITERATURE, HOSPITAL LITERATURE INDEX)?
   a. yes
      If yes, how do the printed versions compare to Knowledge Finder (the system you just used)? (Circle ONE)
         a. easier to use
         b. harder to use
         c. about the same to use
   b. no

7. Have you used MEDLINE (computer version of Index Medicus) before? (Circle ONE):
   a. yes, searched it by myself
   b. yes, librarian processed a search for me
   c. no **(Go on to question 9)**
   d. don't know **(Go on to question 9)**

8. **If yes, you've used MEDLINE,** which do you prefer? (Circle ONE):
   a. computer search, searched on my own
   b. computer search, searched on my own using (name system such as PaperChase, Grateful Med, etc.)_____
   c. online, searched by librarian
   d. Knowledge Finder

9. How often have you used Knowledge Finder? (Circle ONE):
   a. first time
   b. once before
   c. 2-5 times before
   d. 6 or more times

10. Knowledge Finder is provided free of charge to library users. How important a consideration was this in your decision to use this system instead of a computer search of MEDLINE? (Circle ONE):

    a. very important
    b. somewhat important
    c. relatively unimportant
    d. would not have requested a computer search of MEDLINE

11. If Knowledge Finder had not been available today, what would you have done? (Circle ALL that apply):

    a. used a printed version
    b. requested a computer search of MEDLINE
    c. asked a library staff member
    d. asked a friend or colleague
    e. browsed through the stacks
    f. nothing
    g. other (please specify)_____

12. Next time you need this sort of information, what will you do? (Circle ALL that apply):

    a. try Knowledge Finder
    b. try an online version
    c. try a printed version
    d. try another source
    e. other (please specify)_____

13. While using Knowledge Finder, I got help from (Circle ALL that apply):

    a. reference sheet provided with this questionnaire
    b. printed tutorial
    c. user manual
    d. on-screen "HELP"
    e. Apple Tour of the Macintosh
    f. librarian or other library staff member
    g. friend or other users
    h. other (please specify)_____

14. How would you rate the results obtained through Knowledge Finder? (Circle ONE):

    a. sufficient for my needs
    b. I will probably request a computer search by a librarian
    c. helpful, but incomplete; I will continue to look for more information on this topic
    d. not useful at all

15. How many times did you "run" this search (click on the picture of the runner)? (Circle ONE):
   a. 1 time (if you "ran" your search only once, please skip to question 18)
   b. 2-3 times
   c. 4-6 times
   d. 7 or more times

16. Why did you run this search more than once? (Circle ALL that apply):
   a. articles weren't useful
   b. found too little
   c. found too much
   d. adjusted search controls ("relevance filter", "number of articles", "word variants")
   e. abandoned search, but started over again
   f. got help from another person
   g. chose different search terms
   h. other (please specify)_____

17. Which of the following sentences applies to your search session? (Circle ALL that apply):
   a. I changed the free-form topic search statement.
   b. I changed the term selection criteria ("use only", "try to use", "don't use").
   c. I generated new terms using the subject heading thesaurus.
   d. I generated new terms using word dictionary.
   e. I got ideas for new terms from looking at articles.
   f. I thought up new terms on my own.
   g. I did not change my search statement, but I used other features to affect the outcome of my search (please specify)_____
   _____

18. Knowledge Finder searches a limited number of journals for a period of five years. Which of the following enhancements would be MOST important to you? (Circle ONE):
   a. more journals (more than the core of 220 titles)
   b. more backfiles (more than five years)

19. Please circle the number that most nearly charcterizes Knowledge Finder:

Frustrating	1	2	3	4	5	6	Satisfying
Efficient	1	2	3	4	5	6	Wasteful
Gratifying	1	2	3	4	5	6	Disappointing
Correct	1	2	3	4	5	6	Erroneous
Fun	1	2	3	4	5	6	Laborious
Discouraging	1	2	3	4	5	6	Encouraging
Misleading	1	2	3	4	5	6	Credible
Comprehensive	1	2	3	4	5	6	Incomplete
Friendly	1	2	3	4	5	6	Hostile
Confusing	1	2	3	4	5	6	Clear
Beneficial	1	2	3	4	5	6	Worthless

20. Have you ever used a microcomputer (personal computer)?
   a. yes
   b. no

21. If yes, have you ever used a Macintosh computer?
   a. yes
   b. no

22. On the average, how often do you request a computer search in the library (this one or another library)? (Circle ONE):
   a. more than once a month
   b. 7-12 times per year
   c. 1-6 times per year
   d. less than once a year

23. About how often do you use the materials in this library? (Circle ONE):
   a. more than once a week
   b. 1-4 times a month
   c. less than monthly
   d. never been here before

24. Please write down what you were looking for when you began your Knowledge Finder session:

_____

_____

Thank you very much for your participation. Please return your completed questionnaire to the Circulation Desk.

KNOWLEDGE FINDER EVALUATION FORM
FOR THE OFFICE FOR FAMILY PRACTICE

The Knowledge Finder CD-ROM MEDLINE is being tested in the Office for Family Practice by the Library of the Health Sciences-Rockford. We would like you to fill out this questionnaire in order to help us find out how you are using the system, and whether it is useful to you

1. The information I found was (Circle ONE)
    a. what I was looking for
    b. more than I needed
    c. some of what I needed
    d. not useful

2. Have you used an online version of MEDLINE (either yourself or by having a librarian process a search for you? (Circle ONE):
    a. yes, by myself
    b. yes. librarian search
    c. no

3. If yes you've used MEDLINE, which system do you prefer? (Circle ONE):
    a. online, searched on my own
    b. online, searched on my own using (name system such as PaperChase, Grateful Med, etc.)
    c. Knowledge Finder
    d. online, searched by librarian

4. Next time you need this sort of information, what will you do? (Circle ALL that apply):
    a. try Knowledge Finder
    b. go to the library
    c. try an online version
    d. try a printed index (Index Medicus)
    e. nothing

5. How often have you used Knowledge Finder MEDLINE? (Circle ONE):
    a. first time
    b. once before
    c. 3-5 times before
    d. 6 or more times

6. Did you modify your search topic during this session? (Circle ALL that apply):
    a. no
    b. yes, I modified the free-form topic search statement
    c. yes, I used the subject heading thesaurus
    d. yes, I used the word dictionary
    e. don't know

7. Which of the following statements characterizes the results you obtained through Knowledge Finder? (Circle ALL that apply)
    a. The citations plus the abstracts were sufficient for my needs.
    b. I will probably go the library to pursue this question further.
    c. I will probably request an online search by a librarian.
    d. The search on Knowledge Finder was not helpful.
    e. other (please specify):_____

115

8. In your judgment, will the information you obtained through this search affect the care your patient receives? (Circle ONE):
   a. Yes, the information is directly applicable to the situation
   b. Possibly, it is difficult to tell at this point.
   c. Probably not directly.
   d. Definitely not.
   e. My question was not related to a patient care situation.

9. Have you ever used a personal computer (microcomputer)? (Circle ONE)
   a. yes
   b. no

10. If yes, have you ever used a Macintosh computer? (Circle ONE)
    a. yes
    b. no

11. About how often do you request a computer search at UICOM-R or elsewhere? (Circle ONE):
    a. once a month or more
    b. about twice a year
    c. less than once a year

12. About how often do you visit the library? (Circle ONE):
    a. several times a week
    b. 1-3 times a month
    c. about twice a year
    d. once a year or less

13. Knowledge Finder is being provided free of charge during this trial period. How important is cost to you in determining whether to search for information? (Circle ONE)
    a. very important
    b. somewhat important
    c. not important

14. Please use this space to indicate any enhancements or improvements to Knowledge Finder or to note any particular problems you have encountered in using Knowledge Finder.

    _____

    _____

    _____

    _____

Thank you very much for your participation. Please place your completed questionnaire in the envelope next to the Knowledge Finder.

EVALUATION OF

MEDLINE
Knowledge Finder:

THE SYSTEM'S FEATURES, USERS, AND USES AT THE GOOD SAMARITAN MEDICAL CENTER LIBRARY, PHOENIX

By   *Jacqueline D. Doyle*

Good Samaritan Medical Center
Health Science Library
P.O. Box 2989
Phoenix, Arizona 85062

EVALUATION OF MEDLINE KNOWLEDGE FINDER: THE SYSTEM'S FEATURES, USERS, AND USES AT THE GOOD SAMARITAN MEDICAL CENTER LIBRARY, PHOENIX

Introduction

Evaluating MEDLINE Knowledge Finder (MKF) was a new and unique experience for Good Samaritan Medical Center health professionals and library staff alike. While GSMC has many Grateful Med end-users, Knowledge Finder was the Library's first and only CD-ROM experience, the first use of a Macintosh, and the staff's first exposure to "fuzzy" Boolean logic. The evaluation ultimately resulted in an enthusiastic acceptance of a new method for GSMC health professionals to search MEDLINE.

Setting

A community teaching hospital, Good Samaritan Medical Center (GSMC) is the oldest and largest of Samaritan Health Service (SHS), a multi-hospital corporation. The GSMC Health Science Library is based on a 13,000-volume collection located in the Ancillary Building of the medical center. From and with that collection, a staff of 4.2 FTE serve not only the GSMC staff (1,700 physicians, 200 medical residents, 1,500 nurses, and 2,200 allied health professionals), but in addition, the medical staff and employees of Phoenix Children's Hospital (PCH), the Samaritan Corporate Center, and several local and regional hospitals and clinics owned or managed by Samaritan Health Service in Arizona, Utah, Texas and California.

GSMC and PCH, the teaching hospitals on the GSMC campus, offer 8 residency training programs to 200 house staff physicians, clinical sites for undergraduate and graduate nursing programs, and numerous other training opportunities in the allied health professions, including respiratory therapy and pastoral care. Most medical residents are based here, while others rotate among other Phoenix area teaching hospitals. The University of Arizona medical school is in Tucson, over 100 miles away, but GSMC also hosts U of A medical students for 6-week clerkships on a year-round basis.

The Health Science Library staff consists of 1 professional librarian who is the Director, 2 paraprofessional library assistants, and 2 part-time library clerks. During the cooler winter months loyal and hard-working volunteers supplement the paid staff, but that number decreases when the 110+ weather arrives! All staff had basic familiarity with IBM PC/XTs (since IBM is the only PC the corporation supports), but little knowledge of Apple computers and none with the Macintosh. While a conceptual knowledge of microcomputers proved to be helpful in learning the Mac-based system, the transition from IBM and DOS (almost "dirty" words to a Macophile), while at first frustrating and puzzling, was eventually fun and gratifying. One paraprofessional staff member, in addition to the Director, is a trained MEDLINE searcher. This previous knowledge and understanding of the MEDLINE database also proved to be helpful.

In addition to the traditional book and journal collection, library staff provides mediated database search services (about 200 searches are provided for library customers every month); interlibrary services; basic microcomputer training; online end-user training; and library consulting services.

Library staff have been teaching medical and house staff, and medical center employees to do their own MEDLINE searching for the last three years, using a variety of systems. Knowledge Finder is the first experience with CD-ROM, however. PaperChase was the first user-oriented MEDLINE system utilized; GSMC also tested MEDIS when it was available; assisted departments and individuals to obtain their own BRS Colleague passwords; and in the last two years Grateful Med searching has been taught. Most house staff are Grateful Med searchers; one residency has its own NLM password, PC and software. So almost all resident physicians, many nurses and other health professionals have been at least exposed to do-it-yourself searching. Many have actually persisted and continue, after training, to run their own searches. At this point probably the most-used access method is Grateful Med.

The MEDLINE Knowledge Finder work station included a MacIntosh SE, with a 20 mb internal hard disk and one internal 3-1/2" disk drive, a Toshiba T2100 CD-ROM Disc Player, and an Apple Imagewriter II printer. Several instructional pieces were developed for users: a "tips" sheet (3 pages), and a screen print of the search formulation screen menu, with steps 1,2, and 3 highlighted. (See Appendix A and B) The GSMC experience was that users had trouble only at the very beginning of their search process, and again at the "print" point. The goal of the Library staff was to get patrons searching without training, but most requested an orientation. Once they were shown "how to do it," users rarely had to ask for pointers again. At that point, their intuition did kick in! Many searchers became quite proficient with the mouse and were quick to offer their expertise to their colleagues.

MKF's Features

Knowledge Finder uses a probabilistic retrieval mechanism that locates and displays article citations that are *most likely* to be related to the searcher's objective. This point is important for MKF users, and especially significant to trained searchers. The mechanism allows for the inexperience of new searchers by providing article citations containing all or some of the text words entered. Library staff found this "fuzzy" or "soft" form of Boolean logic to be foreign at first.

Access to the MEDLINE database is provided by Aries in two configurations: the *core journal subset* of 220 clinical medicine journals (the Brandon list and the AIM list combined) and the *unabridged* (complete) MEDLINE, one year per compact disc. CDs are available for the unabridged system for the current year, plus nine prior years. The core subset CD contains the current year, plus four prior years. Both configurations are updated quarterly.

The Aries Knowledge Finder software makes the discs easily and immediately searchable by users with little or no experience, and as Mac users are so very fond of saying, is "intuitive." For example, to begin searching, one clicks on the search runner; to see the results of a search, one uses the mouse to click on the eyes icon. To see the abstracts, one clicks on the "big" icon, as opposed to the small or the middle-sized icon. To erase a search strategy, one clicks on the eraser icon.

During this trial period, four updates of the software were received, plus several quarterly updates of the CDs. In June the full unabridged discs arrived, along with version 1.3 of the software and a demonstration/tutorial disk available via Hypercard. Aries also provided a Search Log that records searchers' strategies. This information proved useful in identifying and examining searcher behavior.

The cost of the system as of July 15, 1988 ranged from $895 to $2,295 for the core subset, depending on whether the intended use of the system was personal, institutional or for a network. The cost of the unabridged MEDLINE system ranged from $1,295 to $2,995. The total hardware package ran about $4,000 for the Mac SE, keyboard, mouse, printer, and CD-ROM drive.

Many well-designed screens have been created by Aries (the most frequently used are included in the Appendix). They are: 1) the Welcome/Copyrights Acknowledged Screen; 2) the Search Formulation Screen; and 3) the Articles Retrieved Screen. Aries makes full use of conventional MacIntosh features including pull-down menus, command/key combinations as short cuts, use of the return key in lieu of mouse clicking, etc.

Two methods of searching are available. New users find the quick and easy method to be the "free form topic search." Experienced or more inquisitive searchers can search using MeSH terms. With the free form method, users simply type significant words in the free-form box, and then press the return key. To search via MeSH terms, one must use the mouse to click on the Subject Headings rectangle and then type in the word or words to be searched. Knowledge Finder will then assist the user to locate the legitimate term or terms to search. Searchers can also identify and use sub-headings appropriate to their query. The default search file includes English-language articles only, but one can easily choose to search for non-English language articles as well. Once a search strategy is entered, it can be saved for searches of additional CDs.

Citations are displayed in order of their likely relevance. Three display formats are available, ranging from a short format, including author, title, source, and unique identifier, to the longest format, which includes the above, plus 17 other fields or paragraphs, including the abstract. An on-screen relevance scale indicates the degree of relevancy of each citation.

Features unique to MKF also include the ability to easily narrow or broaden the search formulation by means of sliding a relevance filter; increase or decrease retrieval by indicating the number of articles desired; and search on variant forms of free text words entered.

The Print Format defaults to the long display format, but can be modified by the user to print only those fields desired. (The Display Format Definitions Screen is shown in the Appendix.) Retrieved citations can be downloaded to a print file or a save file which can then be manipulated using Sci-Mate or Pro-Cite.

The excellent MKF documentation is published in a small loose-leaf binder. It is well-written, easy to use, and the installation instructions are clearly stated. A useful 26-page tutorial is found in chapter 3. While library staff used it initially, and its use was recommended to health professionals, few indicated they used the manual at all.

The Aries search transaction log capability permitted library staff to "eavesdrop" on searches run, and to examine the search methods of end-users.

GSMC's Use of MKF

The MacIntosh workstation was placed in the library's main reading room, directly adjacent to the printed *Index Medicus*. This placement proved helpful in convincing users to make the transition to the new system. For security purposes, the system could be available to users only during the library's staffed hours, not during after-hours access.

The system was immediately visible to people entering the library, and its attractive appearance was a distinct draw. In contrast, the public-access IBMs are in the Microcomputer Center, a room not easily seen from the library entrance. Users must check out IBM software from library staff, as only one IBM has a fully-loaded internal hard disk; the others require the use of floppies or Bernoulli cartridges.

For the first three and one-half months, only the Core Journal Subset CD was made available. Once the Unabridged configuration arrived, the additional CDs were left at the workstation for people to load and search, with instructions for their use posted near the computer.

Evaluation of MKF

The system was placed in the public area in mid-March, one week after we received it. Library staff used that first week to experiment and to become comfortable with the Macintosh interface and hardware.

From the first (after printed publicity in both the medical staff and general staff newsletters, word of mouth among residents, and announcements at committee meetings) the system was HOT! Reservations were not accepted; it was "first-come, first-use." It is now apparent that a system of reservations and limiting time is a necessity.

GSMC users reported that MKF was valuable for a number of reasons:

First was its attractiveness and its uniqueness. As previously mentioned, SHS supports and acquires only IBM hardware and software. Only one other hospital department uses a Macintosh. As a result, many people were interested, intrigued, and curious about it. Most didn't realize they were searching a CD-ROM; they figured it was simply another version of Grateful Med or even MEDIS.

Second, users liked having the abstracts easily available. Though they didn't always choose to print them, they appreciated reading them before making their print decision. Only a few users took advantage of the feature for quickly printing all the citations retrieved; most wanted to be selective.

Third, patrons liked getting their results easily and immediately. Although the mediated search service turnaround time goal is 24 hours, that goal is not always achieved. When the Macintosh was available, patrons could sit down and run their searches immediately. Several library users, both nurses and physicians, were seen searching every single day for weeks at a time.

Fourth, new Mac users thought the system just plain fun! They liked the icons, once they got used to them, and the mouse, once they gained the modest amount of hand-eye coordination required. Experienced MKF searchers have begun to go beyond the free-form method to searching with MeSH terms and subheadings.

Fifth, the Mac was of interest because many GSMC health professionals are in the market for a home or office computer, and this gave them the opportunity to evaluate a system other than IBM.

Results of User Questionnaires

A copy of the questionnaire used is found in the Appendix. The results are summarized below; a complete tabulation of results is also found in Appendix C. (114 usable completed forms were collected. One question was answered so erratically that it is not reported.)

The users of the system reflect the same pattern as the library users: About 68% were physicians (almost 50/50 house staff to medical staff), 21% were nurses, and 11% were other health professionals.

The purposes of their search were as follows: 30% Patient care; 30% Research projects; 23% Teaching preparation; 7% Current awareness; 4% of our users were "just curious", and 6% responded that their purpose was "Other," not specified. Again, this is a similar result for the ultimate use of information gathered as a result of a requested mediated database search.

Library staff were concerned that the *core journal subset* would not be enough to adequately fill the needs of GSMC users. Since the Health Science Library journal collection holds over 500 titles, and the core subset only 220, patrons would not be making full use of the collection. As evident below, however, most users didn't feel that way. Most of these surveys were completed prior to use of the full unabridged discs, and most customers were pleased with both the number of journals indexed, and the backfile years covered. However, most library users do not know how large the body of medical literature really is, and this is the probable reason for the voiced satisfaction. Some patrons used the system without consulting either a library staff member, or the manual or tips sheet, and therefore data was not collected about their level of knowledge or about their concerns or complaints. Some users went directly from MKF to the Grateful Med IBM PC and did a second search on their own.

Users were asked to describe the *amount of information found*. Over 46% reported that the amount of information they retrieved was "just right"; 15% said it was more than they needed; 38% said it gave them "some of what they needed"; and less than 1% said it gave them nothing.

The method used by most of our health professionals was what Aries calls "free form" searching. Only 17% used MeSH terms to search, and less than 1% searched by author name.

Users were asked *if they were satisfied* with MKF's ease of use, and to rate its value. Over 97% rated it very easy or moderately easy to use; only 3% said it wasn't easy at all. About 90% rated MKF as very valuable, 10% said it was moderately valuable. 76% reported they would find it useful at their work site.

Anecdotal Reports

Only a very few complaints were voiced by MKF users. Experienced Macintosh users commented that they thought the main screen was a bit busy and confusing. Once they became familiar with it and with the pull-down menus, they seemed to be able to go beyond that initial impression. Two library users have complained about printer noise, and several about its slow speed.

It became evident that inexperienced Mac users were not as intuitive as Mac aficionados say they are. Perhaps they have, as one Mac user stated, MS-DOS mentalities, and will never have the intuition required to become a true Mac hacker. On occasion it was necessary for Library staff to identify even the mouse to some users. Other users succeeded with no orientation at all. Some patrons (not many) simply sat and stared, and just didn't know where to start. Library staff would find them there, thirty minutes later, with no progress made, and a bit too embarrassed to ask for help.

Most anecdotal input received indicated that Library staff should not even consider sending the system back. While use of mediated search services did not decrease during these months (in fact it increased!) some search requests were not submitted for staff completion, and MKF searches were run by the user instead. Many MKF users were new library customers, due to the advertisements and word of mouth, and to the fact that the time period was the traditional college "term paper" time. Spring seems to be the period when the library receives many new users anyway: papers are due, and nursing students who have never used the library at all suddenly find the library useful.

While complex searches requiring multiple term combinations, large "ors" or explosions are virtually impossible, "one-term" searches, or information needs that could be filled with broad overview type of articles were ideal for MKF. Many nurses had no idea how to break down a search request for "articles on everything new in perinatal nursing," but eventually found ways to do so when they performed the search themselves. Requests for "a few good articles" were satisfied quite nicely using MKF.

Most users were not aware of the fuzzy-Boolean-logic difference between a self-run MKF search, and a mediated search of the full MEDLINE file. This became obvious when a MKF user suddenly moved over to printed *Index Medicus*. When queried by library staff, they expressed frustration with large retrieval but were reluctant to complain or ask for help. Some of these people said they just liked to use the indexes to browse, and said they found more that way. They were obviously in the minority.

Librarians/Library Staff Evaluation

Staff experienced both pluses and minuses during the trial period, the pluses far outweighing the minuses. Those requests for quick one-term searches, when run by the patrons themselves, did save some online time and Medical Center expense. The addition of a Mac to existing PC resources enhanced the Library's reputation and clout within the corporation. Although an initial orientation for users with no library research or PC experience was necessary, the staff time was well worth the effort once users became accustomed to helping themselves. The automatic saving and ease of re-running a search strategy on the backfiles CDs was a great plus. The potential of using the Mac for other purposes, such as graphics and other general microcomputer applications is a strength. Library staff found themselves turning away patrons who had other uses in mind.

The assistance and support received from Lyndon Holmes, the man behind MKF, was a great advantage. In spite of the distance and time difference, Dr. Holmes was always professional and helpful in his approach to providing support. He always indicated a willingness to receive suggestions for changes to the system. Each new version of MKF showed valuable improvements and illustrated his willingness to respond to user suggestions.

The few negatives experienced by Library staff included an initial discomfort with icons and with fuzzy Boolean. However, they finally have overcome that ignorance and now feel they can live equally comfortably in both the MS-DOS and Finder worlds. Fuzzy Boolean was a difficult concept to grasp and explain to puzzled users, but is now comfortable and useful. One suggestion would be that the concept behind probabilistic retrieval be described in the MKF manual, especially the method the system uses for rating article relevancy. Some users were especially curious about the relevancy scale.

The limitations of the original core journal subset were felt at this institution since the collection holds many titles not included. It was finally determined that the larger unabridged file would be the system to acquire. An additional file GSMC would find useful on CD-ROM and MKF would be Health, since many mediated searches are run on the latter, and many library users are looking for the administrative and financial aspects of clinical problems and health care delivery.

The appearance of the printouts is still somewhat unsatisfactory, but only to Library staff, not to users. The default feature of always printing the full record unless the print format is changed is a bit of a negative, since changing the format requires a good deal of mouse use. Few users learned to make these changes on their own. Use of the pull-down menus for accessing sub-headings was a similar (but minor) problem.

One problem forwarded to Dr. Holmes was the use of the phrase "Subject Headings" on the search formulation screen, and the phrase "Major/Minor Descriptors" on the citation screen. Use of the same phrase in both screens would assist librarians trying to explain the concept to users and to describe the significance of the subject heading approach to new searchers who are using only the free form technique.

While MeSH term searching is available, and in some ways quite nice, the use of MeSH descriptors for complex searches remains tricky and sometimes impossible. Once Library staff recognized that the primary customer of MKF is the health professional end-user, they better accepted their inability to perform the often-used techniques of professional searchers (such as pre-explosions and "or-ing" several like terms or concepts.) The self-sufficiency of end-users, once they were provided with a brief introduction, far outweighed any complaints.

A searcher must perform two functions before beginning a search. The previous search strategy, if there is one, must be erased. Also the previous print list must be cleared. These tasks were small inconveniences, and some searchers found that they printed not only their citations, but also those saved from the previous searcher. The necessity for performing these operations is not immediately evident to new users; library staff took the time to point out the procedures in order to avoid additional user frustration.

An interesting, new, and often frustrating experience for Library staff was that frequent occasion when a patron had so much fun experimenting that he found herself back at Finder (sort of like being at the C: prompt in the root directory in DOS). Users would then move files around, or re-name them, or sometimes delete the names, or the files altogether. Only one critical (fatal) error was made during the evaluation period, from which staff recovered with difficulty. But even the small crashes required additional time from library staff. These problems will be overcome once they become proficient at using other Mac software to protect MKF from experimenters.

A related problem for this Library is security. The department has 24-hour access for all medical staff. Since it is not staffed a good deal of that time, the system was not left up over night. Naturally, middle-of-the-night searches are often needed, and having the Mac available would be a valuable information service. A more secure workstation will be developed in the near future.

As already mentioned, Samaritan Health Service supports IBM microcomputers exclusively. Therefore, any consultation or help needed by staff had to come from either Aries or other, outside Mac users. The availability of institutional support must be considered before a purchase decision is made. GSMC was fortunate to have Dr. Holmes and other Phoenix area medical librarian Mac users to ask questions, get demonstrations, and generally get the Mac hype. And it worked!

Prior to participating in the evaluation, the GSMC library staff had not taken the time to identify the features and capabilities of the "ideal" CD-ROM end-user system. In retrospect, and with MKF experience, staff now know that such a system would offer both an expert and a novice mode of searching. It would also permit the use of pre-exploded MeSH terms, and permit the "or-ing" of several terms or concepts. An ideal system would also be updated on a monthly basis, and would offer access to more than one database, including such files as Health Administration & Planning, Psychological Abstracts, and one or more of the business files. In addition to bibliographic files, CDs would be available for textual materials such as drug information books, and general medical and nursing textbooks. The GSMC Library staff is hopeful that these features will soon be available on the Aries system.

Conclusions

By mid-summer Library staff had concluded that MKF best meets GSMC's current needs, and had made the decision to acquire the Aries system. After the decision had been made, a welcome surprise was received from the Apple Corporation—a grant of the Macintosh system. While MKF is not likely to entirely replace the mediated search service, library staff members do feel it is an enhancement of library resources and services, and that GSMC patrons and their patients benefit from its use. Coincidentally, the Apple Corporation has identified health care as a new target audience, and relationships between Samaritan and Apple are being established.

Participation in NLM's CD-ROM evaluation was a positive experience for Good Samaritan Medical Center, both for its library staff and its health professionals. A good deal about the information-seeking behaviors of library users was learned, as were new ways to access the MEDLINE file, new ways of processing and managing information, and new ways to better serve the health professionals of Samaritan Health Service.

Tips for Using Knowledge Finder MEDLINE

NOTE: Any time during a search, you may "pull down" the HELP menu from "HELP" at the upper right part of the screen.

For a brief introduction to KF MEDLINE, we suggest you complete the tutorial on p. 3-1 of the KF MEDLINE Manual!

SEARCHING THE MEDLINE DATABASE:

- The main menu ("search formulation") screen will appear. There are three ways to search on KF MEDLINE:

  1. Use the **"free form area"** in the upper left corner box (this is a "quick and dirty" method: gets some results fast.

      • Type the significant words of your topic in this box, leaving spaces between words; eliminate "or," "and," etc. Then press the return key.

  2. Use **subject headings** (this will result in a more precise search.)

      • Click on the Subject Headings box. Type the word or words you wish to find subject headings for, then press return.

  3. Use a **combination** of free text and MeSH terms.

- Use the pull-down HELP menu to find help screens. Click on "HELP" at the upper right, and, holding down the click, pull down the main menu. Release the click on the line you wish to explore.

- Click on the "Search Runner" icon or press Return to begin the search.

- After your search is complete, KFM will let you know how many articles you retrieved.

HOW TO SEE YOUR RESULTS:

- Click on the "EYES" icon to view the citations you've retrieved.

HOW TO PRINT YOUR CITATIONS:

BE SURE YOU HAVE CLEARED THE ARTICLE PRINT LIST (IN THE PULL-DOWN
MENU UNDER "ARTICLES") BEFORE SELECTING THE CITATIONS YOU WISH TO
PRINT! (Then perform the three steps below.)

- To print, click on the Print List Icon for each citation you want
  to print. To print ALL the citations retrieved, and save some time by
  not examining each of them, press the mouse and the command key
  simultaneously while clicking the Print List Icon.

- Press the command key and the P key together.

- At the print menu, use the mouse to click on the DRAFT circle.
  Then click OK to print. Watch the paper to be sure it doesn't
  become jammed.

HOW TO STOP PRINTING:

- Anytime you wish to STOP the printing action, press the command
  key and the " " (period) key simultaneously.

AFTER YOU'VE PRINTED:

- Erase your search strategy and clear your print list for the next
  searcher!

**LET US KNOW HOW YOUR SEARCH WENT, IF YOU NEED HELP, OR
WISH TO LEARN MORE ABOUT KNOWLEDGE FINDER.**

Welcome To Knowledge Finder™
Version 1.408 -- October, 1988

Knowledge Finder allows you to easily and rapidly search biomedical databases stored and distributed on CD-ROM optical disc. These include Unabridged and specialty interest MEDLINE discs.

Bibliographic searching is a combination of science and art. Typically, your results correspond to your experience as a searcher. IF YOU HAVE ANY DOUBTS ABOUT THE COMPLETENESS OF YOUR SEARCH RESULTS, AND COMPLETENESS IS OF PARAMOUNT IMPORTANCE TO YOU, YOU SHOULD SEEK THE ASSISTANCE OF A QUALIFIED, PROFESSIONAL SEARCHER.

Some material in these databases is from copyrighted publications of the respective copyright claimants. Users of the databases are referred to the publication data appearing in the bibliographic citations, as well as to the copyright notices appearing in the original publication, all of which are incorporated by reference.

HINT		FOR ASSISTANCE
Create your own citation layouts with 'Display Formats...' (under the 'Articles' menu).	**Ready to search!** **Acknowledged**	Please contact: Aries Systems Corporation (508) 689-9334

Knowledge Finder™ Search Formulation

Free-Form Topic Search Statement

Search Progress

Search Also/Instead By :

- Subject Heading(s)
- Author Name(s)
- Publication Date(s)
- Journal Title(s)
- Language(s)
- Subject Check Tag(s)

Selected Dictionary/Thesaurus Search Terms

Jan 1984 – Jun 1988 MEDLINE Core Journals

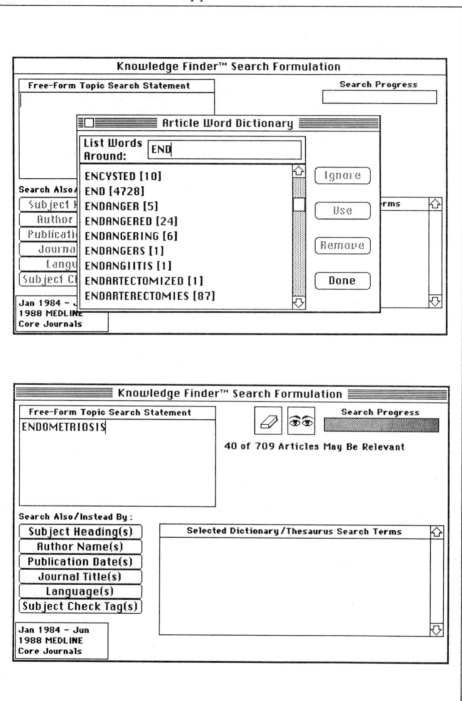

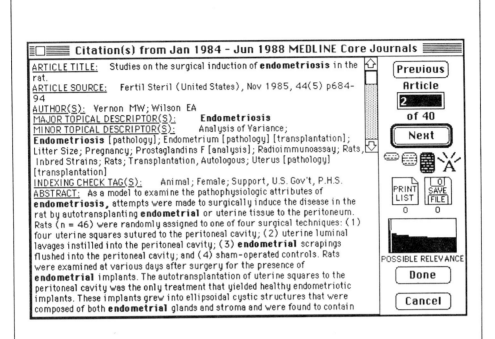

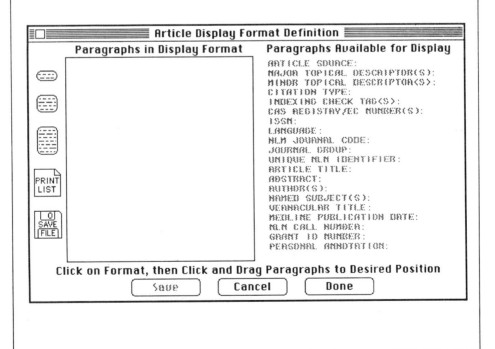

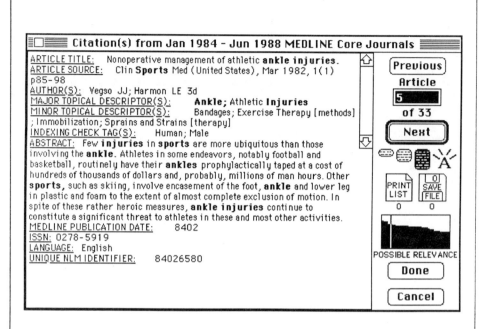

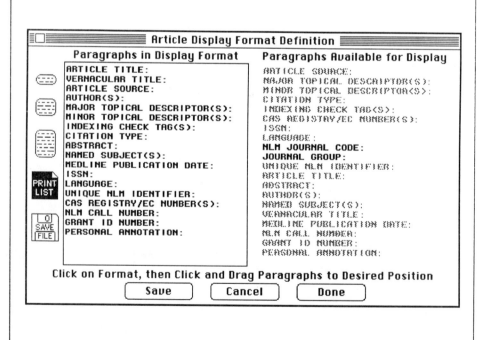

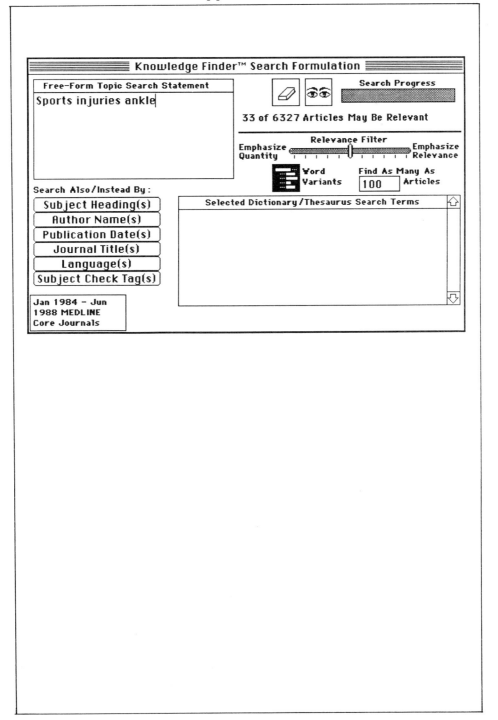

Appendix C

GSMC Library & Microcomputer Resource Center
MEDLINE Knowledge Finder Evaluation Questionnaire

1. How often have you used MEDLINE Knowledge Finder? (circle one)
   - a. First Time   77.3%
   - b. Once before   13.3%
   - c. 3-5 times before   8.0%
   - d. 6 or more times   1.3%

2. How much information did you find? (Circle one)
   - a. Just what I was looking for   46.1%
   - b. More than I needed   14.5%
   - c. some of what I needed   38.2%
   - d. Nothing useful   0
   - e. Other (Specify___ N.A. 1.3%___)

3. If KF MEDLINE had not been available, what would you have done? (Circle one)
   - a. used a print index   42.4%
   - b. used another online system   13.8%
   - c. left a request with a library staff member   27.5%
   - d. asked a colleague   0
   - e. browsed through the stacks   13.8%
   - f. nothing   2.5%
   - g. other (specify___ N.A. 2.5%___)

4. Next time you need this sort of information, what will you do? (Circle one)
   - a. Try KF MEDLINE again   97.3%
   - b. Try a print index   2.7%
   - c. Try another online system
   - d. Try another source
   - e. Other (Specify_____)

5. What method were you using to search the database? (Circle as many as apply)
   - a. by subject(s) - (free text)   56.8%
   - b. by subject(s) - (using MeSH) subject terms)   16.9%
   - c. by author name(s)   .8%
   - d. by journal title
   - e. other (Specify:_____)

6. What was the purpose of your search (Circle as many as apply)
   - a. patient care   30.2%
   - b. case report   1.9%
   - c. presentation/teaching   22.6%
   - d. research project   30.2%
   - e. keeping current   6.6%
   - f. checking a reference   .9%
   - g. planning a course   .9%
   - h. just curious   3.8%
   - i. other (Specify:___   2.8%)

7. Have you used other online systems to access MEDLINE? Circle as many as apply.)
   - a. yes, by myself   19.5%
   - b. yes, the library staff searches for me   35.1%
   - c. no   45.5%
   - d. don't know   (N.A. = 2)

8. If yes, which system to you prefer? (Circle one)
   - a. online, by myself
     1. Grateful Med   53.6%
     2. MEDIS   4.7%
     3. PaperChase
     4. BRS Colleague   3.5%
     5. other (Specify: NLM = 7.1%)
   - b. online, library staff doing the search   28.6%
   - c. other (Specify:_____)

9. KF MEDLINE contains material from the last 4 years. Was this...(Circle one)
   - a. more than I needed   6.4%
   - b. less than I neede   31.9%
   - c. just right   61.7%

10. KF MEDLINE contains articles from 225 English language clinical medical, nursing, and allied health journals Was this...(circle one)
    - a. too many journals   8.8%
    - b. too few journals   16.2%
    - c. just right   61.7%

11. Were the instructions for use of KF MEDLINE adequate?
    - a. yes   100.0%
    - b. no

12. Was the KF MEDLINE manual helpful?
    - a. yes   51.4%
    - b. no   4.3%
    - c. Did not use manual   44.3%

13. What is your primary affiliation (Circle one.)
    - a. Medicine (Speciality:_____)
    - b. Nursing
    - c. Occupational/physical therapy
    - d. Psychology
    - e. Other (Specify:_____)

14. What is your profession? (Circle one)
    - a. physician (attending)   31.5%
    - b. physician (housestaff)   37.0%
    - c. nurse   20.5%
    - d. other health professional   2.7%
    - e. educator   1.4%
    - f. researcher   1.4%
    - g. student   2.7%
    - h. librarian   1.4%
    - i. other (Specify:___   1.4%)

15. Would you find this system useful to you if it was available at your worksite?
    - a. yes   76.0%
    - b. no   14.0%
    - c. undecided   10.0%

16. Overall, how would your rate KF MEDLINE's ease of use?
    - a. very easy   67.1%
    - b. moderately easy   30.1%
    - c. not at all easy   2.8%

17. Overall, how would you rate KF MEDLINE's value?
    - a. very valuable   89.9%
    - b. moderately valuable   10.1%
    - c. not at all valuable   None

THANK YOU VERY MUCH!! PLEASE RETURN THIS FORM TO THE GSMC LIBRARY.

EVALUATION AT

THE UNIVERSITY OF ROCHESTER OF

BRS COLLEAGUE DISC:

A MEDLINE CD-ROM PRODUCT

By *Kathryn W. Nesbit*
Julia Sollenberger

Edward G. Miner Library
School of Medicine and Dentistry
University of Rochester
601 Elmwood Avenue
Rochester, NY 14642

EVALUATION AT THE UNIVERSITY OF ROCHESTER OF BRS COLLEAGUE DISC: A MEDLINE CD-ROM PRODUCT

INTRODUCTION

Whenever the staff of a library considers a new product or service in the hope of enhancing the library's value to its clientele, the ideas and opinions of two groups — the staff members and the users — become immediately relevant. While soliciting input from the staff is usually an informal process, more formal surveys are often necessary to collect representative data from patrons. The benefits of such surveys can move beyond mere information gathering to serving a public relations function, especially if that new product or service is available to the users on a trial basis. Such was the case with the Colleague CD-ROM MEDLINE evaluation project at the Edward G. Miner Library. Patrons searched enthusiastically and completed their questionnaires willingly, hoping all the while that this trial period would never end! The opinions and ideas collected from the users, as well as staff observations of the end user search process, have provided valuable information as the Library was making its decision regarding in-library access to free CD-ROM searching.

BACKGROUND

The Edward G. Miner Library serves the faculty, residents, researchers, staff and students of the University of Rochester's School of Medicine and Dentistry and School of Nursing, as well as the staff of the Strong Memorial Hospital. In response to strong patron interest and a desire to expand its user education program, the Library has developed MEDLINE end user training programs for both the BRS Colleague online search system and PaperChase. The primary objective of these programs has been to produce end users who are able to search efficiently and who have a basic understanding of MeSH headings and strategy design. The Library's user education programs have been enthusiastically received by the attendees and new courses are being planned.

Since 1985, the Colleague course has been taught in both twenty-hour and nine-hour versions, the longer course being an elective for medical and graduate students while the shorter evening course is for faculty, residents and fellows. Hands-on exercises are incorporated into both versions to help master the arts of finding MeSH headings, building a search strategy and using the appropriate Colleague commands. As of July 1988, a total of 90 faculty, residents and staff have completed the short course and 40 medical and graduate students the long course. After finishing the course the students have access to subsidized Colleague searching in the Library. Faculty, residents and staff can take advantage of the Library-sponsored Colleague Group Account.

With the Library's Colleague training program firmly established and the librarians' expertise well known within the Medical Center, the Reference staff was approached in the summer of 1987 about the possibility of teaching the entire class of third year medical students to search MEDLINE. With only a brief amount of time allotted for teaching, the librarians selected PaperChase as the most user-friendly of the end user systems. Using PaperChase, a menu-driven system that maps textwords to MeSH headings, minimally trained user can retrieve highly relevant citations without previous knowledge of MeSH, a feature that makes PaperChase one of the easiest systems to teach. In September of 1987, 100 medical students learned to use PaperChase during a one and a half hour lecture followed by a one hour individual hands-on practice session. A PaperChase terminal was set up in the Library for students to use. In addition to medical students, PaperChase instruction has been given to 56 residents in the Departments of Medicine, Neurology and Anesthesiology. In all cases, the residents have access to a departmental PaperChase terminal.

With the experience gained from the Library's teaching efforts, the staff established criteria for evaluating and selecting a MEDLINE CD-ROM search system. Having searched on PaperChase, both patrons and librarians noted the usefulness of automatic mapping of textwords to MeSH headings as well as transparent use of Boolean operators. Both of these features aid the novice user by increasing the chance of finding more relevant citations. Also, since PaperChase automatically searches plural as well as singular forms of a word and tries to find the closest terms related to a misspelled word, textword searching techniques are not dependent on end user skill. In general, PaperChase does not expect the user to know how to search — how to use MeSH headings, how to enter commands, or how to truncate textwords. It helps the searcher move through the process one step at a time and is more forgiving of users' errors.

The librarians' expectations for a CD-ROM product were heightened after seeing the capabilities of a truly user-friendly system. The most beneficial system would be self-explanatory and require little training or assistance from the reference librarians. It must also be sophisticated enough to satisfy advanced end users who want features such as downloading and tree explosions. The Library staff hoped to use this evaluation project to determine how a MEDLINE CD-ROM product would complement current offerings to end users, how end users actually search on such a system and how successful they are at retrieving what they want.

SYSTEM FEATURES

The focus of this study was the BRS Colleague MEDLINE CD-ROM product. This system contains the English language portion of the MEDLINE database for the years 1985-1987, with each year (including abstracts) available on a separate disk. Halfway through the trial period the January-May 1988 update disk was received. The Colleague CD-ROM search system is similar in appearance to its online counterpart. In order to manipulate the system, the end user must know how to enter the Colleague commands. Retrieval is enhanced by searching for an unqualified term in all fields, including double-posted words in MeSH headings (e.g. "heart" will retrieve any MeSH heading with the word "heart" in it). If the user types in a phrase, Colleague assumes adjacency of the terms which simplifies textword searching. Unlike Colleague online, the CD version cannot automatically search plurals of a textword or correct for variant British and American spellings. It cannot distinguish a single word MeSH heading; for example, "anemia.de." will retrieve any heading containing the word anemia such as ANEMIA, APLASTIC.

At the beginning of each CD-ROM session online help for learning or reviewing the system capabilities is available from either the Tutorial or Quick Start option. Once a search is under way there are help screens for the users as well as a command line at the bottom of the screen listing the command words. The user of Colleague CD-ROM can download the search retrieval onto a floppy disk as well as save a strategy to be executed on the next year/disk. At the time of this study, the BRS search software did not provide the capability of searching several years simultaneously.

METHODOLOGY

In order to assess the impact of a MEDLINE CD-ROM product on the Library and its users, the Library conducted a formal survey using a three-page questionnaire and analyzed the data with dBase III Plus and SPSS statistical software (See Appendix A). Questionnaire responses indicated not only who used the CD-ROM but also why they were using it, what they were looking for and whether or not they had found it. Patrons' attitudes towards this new technology were also assessed. After trying the CD-ROM, would those end users with access to an online search service prefer their online system or CD-ROM?

On April 7, 1988 the CD-ROM work station was set up so it was the first thing patrons saw upon entering the Library. Signs announcing the trial project and the hours for the CD-ROM were posted near the machine. It was available 8:45 am - 4:30 pm Monday through Friday and on Saturdays from 11 am - 4 pm, with the possibility of expanding the hours later in the study. Due to heavy use and patrons' suggestions, a sign-up sheet was instituted on April 20th. A schedule of 10 forty-five minute sessions was designed for each weekday. Patrons were allowed one time slot per day with reservations taken only one day in advance.

Questionnaires were placed near the work station along with a drop-off box for completed forms. Users were asked to fill out a form every time they used the search system. A two-page instruction sheet written by the Reference staff presented the basics of searching on the Colleague CD-ROM (See Appendix B). At the start of each day the system was booted with the 1987 MEDLINE disk in place. The librarian on duty at the Reference Desk was available upon request to help CD-ROM users. With the exception of checking in and out of older years/disks at the Reference Desk, patrons were left on their own to learn the system. As the work station was only 20 feet away from the Reference Desk, the librarian on duty was able to monitor CD-ROM use. The staff kept a record of questions and help given to the end users along with the amount of time spent on each encounter. The librarians were concerned that this new service would require substantially greater assistance to patrons than current staffing could provide.

During the third week of June, the CD-ROM work station was set up in the Operating Room area of the hospital for three afternoons. The station was attended at all times by a reference librarian. In order to enter the sterile area the librarians were required to don surgical scrubs, a new experience to be sure! In this clinical environment the CD-ROM was available to the faculty, residents and nursing staff of the Departments of Anesthesia and Surgery. Because the staff in this area are on-call for most of the day, their access to the Library is restricted. Several months ago, in an effort to improve their access to information, the Education Librarian instructed the Anesthesia residents and staff in the use of PaperChase; the residents have since been issued passwords for searching on a terminal in the residents on-call room. Members of this group seemed likely candidates for utilizing CD-ROM in a clinical setting

RESULTS

Who Used the CD-ROM

Questionnaires and data on reference staff activity were collected from April 7 through June 7, 1988. The work station was kept in place until June 17th. There were 200 completed questionnaires including 40 with a fourth page of supplementary questions. Of the 200 respondents, 124 were first time users, 32 second time users, 31 had used it 3-5 times and 13 more than five times. The 83 searches saved on the station's hard disk by those end users who wanted to rerun a search strategy on another year/disk provided a second source of information. The sign-out sheets for exchanging the disks indicated how many people used more than one year/disk. The daily reference records detailed time spent on various questions and problems related to the CD. Finally, the reservation sheets showed that 362 people signed up for a time slot. From all of this data it is estimated that more than 525 end users tried the Colleague CD-ROM search system during the two and a half month trial period.

The CD-ROM was used by all segments of the Library's patron population (see Table 1). Comparing the numbers of users of the CD-ROM to the Library's subsidized online search service shows that a *larger* percentage of fellows, medical and graduate students used the CD-ROM. On the other hand a *smaller*

Table 1
Use of Librarian-mediated search service versus CD-ROM

POSITION	% used search service*	% used CD-ROM	Difference
Faculty	42.0	22.0	-20.0
Resident	10.0	9.0	-1.0
Fellow	15.0	24.5	+ 9.5
Staff	10.0	7.0	- 3.0
Medical Student	5.0	11.5	+ 6.5
Nursing Student	6.0	4.5	- 2.5
Graduate Student	8.0	18.0	+10.0
Other U of R	1.0	3.0	+ 2.0
Non U of R	3.0	.5	- 2.5

(* 1987 statistics)

percentage of faculty members used the CD-ROM compared to the online search service. As the librarian-mediated search activity rose 13% over the same time period last year, it appears that a different set of users is attracted to the CD-ROM; those with limited financial resources, perhaps, or those who prefer not to explain their search topic to a librarian. Several users expressed the latter view in the written comments section of the questionnaire, saying that sometimes they just do not know exactly what they are looking for and are embarrassed to explain that to a librarian.

Easy to Use?

Even though 72% of the CD-ROM users had never received any formal search training, they considered Colleague CD-ROM easy to use. Of the first time users, 97% considered it easy to learn and 98% considered it easy to use once they had learned it. Only 12% indicated that they needed *no* help in learning the system, as they either had prior experience with another system or because of native intelligence (the "learn from your mistakes" theory of life). The various search aids were most often used in combination. Three quarters of the respondents used the instruction sheet prepared by the Library staff and half tried the online help from either the Tutorial, Quick Start or help screens. Even with all of this assistance, 30% of the users sought help from the reference librarians whether they were first time or experienced users.

Nearly all of the end users (94%) considered that their search had been completed within a reasonable amount of time regardless of how long they spent on the system. Though half of them searched for less than 20 minutes, one third spent more than 36 minutes on the system. Only 18% spent under ten minutes. A possible explanation for the variation in searching times could be the purpose of the search. Many patrons were looking for research information rather than just a few articles. (Full details of the purposes of the searches appear in the next section.)

The end users had two ways to capture their retrieval. They could either use the printer to create a paper copy or download it to their own floppy disk: 83% chose the printer and only seven people tried downloading. There were 18 people who did not print, download, or even write down citations on a piece of paper, yet only five indicated that they did not find useful citations and another six tried the system only out of curiosity. This leaves seven people who must have memorized the citations from the screen(!).

Even though the users considered the system easy to learn and to use, they did encounter problems with it. The first stumbling block for many was the concept of entering a one or two letter code instead of the entire command word. This was complicated by the command line that appears at the bottom of the search screen showing the entire command word with only the code letters capitalized (i.e. Search PurGe DisK). Users were to conclude that they should type only the upper case letters. This was not the case, however, and when novices would type in the whole word Colleague would search it as a textword. Then, when a search became cluttered with these mistakes, there was no way to purge or erase individual search statements. According to BRS Colleague, the distinction of the one or two letter codes in the command line is much more apparent if a color monitor is used.

The patrons also had problems using the print command. The last query of the print command sequence is "Enter y to confirm your printer is ready, otherwise strike RETURN." Many people did not read this correctly and pressed the enter key only to be returned to the search mode without printing anything. This caused confusion for many novices. It also became evident that there was no way to stop or escape once the printer had started. A librarian had to reboot the system in order to stop the printer. A truly unique printing problem was experienced by one person who instructed the system to print citations numbered 105-9. Colleague started at 105 and then printed in reverse order to number 9. When the user noticed what the system was doing, the librarian had to reboot and the search was reentered.

Patrons experienced other problems with the system. The Colleague CD-ROM has an interrupt feature for aborting a search statement while the system is searching for it. This Crtl & Q command did not always work properly. Sometimes the system would beep when those keys were pressed even though it was an option on the screen. Occasionally the keyboard would lock and require that a librarian reboot the system.

Changing disks to search the older years also caused some difficulties. The more enterprising patrons simply removed the CD-ROM disk without reading instructions. Colleague does not allow one disk to be removed and another inserted unless the appropriate Change command sequence was used. If done improperly the librarian would once again have to reboot the system. The reference librarians soon learned to ask patrons whether they had used the Change command before exchanging disks with them. Also the repeated handling of the disks caused them to get dirty and scratched. Two of our test disks malfunctioned after heavy use.

What Were They Looking For

By an extremely wide margin end users were looking for subjects (96%) rather than authors (15%). More than three quarters of the people doing author searches were searching by subject as well; patrons searched for authors known to be working in the field. The respondents needed the information because they were working on a research project (60.2%), on a paper or report (43.5%), on keeping current in the literature (26%), and on patient care (only 10.5%). A third of the researchers were also using the CD-ROM as a current awareness tool and a quarter of them were working on a paper or report. Nearly half of the patient care users were also writing a paper or a report; these may have been residents preparing for a rounds presentation.

In general people were satisfied with the citations that they found using the CD-ROM (see Table 2). The majority of the patrons (58%) found what they were looking for and another 12% found more than they needed. A third, however, found only *some* of what they needed, which could be considered a measure of dissatisfaction with the system.

The number of citations retrieved by patrons was more diversified than expected. Many patrons needed more than just a few good articles to satisfy them. While half of them found fewer than 25 citations, a quarter found more than 75 articles (including 12% who found over 150). It is interesting to correlate patron satisfaction with the number of articles retrieved. Eight end users

Table 2
PATRON SATISFACTION WITH RETRIEVAL

	Responses	%
The information I found was:		
What I was looking for	111	57.8
More than I needed	23	12.0
Some of what I needed	60	31.3
Not useful	5	2.6
Other	2	1.0
Total =	192*	100.0

Respondents could choose more than one answer.

retrieved a large number of citations (more than 150) and still found only some of what they were looking for. Another person with a retrieval of more than 150 articles did *not* find what he was looking for. Yet another with a very small retrieval (5 articles) felt he had more than he needed!

Half of the patrons used one year/disk for their search and only 8% tried all three disks. During April and May of 1988 when the Colleague CD-ROM covered the years 1985-87, 30% of the patrons were not satisfied with the time span. Though many of the users wanted both more current and older information, 76% of these unsatisfied end users indicated they wanted a system to cover the years prior to 1985. The small number of people who actually used the older years could be related to the inconvenience of changing the disks, or perhaps the users' not knowing that other disks existed even though signs were posted.

The inability of end users to find the information they needed might have several explanations. It could be linked to the number of years searched. Almost half of the users who found only *some* of what they wanted searched just one year of the file (though 51% of those who did find what they were looking for also searched just one year/disk). Another reason for end users not finding the information they sought could be the manner in which they searched. A review of 83 saved searches (see Table 3) revealed an obvious lack of searching sophistication or even understanding of basic principles. (This is even more disturbing when one considers that patrons who had figured out how to save a search were probably a more knowledgeable group of searchers.)

Table 3
HOW SEARCHES WERE CONSTRUCTED

TEXTWORDS

Only textwords	14	17%
Textwords Anded	21	25%
Textwords with MeSH	29	35%
	64	77%

INDEXING TERMS

MeSH headings	32	38%
Subheadings	1	1%
Majored headings	1	1%

OPERATORS

AND	59	71%
OR	8	10%
WITH	8	10%

The average saved search had eight search statements and used textwords as part of the strategy. Nearly a quarter of the searches had three or fewer statements, though one search by a graduate student who had taken the Library's 20-hour Colleague class had 47 search statements!

Those who searched just textwords without using any operators were treating the system as if it were a printed index, looking under one entry at a time. They were probably not aware of the power of Boolean operators for refining a search. It was gratifying to see the number of patrons who did search with MeSH headings, usually in combination with textwords. The very small number using a Boolean OR, however, was surprising. Even fewer people used the more sophisticated options such as truncation, majoring a MeSH heading or searching with subheadings. For trained searchers the thought of textword searching without truncating terms or using the Boolean OR is somewhat alarming. It must be remembered, however, that nearly three quarters of the people who used the CD-ROM had had no formal search technique training.

Problems that patrons had manipulating the system also appeared in their saved searches. About a quarter of them had trouble entering a command, especially "execute" (13%) and "display/print" (11%). Eighteen (22%) of the saved searches had at least one term that was not found in the dictionary, though ten of the searchers were able to select a term from the index when this happened.

Patrons' Future Use of CD-ROM

Most of the end users would use the CD-ROM to answer their questions in the future. Respondents who indicated they would have used a printed index if there had been no CD-ROM available were especially interested in the future use of CD-ROM; 87% of those potential index users would now rather use the CD-ROM. Whether people had to pay or not did not seem to influence their new preference for the compact disk. Surprisingly, everyone is cost conscious whether the money is coming out of their own pocket or not. Patrons stated that they *would* use the CD-ROM as a possible alternative to paying for a search. None of the people who had to pay for their own searches would pay for a search if the CD-ROM was free.

Even end users who do their own online searching are going to add searching the CD-ROM to their information seeking behaviors. One patron said that he would use it to test a search strategy before going online and being charged for it. For those who still prefer their own online searching to the CD-ROM, primary reasons were the greater time span available online and the ability to search in their own office or home.

CD-ROM's Impact on the Library and Library Staff

From the daily activity sheets, the staff estimates that an average of 30 minutes per day was spent on the CD-ROM, including set up and take down. This seems rather low, probably due to librarians forgetting to record each and every encounter. There is no record of the time spent on major breakdowns, including a bad disk that had to be replaced by BRS. With the staff's familiarity with Colleague online and the similarities of the CD-ROM version to it, the librarians quickly learned to use the system and discovered some of its tricks. Library staff did spend time writing a two-page sheet of instructions that end users could take away and read.

Half of the staff's time was spent on brief questions lasting less than two minutes. The reference staff had been concerned that they would have to spend considerably more time hand holding and teaching people than was actually the case. Only 15% of the librarians' time was spent on strategy questions and 9% on helping first time users. Patrons were willing to invest their own time to learn the system using the online help or instruction sheet. However, 30% of the CD-ROM users did receive help from the librarians. Staff spent time exchanging disks (32%), rebooting the system (6%), and helping with command problems (7%). With these difficulties being so prevalent, Library staff decided that CD-ROM availability could not be expanded beyond the regular Reference Desk hours. The evening student workers at the Circulation Desk could not be expected to deal with these CD-ROM problems.

CONCLUSIONS

The success of the CD-ROM trial project in the minds of the end users was overwhelming and their enthusiasm for free self-service searching astounding. One user called it "the greatest thing since Dewey Decimals!" CD-ROM seems to fulfill a need for those patrons who want to search independently of library staff. "Using it [CD-ROM] yourself, you can try different search titles... saves having to explain all [of the search topic] to the librarian" was one patron's written comment. The incredible popularity of the was clearly demonstrated by the fact that 83% of the users had to reserve a time slot for searching. It is apparent that the Library will need more than one work station in the future.

Patrons did have ideas for improving the CD-ROM system. The majority of the users wanted the ability to search several years at once (87.5%) and to have online assistance in finding appropriate MeSH headings (70%). They also felt strongly that the system should allow downloading of the retrieval (50%), and that abstracts should be available online (58%) both of which Colleague provides. Though end users were not queried whether they would be satisfied with a smaller MEDLINE subset, it seems doubtful that they would be, judging from their interest in searching the years prior to 1985.

A group of sophisticated users suggested that MEDLINE should be made available on one of the University's main frame computers. Several wanted the capability to dial in to a local MEDLINE system. They also felt that several people should be able to search simultaneously. One patron sent in an advertisement for a V-Server which allows the CD-ROM player to be accessed through a VAX computer! While this option would address the dial-in concept, it still would not permit several users to search at the same time. (BRS did not support such hardware configurations as of July 1988.)

Though they were very pleased with the patrons' acceptance of the CD-ROM, the librarians still had reservations about the Colleague MEDLINE CD-ROM product. The major criterion of the Reference staff, that users be able to search effectively with little assistance from the librarians, was not met. The system did not allow the patrons to be totally self-sufficient searchers. One reason for so much staff assistance was the security problem of the alternate years/disks. The staff felt it was unacceptable, even foolhardy to leave the extra disks unattended. The user-friendliness of the system was also a concern. Patrons' problems with manipulating commands demonstrated the need for a menu-driven system for novices (one that could easily be overridden by more experienced users). Perhaps most significant, however, with the large percentage of end users who rely on textword searching, is the capability of a MEDLINE search system to map textwords to MeSH headings. Search systems should be capable of making the power of MeSH more easily accessible to the end user who searches MEDLINE.

No matter how user-friendly or menu-driven or "automatic" a system may be, librarians will still need to develop brief training sessions to teach end users basic search techniques and strategy design. It would be helpful if CD-ROM producers could provide a floppy disk tutorial that covered some of these basic concepts as well as the uniqueness of MeSH headings, the cornerstone of MEDLINE. With the tutorial on a floppy disk the novice could learn the system on a separate microcomputer rather than monopolizing the CD-ROM work station. If a vendor-produced tutorial disk is not available, then appropriate handouts should be provided since patrons seem to want instructions to read before their search session as well as during the search.

SUMMARY

The information gathered during this MEDLINE CD-ROM evaluation project at the Edward G. Miner Library has come from both Library staff and patrons. The opinions, ideas and observations of both groups have been valuable in establishing criteria for the CD-ROM "system of choice" and for developing policies and procedures regarding use of a CD-ROM product in the Library. Even with its current limitation of a single user per work station, a CD-ROM database system offers an exciting new mode of access to end user bibliographic searching. Rather than replacing either the librarian-mediated or user-friendly online search services, CD-ROM searching is a welcome additional service which the library can provide to a group of users who, for lack of funds or willingness to disclose their search topic to a librarian, have not previously taken full advantage of the wonders of computerized retrieval.

Appendix A-1

Edward G. Miner Library - University of Rochester
MEDLINE CD-ROM QUESTIONNAIRE

Please help us evaluate this MEDLINE CD-ROM product from BRS
COLLEAGUE. Your input regarding its usefulness is vital as we make
purchase decisions. We may look at other MEDLINE CD-ROM products to
compare with this one in the future.

<u>Check the appropriate box for each answer</u>. In some cases check all
answers that apply. Put your completed form in questionnaire box.

1. What is your position at the University of Rochester?

[] Faculty   [] Medical student   [] Other:
[] Resident   [] Nursing student   _____
[] Fellow   [] Graduate student   [] non-affiliate
[] Staff   [] Undergraduate   of U of R

2. How often have you used this BRS Colleague MEDLINE CD-ROM?
        [] a. first time   [] c. 3 to 5 times
        [] b. second time   [] d. 6 or more times

3. I was looking for articles: [] a. on a subject
                                  [] b. under a title
   CHECK ALL THAT APPLY.   [] c. by an author
                                  [] d. in a specific journal
                                  [] e. other _____

4. I needed the information for: [] a. patient care
                                  [] b. a paper or report
   CHECK ALL THAT APPLY.   [] c. research project
                                  [] d. keeping current
                                  [] e. to check a reference
                                  [] f. teaching/planning a course
                                  [] g. not needed, just curious
                                  [] h. other _____

5. My search produced _____ articles.
   [] a. 0-5   [] b. 6-25   [] c. 26-75   [] d. 76-150 [] e. over 151

6. The information I found was: [] a. what I was looking for
                                 [] b. more than I needed
                                 [] c. some of what I needed
                                 [] d. not useful
                                 [] e. other _____

7. Was this BRS Colleague CD-ROM easy to learn? [] yes   [] no

8. Was it easy to use once you had learned it?   [] yes   [] no

9. I spent _____ minutes on this search.
        [] a. 0-10   [] b. 11-20   [] c. 21-35   [] d. over 36

147

MEDLINE CD-ROM QUESTIONNAIRE page 2

10. Was the search completed within a reasonable amount of time?
[] yes   [] no

11. Did you print or download any of the citations from your search?
[] a. yes, I printed them on paper.
[] b. yes, I downloaded them on to a disk.
[] c. yes, I copied off the screen by hand.
[] d. no, I did not.

12. Was the time span covered by the CD-ROM MEDLINE sufficient for your needs? There are 3 discs; one for 1987, 1986, & 1985.
[] a. yes, I used one year's worth (= 1 disc)
[] b. yes, I used two year's worth (= 2 discs)
[] c. yes, I used all three years (= 3 discs)
[] d. no, the time span was not sufficient.

13. If your answer to 12 was NO, what time span would meet your needs? CHECK ALL THAT APPLY.
[] a. more current than 1987   [] b. older than 1985

14. If you checked 13b, what time span would you need?
[] a. 1983 +   [] b. 1978 +   [] c. 1966 +

15. What kind of assistance did you need to learn to use this MEDLINE CD-ROM ?   CHECK ALL THAT APPLY.
[] a. Instructions next to the machine
[] b. Quick start information on disc
[] c. Tutorial on disc
[] d. Help screen during the search
[] e. Received assistance from a Librarian
[] f. Received assistance from a friend
[] g. Needed no help because of familiarity with other CD-ROM packages or online systems
[] h. Needed no help - learned from my mistakes

16. If this MEDLINE CD-ROM had not been available today, what would you have done?
[] a. used printed Index Medicus, International Nursing Index, or other indexes.
[] b. done my own search online using Colleague, PaperChase or other system
[] c. asked a Librarian for help or requested a computer search
[] d. asked a friend or colleague
[] e. browsed through the stacks
[] f. nothing
[] g. other _____

17. I have access to MEDLINE on these online systems:
[] a. PaperChase
[] b. BRS Colleague
[] c. Grateful Med
[] d. through the librarians only
[] e. I do not have access to any online systems.
[] f. other _____

MEDLINE CD-ROM QUESTIONNAIRE page 3

18. In the future, my preferred method of finding articles will be:
    [] a. this MEDLINE CD-ROM product
    [] b. PaperChase
    [] c. BRS Colleague online version
    [] d. other online system (e.g. Grateful Med)
    [] e. to have a librarian do the search for me
    [] f. use the printed Index Medicus, International Nursing
        Index or other indexes.
    [] g. other _____

19. If your answer to 18 was b,c or d, why do you prefer an online
    system over this MEDLINE CD-ROM? CHECK ALL THAT APPLY.
    [] a. I can do my searches in my office/department/home.
    [] b. The online system is faster than the CD-Rom.
    [] c. I can search more years at once online.
    [] d. The online system has features which make it more
        powerful to use.
    [] e. other_____

20. Have you ever attended a training session offered:
    [] a. by the Library on PaperChase
    [] b. by the Library on BRS Colleague
        [] 9 hour evening course
        [] 20 hour course
    [] c. by representative of PaperChase/Colleague/vendor
    [] d. Learned from a friend
    [] e. other_____

21. Who pays for your searching?
    [] a. I pay for searches out of my own pocket.
    [] b. I use a grant or account number to pay.
    [] c. Someone else pays for my searches.
    [] d. other_____

22. Would you use this CD-ROM in the library as an alternative to
    paying for searches?
             [] yes   [] no   [] sometimes

23. Please give us any additional comments about this BRS Colleague
    CD-ROM product.

    _____

    _____

    _____

    _____

(optional) Name_____ Phone_____

PLEASE RETURN YOUR COMPLETED QUESTIONNAIRE TO THE BOX IN THE LIBRARY.

Edward G. Miner Library
MEDLINE CD-ROM Questionnaire Part II

Please help us evaluate this MEDLINE CD-ROM product. With this
questionnaire we are interested in how you are using this system to
find information.

Check the appropriate box for each answer. In some cases check all
answers that apply. Put your completed form in questionnaire box.

1. Did you reserve a time slot to use this equipment?
   [] a. Yes, I reserved a time slot for today.
   [] b. Yes, I signed up for my reserved slot yesterday.
   [] c. No, I did not. The chair was empty so I sat down.
   [] d. No, I waited for someone to finish before I could use it.

2. Which of these did you do in your search today?
      CHECK ALL THAT APPLY.
   [] a. Just typed appropriate words.
   [] b. Used Medical Subject Headings (HEART-NEOPLASMS, HEART.de.)
   [] c. Connected concepts using an AND
   [] d. Connected concepts using an OR
   [] e. Used a subheading (1 with di)
   [] f. Made a subject heading the major point of the article.
         LUNG-DISEASES.mj., ASPIRIN.mj.
   [] g. Searched for an author or journal title.

3. Which features do you want in a MEDLINE CD-ROM product?
      CHECK ALL THAT YOU WOULD WANT.
   [] a. Ability to search more than one year at a time.
   [] b. Must have abstracts of articles available.
   [] c. Have more than just English language journals.
   [] d. Have only English language journals available.
   [] e. Online help finding appropriate Medical Subject Headings.
   [] f. Ability to download on to a floppy disk.
   [] g. other_____
         _____

Appendix B-1

MEDLINE ON CD-ROM from BRS COLLEAGUE

This MEDLINE CD-ROM contains the English language articles from the MEDLINE database for the years 1987, 1986, and 1985. Each year is on a separate disc. (See Section E for using more than one disc for your search.)

Basic instructions are given here to get you started. Remember for more detailed help consult the Tutorial program on the system.

The system will start with a couple of screens explaining this system. The QUICK START and TUTORIAL options will give you more detailed information. Your search will start at
   ENTER TERMS HERE
   SEARCH 1-->

A. Searching by Subject
      The best way to look for a subject is to use the same Medical Subject Headings (MeSH) that you would in Index Medicus. Remember to press the Enter key after you finish typing in order to send it to the system.

      For a multiple word MeSH heading type heart-neoplasms
         The hyphen between the words will make your search go much faster.
      For a single word MeSH heading type heart.de.

      To search a phrase simply type in the words and press the Return key. Search 1 : toxic shock syndrome
      To be more precise qualify your terms to the Title (ti) and/or Abstract (ab) fields.
               blue nevus.ti. will retrieve this phrase
               only when it appears in a title of an article.

B. Combining terms using AND, OR and WITH
      There are several ways to combine your search statements with the Boolean operators (AND and OR) and a positional operator (WITH).

      1. AND - Using this BOOLEAN operator means that both of your terms must appear in the same citations.
         For example:
            Search 3--> 1 and 2
            Search 2--> adolescence.de.
            Search 1--> acquired-immunodeficiency-syndrome
         Search statement 3 will retrieve articles that talk about both AIDS and adolescents.

      2. OR - Using this BOOLEAN operator means that either of your terms will appear in the citations.
         For example:
            Search 1--> HTLV or HIV
         Search statement 1 will retrieve articles that talk about either HTLV or HIV.

151

B. Combining your terms continued
    3. WITH - Using this positional operator means that your
       terms will appear in the same sentence. For example:
         Search 1--> duchennes with dystrophy
       This search statement will retrieve articles that have
       Duchennes and dystrophy in the same sentence in either
       the title or abstract. It will retrieve the phrase
       Duchennes muscular dystrophy.

C. To print your citations
    Use the P command to have your citations printed on paper.
    If you have problems with the printer report them to the
    Reference Desk.

D. To display your citations on the screen
    Use the D command to have your citations appear on the
    screen.

E. To repeat your search on another year's worth of Medline:
    (There are 3 years available 1987, 1986 and 1985)   The
    other discs are available at the Reference Desk.
   1. Use the SV command and give your search a name.
   2. Use the C command
   3. Type Mesh
   4. On the CD player, press the RUN key to turn it off and
     press the lid to open it.
   5. Remove the CD disc and take it to the Reference Desk.
     You will be able to sign out another year's disc.
   6. Insert the new disc, close the lid and press RUN key on
     CD player.
   7. Press enter to start up the new disc. It will show you the
     beginning screens. Press enter to continue.
   8. At Search 1--> Type EX and give the name of your saved
     search.
     The system will now run your strategy on this CD.
   9. Once you have finished with this disc, repeat steps 2-7,
     leaving the 1987 disc in the player for the next person.

F. To correct a typing error
    Use the backwards arrow or backspace key to move cursor
    back to the mistake. Then retype the word correctly.

G. To end your search
    Use the Q command to end your search and prepare the system
    for the next user.

H. Commands - TYPE IN THE 1 OR 2 LETTERS (not entire word)
    S = Search   To search for terms in database
    D = Display   To display citations on the screen
    P = Printer   To print citations on the printer
    H = Help   Gives specific help on using the system
    Q = Quit   To Sign off system
    SV =Save   Saves your search strategy
    EX =Execute   To execute a previously saved search
    PG =Purge   To erase a saved search
    DK =Disk   To capture citations to floppy diskette
    C =Change   To change to a different year of MEDLINE
                (Save your strategy first - see Section E)

EVALUATION OF

BRS COLLEAGUE CD-ROM

AT UNC-CH HEALTH SCIENCES LIBRARY

By   *Merry Lynn Bratcher*
Dee Marley
Cindy Rhine
Nidia Scharlock
David Talbert
Cathryn White

Health Sciences Library
University of North Carolina
at Chapel Hill
P. O. Box 7585
Chapel Hill, NC 27514

EVALUATION OF
BRS COLLEAGUE CD-ROM
AT UNC-CH HEALTH SCIENCES LIBRARY

Introduction

The Health Sciences Library at the University of North Carolina at Chapel Hill was a NLM test site for BRS Colleague Medline on CD-ROM. We modified the questionnaire provided by NLM in order to evaluate this product (see Appendix A). This report is based on an analysis of the questionnaire, on comments from users, and on observations of staff members involved in the study.

Equipment and Staffing

On April 12, 1988 the library opened its Electronic Information Center (EIC). This Center included equipment and staff support for users to search BRS Colleague Medline on CD-ROM. The CD-ROM software was loaded on an IBM XT which was connected to a Philips CD-ROM player. A Hewlett Packard Think-Jet printer was also available. Originally, users signed up in person for thirty-minute appointments between the hours 9:00 a.m. to 1:00 p.m. Monday through Friday. However, it soon became evident that half-an-hour was insufficient time for users to enter their search strategy and print or download their results. Forty-five minute appointments also proved to be inadequate, and we have now implemented one hour appointments. If a user does not show up within ten minutes of his appointment the time may be given to a walk-in requestor. The Center hours have been expanded to include Monday through Thursday evenings from 6:00 to 9:00, Saturdays from 9:00 a.m. to 12:00 p.m. and 2:00 p.m. to 6:00 p.m., and Sundays from 12:00 a.m. to 7:00 p.m. Length of appointments and hours of system availability influenced our belief the Center needed to be staffed.

Although BRS Colleague was user-friendly and provided an online tutorial and online help, we felt users would have a more positive experience if assistance was provided. Staffing was a critical element in developing the Center. Currently, the Center is staffed twenty hours a week by a para-professional or by a support staff volunteer. These staff members have undergone an extensive two-week training program which provided instruction in MeSH, search strategy formulation, interview techniques, and system mechanics. In addition to didactic presentations, staff found it helpful to practice using the system by searching sample questions. Librarians at the Information Services Desk provided assistance with difficult questions.

An analysis of our users' comments showed that the majority felt assistance was needed, at least for the first time. This was especially true for users who were not familiar with computers. EIC staff noted that users needed more help formulating search strategies than help with system mechanics. To help users with search strategy a worksheet was developed, and users were encouraged to complete it before their appointments. With staff guidance, users were able to identify correct MeSH terms and subheadings and modify their retrieval to meet their specific needs. To further evaluate the need for assistance and to meet users' requests for more hours to search, we began opening the Center on evenings and weekends with no formal assistance. First-time users were encouraged to sign up during the morning when the Center was staffed. Evening users and those who declined assistance were referred to written documentation. Even though users searching in the evening expressed satisfaction with their retrieval, our experience with assisted search strategy formulation led us to believe unassisted users did not realize the full potential of the system.

Documentation

Written documentation consisted of a printed version of the tutorial and a short "cheat" sheet. The tutorial was reproduced with each section on a separate page. A table of contents was made and an additional section on how to search for journal titles was developed. The documentation was organized in a tabbed notebook and placed next to the terminal. Users' requests for a quick reference sheet prompted the development of a two- page handout which allowed users to easily determine how to enter a specific command (see Appendix B). Since most users did not wish to use search time to read through the online tutorials, BRS should consider producing a user manual and a quick reference guide similar to the one for BRS Colleague online. To date, we have not provided formal training sessions for users. Adequate documentation and staff assistance held mechanical problems to a minimum.

Trouble Shooting

Other institutions reported users placing the CD-ROM disk in the floppy disk drive and other problems with computers, players, and printers. It is our belief that the high level of staffing helped prevent system problems and downtime. During the evening hours, more problems were reported. The reπference librarian on duty dealt with these problems. Primarily, these consisted of error messages and were corrected by turning the computer off and restarting the system. Requests for system improvements were more numerous than problems, however.

Suggested Improvements

In terms of improvements our primary request would be to see BRS add the ability to explode MeSH terms. Other system improvements follow in order of priority:

1. Emphasize importance of searching with MeSH terms. It would be useful if the software could map free-text words.

2. Extend database coverage back to 1966.

3. Provide monthly updates.

4. Provide the capability to automatically print or download the search strategy with the citations.

5. Extend the break command to the print function.

6. Include non-English citations.

7. Produce a core and comprehensive database.

8. Provide written documentation.

Valuable System Features

Users found certain system features to be particularly valuable. The features our users found useful were:

1. The ability to download retrieval

2. The availability of online abstracts

3. The save and execute commands

Users and User Satisfaction

"Who were our users", "what were they looking for", and "how successful were their searches" were questions answered from data collected in the questionnaire. *A total of two hundred and forty-four users* accessed BRS Colleague between April 12, 1988 and June 30, 1988. The majority of our users were graduate students, followed by faculty and staff. These figures reflect the fact that the system was offered primarily at the end of the semester and during the early summer. Once the fall semester begins we expect to see an increase in the number of students. Users were accessing the system primarily for information to support research and publication. Almost all of the users were looking for information on a subject. Users were able to locate at least some of the information they were looking for. The vast majority felt that searching the system was easier than using print indexes. The next time users needed information the majority would return to use the CD-ROM system. The fact that the system was free was of great importance to most users. User satisfaction and desire to return has not yet had a discernable impact on the library's fee-based online search service.

Fee-based online searches did not decrease as an effect of a free CD-ROM service. At times, online search librarians referred users to the Center and at times Center staff referred users to the online search services. We will continue to monitor the impact of CD-ROM on our fee-based service.

We did not have the opportunity to place the system in a clinical setting. However, we are investigating the possibility of working with medical school faculty to place CD-ROM systems in the hospital for use by residents, nurses, and students.

Future Plans

In the future, we will definitely continue to offer a CD-ROM Medline product. However, BRS Colleague may not be the product to which we subscribe. We will choose a system that:

1. Provides the ability to explode now or in the near future

2. Has companion databases using the same search interface

3. Provides discounts for multiple subscriptions

4. Provides monthly updates

5. Covers more years

6. Offers a comprehensive and core database

Due to the popularity of the system we plan to purchase two Medline subscriptions. We also plan to add other CD-ROM databases such as NTIS and, when they become available, NurseSearch and International Pharmaceutical Abstracts.

Appendix A-1

```
        BRS COLLEAGUE MEDLINE CD-ROM EVALUATION QUESTIONNAIRE


Instructions

This BRS Colleague MEDLINE CD-ROM system is being tested by the
Health Sciences Library.  We would like you to fill out this
questionnaire in order to help us find out who is using the
system, and how useful it is to you.  Thank you!

                HEALTH SCIENCES LIBRARY AT UNC-CH

ABOUT YOURSELF
1.    My status at UNC-CH is:
             (circle one)
      a.   faculty
      b.   staff
      c.   medical or dental student
      d.   graduate student
      e.   undergraduate student
      f.   fellow/post doc
      g.   intern/resident
      h.   other_____


2.    I need this information for:
             (circle ALL that apply)
      a.   patient care
      b.   teaching or planning a course
      c.   a course paper or report
      d.   writing for publication
      e.   research
      f.   keeping up on a topic or subject
      g.   thesis or dissertation
      h.   other_____
      i.   just curious
      j.   to check a reference

3.    I was looking for articles:
             (circle all that apply)

      a.    by an author

      b.    under a title

      c.    on a subject

      d.    in a journal

      e.    other_____
```

4. The information I found was:
        (circle ALL that apply)

   a.   what I was looking for

   b.   more than I needed

   c.   some of what I needed

   d.   not useful

   e.   other_____

5. Have you used any of the printed publications produced from the MEDLINE system (e.g. INDEX MEDICUS, the INTERNATIONAL NURSING INDEX, the INDEX TO DENTAL LITERATURE, or the HOSPITAL LITERATURE INDEX)?
        (circle ONE only)

   a.   yes

   b.   no

   c.   don't know

6. If "yes", how does BRS Colleague MEDLINE CD-ROM compare to the printed versions?
        (circle ONE only)

   a.   easier to use

   b.   harder to use

   c.   about the same to use

   d.   other_____

7. Have you used an online version of MEDLINE (either yourself or by having a librarian process a search for you)?
        (circle ONE only)

   a.   yes, by myself

   b.   yes, librarian searched MEDLINE for me

   c.   no

   d.   don't know

8. If "yes, I've used online MEDLINE", which system do you prefer? (circle ALL that apply)

   a. online, doing my own search

   b. BRS Colleague MEDLINE CD-ROM

   c. online, librarian search MEDLINE for me

   d. don't know

9. If this MEDLINE CD-ROM system had not been available today, what would you have done? (circle ONE only)

   a. used a printed version

   b. done my own online search elsewhere

   c. asked a library staff member to do an online search

   d. asked a friend or colleague for information

   e. browsed through the stacks

   f. nothing

   g. other_____

10. Next time you need this sort of information, what will you do? (circle ALL that apply)

    a. try BRS Colleague MEDLINE CD-ROM

    b. try a printed version

    c. have a librarian do an online search

    d. do my own online search

    e. other_____

11. BRS Colleague MEDLINE CD-ROM is provided free of charge to library users. How important a consideration was this in your decision to use this system, instead of an online version of MEDLINE for which there is a charge?
       (circle one)

    a. very important

    b. somewhat important

    c. relatively important

d.   would not have used an online version of MEDLINE

12.   How often have you used BRS Colleague MEDLINE CD-ROM?
        (circle ONE)

   a.   first time

   b.   once before

   c.   3-5 times

   d.   6 or more times

13.   BRS Colleague MEDLINE CD-ROM contains information from the
      years 1985-1987. What years did you search?

      _____

14.   Enter ONE only (on the following 5 point scale) for
      questions a through g.

SCALE: A   B   C   D   E
        Strongly   Strongly
         Agree   Agree   Neutral   Disagree   Disagree

a.___Help screen instructions on BRS Colleague MEDLINE CD-ROM
     were sufficient for my use.

b.___ The speed at which the computer responds is satisfactory.

c.___The BRS Colleague MEDLINE CD-ROM tutorial helped me to use
     the system.

d.___Changing BRS Colleague MEDLINE CD-ROM discs is easy.

e.___The time span covered by BRS Colleague MEDLINE CD-ROM was
     sufficient for my needs.

f.___Overall, I found BRS Colleague MEDLINE CD-ROM easy to use.

g.___It was necessary to have assistance from library staff when
     I used the system.

Additional comments:

BRS Quick Reference Guide

ONLINE HELP

You can request online help at any point.

    SEARCH 1-->h (then press enter)

If you choose **h** after you have entered a command, the help screen will explain that particular command.

SEARCHING

Enter your search at any
SEARCH > prompt

The system will re-display your search with the number of documents in the database that contain these terms, and prompt you for your next search:

Current Search:

    Search 1--> Smokeless Tobacco
    21 documents

    Enter Search Terms:
    Search 2 -->

You can enter MeSH descriptors or free text terms.

MeSH   i.e. hypertension.**de.**
free text   i.e. high blood pressure
              (assumes adjacency)

CONNECTORS:
AND, SAME, WITH, OR, NOT
(Refining your search)

    Search 1-->hypertension.de. **and**
    exertion.de.   1,149 documents
    and retrieves articles in which BOTH
    terms appear

    Search 1-->hypertension.de. **or**
    exertion.de.   44,787 documents
    or retrieves articles in which EITHER
    term appears

    Search 1-->hypertension.de.
    same exertion.de.   856 documents
    same retrieves articles in which terms
    appear in the same field

    Search 1-->hypertension.de.
    with exertion.de.   336 documents
    with retrieves articles in which terms
    appear in the same sentence

    Search 1-->hypertension.de. **not**
    exertion.de.   29,471 documents
    not retrieves articles in which one
    term appears; excludes all articles with
    the second term

Use **NOT** with EXTREME CAUTION you might exclude a pertinent article

DISPLAYING

To see, on your screen, some or all documents found from your search

    Search 3--> **d**

then respond to the prompts that follow

Choices for display format:

TI (title)   Title field displayed

B (brief)   Accession number, author, title, journal, publication date, volume/issue, and page numbers

M (medium)   Information from the brief format plus other information such as descriptors

L (long)   The full citation with abstract (if available)

TD (tailored)   You can select any field to be displayed by entering the 2 letter field abbreviations separated by commas (e.g. au,ti,so,ab)

To see the previous document, type in the document number.

PRINTING

To print your search results to paper

    Search 4--> **p**

You will then be prompted to enter the following:
-search number to print
-format
-numbers of the documents to print

enter **Y** to confirm your printer is ready

TRUNCATION

You can search for a single word stem with variant endings by entering the word stem followed by a dollar sign ($)

    Search 4--> **hernia$**
    will retrieve hernia, hernias, herniation, herniated, etc.....

You can limit the possible variations retrieved by placing a digit after the dollar sign

    Search 4--> **hernia$3**
    will not retrieve herniation

BRS Quick Reference Guide

FIELD QUALIFICATION

You can enter search words with the limitation that the words must appear in a specific field

Search 5--> **hemophilia.ti.**
will retrieve hemophilia in titles only

Search 6--> **hemophilia.ab.**
will retrieve hemophilia in abstracts only

Search 7--> **hemophilia.mj.**
will retrieve hemophilia as a Major descriptor only

Search 8--> **N-Engl-J-Med.so.**
will retrieve articles in New England Journal of Medicine

Search 9--> **Davis-W$.au.**
will retrieve articles by W. Davis, W.S. Davis, Walter Davis, William Davis, etc.

COMMAND STACKING

Using command stacking allows you to enter more than one command at a time

Search 4--> **d;3;b;1-5**

d = display command
3 = search number
b = brief format
1-5 = numbers of documents to be displayed

DOWNLOADING TO DISK

Use this option only if you have a DOS formatted diskette available to capture the information

Search 5--> **dk**

You will then be prompted to enter a four-to-eight character name (to avoid confusion use your last name)

You will then be prompted to specify the following:
-search number
-format
-numbers of the documents to download

The system will tell you when to remove the diskette

SAVING A SEARCH

Use this option when you want to do the same search in another year of the database

After you have entered your search strategy, you can save it by entering **SV** at the next search prompt

Search 6--> **sv**

Enter Four Character Name for Saved

Search Search 7--> **exer**

CHANGING YEARS OF THE DATABASE AND EXECUTING A SAVED SEARCH

After saving a search, you can change to another year of the database and execute the search

Search 7--> **c**

Enter Database Label (MESH)--> **mesh**

Follow system prompts to change disks

After changing disks, you can execute the saved search

Search 1--> **ex**

Enter four character name of saved search to execute

Search 2--> **exer**

SUMMARY OF COLLEAGUE COMMANDS

ST The stem command allows you to enter a term and see an alphabetical listing of terms that begin with that word stem.

D The display command tells the system to display your search results displayed on your screen.

P The print command allows you to print your search results to paper.

SV The save command allows you to store your search strategy in the computer. At any time during the month you saved the search you can retrieve it to run it in other years of the database.

EX The execute command allows you to rerun the saved search.

DK The disk command allows you to download your search results to a diskette.

C The change command allows you to change disks.

H The help command shows you the online help screens.

Q The quit command gets you out of the BRS/CD system.

R The review command shows you your full search strategy.

ls 0623 BRS quick reference guide

163

EVALUATION OF

BRS/COLLEAGUE
CD-ROM MEDLINE

IN AN ACADEMIC MEDICAL CENTER
LIBRARY AND IN A CLINICAL SETTING

By *Beth Carlin*
    Suzy Conway
    Kathy Gallagher
    Linda Hulbert
    T. Scott Plutchak

Medical Center Library
St. Louis University
1604 South Grand
St. Louis, MO 63104

Evaluation Of
BRS/Colleague CD-ROM Medline
In An Academic Medical Center
Library And In A Clinical Setting

Introduction

The "hot" technology in libraries these days is CD-ROM. Journals and journal articles devoted to the topic are rapidly proliferating. Most of the information contained therein is descriptive of the technology, rather than evaluative of specific products [1-3]. However, there is a great deal of current interest in such evaluation, and during the time that the study described in this paper was undertaken, a number of these evaluations resulted in published reports [4-5].

As a participant in the National Library of Medicine's evaluation of CD-ROM MEDLINE products, the St. Louis University Medical Center Library was interested in investigating what effect bringing a CD-ROM system into the Library would have on our current online search service as managed by the Reference Department. Specifically, we wanted to know whether or not the CD-ROM system would appeal to a different clientele from that presently using the search service.

Methods

In the Fall of 1987, the Library evaluated the Compact Cambridge MEDLINE and MICROMEDEX CD-ROM systems. The questionnaires and study design used during these evaluations were modified for use during the BRS evaluation.

For the BRS study (which took place in the Spring of 1988), a CD-ROM workstation was set up near the circulation desk in the Library where it would be clearly visible to people entering. Flyers were widely distributed throughout the Medical Center during the month before the evaluation began. A banner at the entrance to the Library proclaimed: "Free MEDLINE Searching." The system was available on a walk-up basis from early April through early June. A stack of questionnaires was left next to the workstation with signs asking that they be filled out (for example, See Appendix A). Since the BRS system is advertised as being "user-friendly," we offered no initial instruction. A short user guide provided by BRS was left by the terminal, and staff were available to answer questions. A copy of *NLM's Medical Subject Headings* (MeSH) was placed near the terminal.

As a subsidiary study a second CD-ROM workstation was set up in the Internal Medicine conference room of the University Hospital for four weeks during April and May. A notice sent to all Internal Medicine faculty by the Department chair announced the availability of that workstation. No other advertising was done and no support was provided by Internal Medicine personnel. Questionnaires were placed in the Internal Medicine conference room with the telephone number of the Library's Reference Department.

During the period of the study, all individuals who came to the Reference Department requesting an online search were asked to fill out a short questionnaire which gathered information concerning their knowledge and use of the CD-ROM product (See Appendix B).

In addition to gathering information by means of the questionnaire, the project team members kept informal notes about their experiences and held regular meetings to discuss the management issues which the technology raises.

Results

One hundred and fourteen questionnaires were returned by individuals who used the workstation in the Library. Fifty-nine percent identified themselves as Medical Center students, 21% as faculty, and 16% as residents or fellows. The remainder included non-medical center personnel and Library staff.

Only nine questionnaires were filled out in the Internal Medicine conference room (3 faculty, 6 resident/fellows). Since the reference staff was in daily contact with the people using the system there, we were able to obtain anecdotal information.

As mentioned, most studies of CD-ROM technology to date have focused on user satisfaction. We were interested in this area as well, although based on the information of other researchers, we were pretty sure what we'd find. In short, everybody loved it. On a scale of 1 to 5, the average satisfaction rating overall was 4.3. We examined the satisfaction rating according to various categories of respondents (for example, patron identification, amount of previous experience, willingness to pay for the search, anticipated amount of use of such a system if it were made permanently available). However, for no categorization was there a significant difference in the average satisfaction or ease of use ratings. No matter who was using the system, what they were using it for, or what their specific experience with it was, everyone rated the system highly both for overall satisfaction and for ease of use.

Few difficulties were reported. Two questions addressed possible problem areas, one focusing on use of the system and the other on the data retrieved. In the former category the most commonly reported problem was difficulty switching disks, followed closely by selecting and entering search terms, and printing. The problem with switching disks is particularly acute with BRS since it is very important that users follow the instructions exactly. Many of our patrons did not and the BRS system gives no error messages to indicate when disks have been switched improperly. The major problem with the retrieval was insufficient years covered, followed closely by not finding enough citations (this last may indicate a misunderstanding of the amount of data contained on each disk). Overall, 49% of the respondents reported some kind of problem using the system and 27% reported some dissatisfaction with the search results.

In addition to problems identified by users, the study team identified a number of other areas of particular concern: the lack of "explode" capability, the need to hyphenate MeSH headings, the length of time required for subheading searches, and an insufficient "stop-word" list.

We were particularly concerned with how such a system in the Library might affect requests for online searches. One approach toward this question was to attempt to gauge the level of previous online experience among the respondents to see if the CD system was appealing primarily to our current online search service users, or was drawing in people who had no experience at all with online searching. Of the 122 respondents who answered the level of experience question, 22% indicated that they had no searching experience whatsoever. Forty- three percent indicated that they had had a search performed by an intermediary. Thirty-five percent had done searching themselves either directly online or by using some sort of user-friendly front-end system. One may assume that most of those in the latter group also had had a search performed by an intermediary at some time, but this information is not reflected in the questionnaires.

Among the three large groups of users, students reported the highest percentages of both those without experience and those who had done searching themselves (27% and 43% respectively). Residents/fellows showed the highest percentage of those having had a search performed for them (65%). Interestingly, everyone from this group who reported that they did their own online searching used some kind of user- friendly system. Fourteen percent of faculty members and 15% of students indicated they did online searching without a user-friendly system. Eleven percent of faculty and 17% of residents/fellows indicated no searching experience whatsoever, illustrating that among all three groups the CD-ROM system reached a significant number of individuals who had not previously made use of MEDLINE in any form. The questionnaire did not ask whether or not any of these individuals were *Index Medicus* users.

Questionnaires were ranked according to what mode of access the respondents would prefer in the future compared to what their previous level of experience was. Twenty-eight percent of those who had no previous searching experience indicated that they would prefer to do all of their searching on CD-ROM. Forty-seven percent of those who said they did their own online searching said they would prefer CD-ROM. Fifty percent preferred having both options available. Only 3% of the total indicated that they would prefer to have all of their searching done by a librarian.

Since the question of economics is of great importance to libraries, respondents were asked two questions relating to money: first, did they think the Library should commit funds to support CD-ROM (the questionnaire pointed out that such a subscription would be equivalent to the average cost of eighteen journal subscriptions), and second, would they be willing to pay a fee for use of the system, and if so, how much. Seventy-six percent of the total respondents felt the Library should commit funds to such a system. The total was highest among students (90%) and lowest among residents/fellows (65%). Eight percent of the total were undecided, with several pointing out that the question was "loaded" because of the reference to journal subscriptions. Sixty-eight percent of the respondents indicated they would be willing to pay a fee, with faculty being most willing (91% of the faculty who answered the question said they would be willing to pay a fee). Residents/fellows were least willing to pay (53%), with students midway between those two groups (77%).

Of those who said they were willing to pay a fee, nearly all indicated the $1.00 to $5.00 range. There were eight respondents (10% of those who indicated willingness to pay) checking the $5.00 to $10.00 range and none higher. Several added comments suggesting that charges be made according to time rather than per search, pointing out the difficulties in determining exactly what a search entails.

Respondents were asked how often they would use such a system if it were in place in the Library. The majority of responses were once a week or once a month. Those who felt they would use the system weekly were significantly less willing to pay a fee (66% indicating they would be willing), than those who said they would use it monthly (78%).

At the site in the Internal Medicine Department the lack of support was a clear problem, as was the lack of publicity on the part of the department. The responses to the few questionnaires showed that users of the system preferred to have it available in the department. However, we found no evidence that they would be more likely to use the system there than in the Library (a ten-minute walk from the department). Indeed, those faculty who were likely to send their secretaries to the Library for searches were just as likely to send them to the conference room. We received panicked calls from individuals placed in this situation for whom the lack of close support was a serious problem. Our experience here suggests that without a strong push on the part of those introducing the system to a clinical department those individuals who are likely to use the system in the Library will use it in the department, but few additional users will be added. Simple proximity, without training and support, is not sufficient inducement to use the system.

Thirty-six questionnaires were filled out in the Reference Department by people requesting online searches during this period. A large portion of requests for searches done in the Reference Department come in by phone and these callers were not asked about CD-ROM.

Seventy-eight percent of the people who answered this questionnaire had not used the CD-ROM system before coming to the Reference Department for that search. The most common reason given for not using the CD system was a need for either older or more current information, although not knowing how to use it or not being aware it was there also were frequent responses. Several respondents mentioned the need for human assistance as their reason for coming to the Reference Department for their search. When asked why they came to the Reference Department for a search after having used the CD-ROM, the concern over years covered was the reason given by half of the respondents. Several people indicated that they hadn't been able to find what they wanted on the CD-ROM or that they needed other reference assistance.

Discussion

It became apparent very quickly, not only from the questionnaires but from discussion with patrons that on the basis of user demand alone, CD-ROM MEDLINE was here to stay. In fact, by the end of the study, the Library had made the decision to enter two subscriptions to BRS/COLLEAGUE CD-ROM MEDLINE. The study raises more questions than it answers, however, about how to best manage the technology and how to be sure that it is best serving the needs of the Library's clients.

For instance, the satisfaction question is a double-edged sword. Patrons clearly like the system and are generally satisfied with the results that they obtain. However, personal observations and discussions with patrons indicate that many of those satisfied users are not using the system efficiently and may in fact, be grossly misinterpreting their results. Satisfaction, in other words, is a poor gauge of quality and value. Many patrons do not understand the limitations of this product database in terms of year and journal coverage. They may think the search is much more comprehensive than it is. A lack of understanding of MeSH and indexing principles leads many users to enter terms inaccurately, leading to search results that are skewed, incomplete, or replete with false drops. A dissatisfied user who comes and asks for help poses less of a concern than a user who is unaware there is a problem and leaves satisfied. One might assume that making use of the HELP instructions would enhance one's facility with the system, but the large proportion of the system's users who did not take advantage of them were no less satisfied than those who did.

The primary cause of dissatisfaction is the number of years covered. Most patrons who commented indicated a preference for a minimum five- year time span. Since problems with switching disks also ranked high, this need presents obvious problems for manufacturers. The "jukebox" concept (in which either several CD-drives are linked, or one drive supports several discs) may resolve this from the technical end, but it increases the financial burden. Clearer instructions and context- sensitive help screens for users changing disks is also necessary. (We had at least two cases in which users inserted the CD disc into the floppy disk drive.)

The study allows us to make a few cautious predictions about the effect that making CD-ROM MEDLINE available is likely to have in the Library. In regard to the question we initially asked, would such a system appeal to a different clientele from those using the current search service, the answer is a qualified yes. A significant number of people using the CD-system had never used online search services; a significant number of people using the mediated search service showed no inclination to use the CD-ROM. This has several implications. Our experience leads us to believe that many of the individuals using CD- ROM will require reference assistance, both in terms of dealing with the system itself and in requesting online searches for those questions which are beyond their abilities or the capabilities of the CD-ROM system. From this standpoint the CD system may increase the overall pool of mediated search service clients. The study provides little evidence to support the proposition that the CD-ROM system will siphon off a significant number of online search requests. While some people will attempt to do all of their searches on CD-ROM, a significant majority in all categories indicated that they want both options available in the Library. This suggests that even avid fans of CD-ROM anticipate the need for mediated searches.

The Reference Department is currently investigating options for providing some formal classes in using the system in order to minimize the number of on-call demand hours that will be required of them. Although the system received high marks for ease of use, it is patently obvious that a significant number of patrons will require human assistance at some point during their search, particularly in the areas of selecting search terms and understanding the capabilities of the system. In addition, some fundamental comprehension of the structure of the MEDLINE database is imperative.

The experience in the Internal Medicine setting highlighted this problem. From discussions with those using the system there and from our own observations, it was clear that the distance of the conference room from reference support staff inhibited effective use. Faculty and residents who were inclined to make use of the system preferred having it closer to them, but they would have come to the Library if need be. Those individuals who said they would rarely use the system in the Library did not indicate they would use it any more often in the Internal Medicine conference room. The lack of support was a serious problem for those who did use it. Although the paucity of formal responses received makes any numeric judgments suspect, it is worth noting that all of the system problems cited dealt with entering and selecting terms, as well as the fact that 2 of the 9 respondents said that they would prefer to have a reference librarian do their searches.

The financial question remains ambiguous. We suggested, although we did not state outright, that it might be necessary to cut journals in order to support the CD-ROM system. Even with that veiled threat, the mandate to commit Library funds is clear. Although there is also a marked willingness on the part of the majority of respondents to pay for individual searches we plan to make the system available free of charge.

Conclusion

As has been the case in every other study, formal or informal, published or unpublished, of which we are aware, the CD-ROM system was enthusiastically received by the Library's clients. The advantages of timeliness, direct interaction with the system, and the ability to work on one's own all lead to a strong feeling of satisfaction with the searches obtained this way. For this reason alone, it appears to be a technology that will find a place in today's libraries as long as the market continues to support it.

However, there is yet no convincing evidence for the overall increased utility of such "end-user" systems over current mediated online services or searches made using paper copy tools in meeting the information needs of health professionals and students. While it is obvious that some very savvy users are making excellent, productive use of such systems, it is also apparent that an uncomfortably large number of users have little concept of the contents of the database or of effective ways to search it. It was apparent from our discussions with users that many were completely unaware that this system was the same MEDLINE as was searched by reference librarians in the Reference Department and that it bore any relationship at all to *Index Medicus*. This is not a problem with the search interface as much as it is a lack of intellectual understanding of the contents of the database and the types of questions which may suitably be put to it.

Our concern with these questions has led us to think long and hard about our approach to training and to developing an understanding of the intellectual structure of the database being searched. It has caused us to examine our own assumptions about "good" versus "bad" searches and to attempt to devise ways that will help insure that the users of these systems have a solid understanding of what they can reasonably expect to obtain and how they can usefully evaluate the retrieval that they get. (We also noted that these are questions that we rarely asked ourselves when we showed users the fundamentals of searching *Index Medicus*.)

The Internal Medicine experience underlined all of these concerns. It is clear to us that to be useful in a clinical setting, CD-ROM must be introduced with the full, on-going support of the department as well as strong training, support and public relations directed to the potential clientele. "User-friendly" is a potentially misleading term — it should not lead us to think that these systems can simply be dropped into the doctor's office and thereby revolutionize the practitioner's information seeking behavior.

The financial impact of CD on the Library is uncertain. It is unlikely that the Library's online costs will drop sufficiently to cover the CD subscription (particularly since demand necessitates more than one workstation). The current decision not to impose user charges for the CD system results in another substantial budget item to cover.

It appears that the overall effect of CD-ROM MEDLINE is to continue to broaden the range of tools available to the Library's clientele for use in accessing the medical literature. As with most new technologies, it will not replace any previous option. Further study is needed for us to determine definitively what niche this particular technology will most beneficially occupy.

References

1 Helgerson LW. CD-ROM search and retrieval software: the requirements and the realities. *Library Hi Tech* 4(2):69-77 Sum 1986.

2 Miller DC. Evaluating CDROMS: to buy or what to buy? *Database* 10(3):36-42 Jun 1987.

3 Peters C. Databases on CD-ROM: comparative factors for purchase. *The Electronic Library* 5(3):154-60 Jun 1987.

4 Glitz B. Testing the new technology: MEDLINE on CD-ROM in an academic health sciences library. *Special Libraries* 79(1):28-33 Win 1988.

5 Capodagli JA, Markikian J, Uva PA. MEDLINE on compact disc: end-user searching on Compact Cambridge. *Bull Med Libr Assoc* 76(2):181-5 Apr 1988.

Appendix A

ST. LOUIS UNIVERSITY

MEDICAL CENTER LIBRARY

PLEASE FILL-OUT THIS QUESTIONNAIRE TO HELP US EVALUATE THE FOLLOWING COMPACT DISK SEARCHING SYSTEM

BRS/COLLEAGUE DISK MEDLINE

1. Are you a
____ faculty member   ____ library staff
____ resident/fellow   ____ non-medical center client
____ student   ____ other medical center personnel
____ (Please specify)_____

2. What experience do you have with online searching?
____ had a search done but did not see it performed
____ present while my search was done by a librarian
____ do my own online searching with my PC at work or
at home (Please specify which database(s)_____
_____
____ used a user-searchable (friendly) or front-end
online search system (for example, BACS/Medline,
Sci-Mate, Paperchase, Quicksearch, Cambridge
Medline etc.)
____ no online searching experience whatsoever

3. How useful did you find the HELP instructions when you
used the BRS/COLLEAGUE DISK MEDLINE system? CHECK HERE
IF YOU DIDN'T USE THE HELP INSTRUCTIONS. ____
CIRCLE the number which best describes your answer

1	2	3	4	5
not-at-all		somewhat		very
useful		useful		useful

4. How easy was the BRS/COLLEAGUE DISK MEDLINE system to
use? CIRCLE the number which best describes your answer

1	2	3	4	5
not-at-all		somewhat		very
very easy		easy		easy

5. Please indicate if you encountered any of these problems
while searching the BRS/COLLEAGUE DISK MEDLINE system.
____ I had difficulty switching disks
____ I had trouble selecting search terms
____ I didn't understand how to enter search terms
____ I had problems printing my results/answer
____ other (please specify)_____
(Room for additional comments on back)

6. How satisfied were you with the results of your search
on the BRS/COLLEAGUE DISK MEDLINE system?
CIRCLE the number which bests describes your answer.

1	2	3	4	5
not-at-all		somewhat		very
satisfied		satisfied		satisfied

(ROOM FOR ADDITIONAL COMMENTS ON BACK)

7. If you were not satisfied with your search results please
select a comment.
COMMENTS:
____too much information to sift through
____I did not find enough citations
____I found too many citations
____the citations I found were not
relevant to my question
____insufficient number of years (please specify years
desired)_____
____other (please specify)_____
(Room for additional comments on back)

8. How will you use the results of your search?
_____
_____
_____
_____
_____

9. Now that you have used the BRS/COLLEAGUE DISK MEDLINE
search system would you
____prefer doing your own searching on BRS/COLLEAGUE
____prefer to have a reference librarian do your
searches for you.
____prefer to have both options available in the library

10. If the library made available the BRS/COLLEAGUE DISK
MEDLINE searching system, how often would you use it?
____ daily   ____once-a-month
____ once-a-week____once-a-year ____never

11. Do you want the Library to commit funds to the
BRS/COLLEAGUE DISK MEDLINE search system considering that
the annual subscription cost to BRS/COLLEAGUE DISK
MEDLINE is equal to the average cost of 18 journal
subscriptions.

yes_____   no____

12. Would you be willing to pay a fee for use of the
BRS/COLLEAGUE DISK MEDLINE search system?

yes____   no____

If yes, what amount
____$1.00-$5.00 per search
____$5.00-$10.00 per search
____$10.00-$15.00 per search
____$15.00+ per search

QUESTIONNAIRE FOR MEDIATED SEARCH USERS

ST. LOUIS UNIVERSITY MEDICAL CENTER LIBRARY

Please fill out this questionnaire prior to your mediated online search.

1. Have you used the BRS Colleague Disk MEDLINE searching system ?

yes_____   no_____

2. If you have used the BRS Colleague Disk MEDLINE searching system, did this influence your decision to ask for a mediated search?

yes_____   no_____

3. Please explain why you chose to ask for a mediated search after having used the BRS Colleague Disk MEDLINE searching system?

_____
_____
_____

4. If you didn´t use the BRS Colleague Disk MEDLINE searching system, why not?

_____
_____
_____

5. How will you use the results of your mediated search?

_____
_____
_____

Any other comments would be appreciated:

_____
_____
_____
_____
_____

Please leave this questionnaire with the Reference staff or send it back to the Medical Center Library when you have completed it. Thanks!

EVALUATION AT

THREE ACADEMIC MEDICAL LIBRARIES

OF

Compact Cambridge
MEDLINE

By   *Nancy K. Roderer*
Susan Barnes
Columbia University
Health Sciences Library
701 W. 168 St.
New York, NY 10032

Terry Ann Jankowski
University of Washington
Health Sciences Library, 5B-55
Seattle, WA 98195

EVALUATION AT
THREE ACADEMIC MEDICAL LIBRARIES OF
COMPACT CAMBRIDGE MEDLINE

Section 1. Introduction

The National Library of Medicine's study of compact laser disc-based MEDLINE systems, in progress for almost two years and encompassing a wide range of geographic locations and user populations, has enabled the collection of a wealth of data regarding compact disc system use and acceptance. This data collection has been well-timed to occur while compact disc (CD) MEDLINE systems are still new and rapidly evolving.

As part of this nationwide study, Cambridge Scientific Abstracts placed Compact Cambridge MEDLINE workstations in the Columbia University Health Sciences Library, the University of Washington Health Sciences Library and Information Center, and the Tufts University Health Sciences Library. These three academic institutions were responsible for maintaining and publicizing the systems, training library staff and users, administering questionnaires, and providing information and statistics regarding library services. The questionnaire results, combined with the libraries' statistics and other information, provide an initial picture of some of the effects of introducing a new technology into the biomedical information gathering process. This report presents evaluation results for Columbia and Washington, the two sites which collected online survey information.

The specific purposes of the Compact Cambridge MEDLINE study were:

1. To study characteristics of Cambridge MEDLINE users;

2. To study these users' acceptance of the system;

3. To assess the impact Cambridge MEDLINE may have on library services and information retrieval;

4. To provide feedback and suggestions to Cambridge Scientific Abstracts.

In addition, the National Library of Medicine wanted to generalize this information to a description of Cambridge use at three sites. Columbia also wanted to use this information in its study of all MEDLINE use at the Columbia-Presbyterian Medical Center, the overall goal of which is to identify the options preferred by the medical center's various user groups.

Environment: Columbia University Health Sciences Library

The library serves the schools of medicine, dentistry, nursing, and public health, allied health education programs, the Presbyterian Hospital, and other health care, instruction, and research programs. A private library open only to Columbia affiliates, it is located on the Columbia-Presbyterian Medical Center campus across the street from the hospital and medical and dental schools, and one block from the schools of nursing and public health. The medical center is 2 1/2 miles north of the main Columbia campus.

The library provides mediated MEDLINE searches on a cost-recovery basis. Since December 1987, the library has provided access to MEDLINE via its online catalog, which contains the most recent eighteen months' worth of MEDLINE references. Since the beginning of its participation in the Cambridge MEDLINE evaluation, the library has also provided access to MEDLINE on compact disc near the Reference Desk. Access to two other compact disc systems, PsycLIT and Cancer-CD, is available in the same area, and is funded by a Pew Foundation grant. Another Cambridge MEDLINE station, funded by the same Pew grant, is located in the School of Nursing's computer center. In addition to its online services, the library maintains subscriptions to many printed indexes, including *Index Medicus*.

Many end-users maintain individual accounts with BRS, NLM, DIALOG, and PaperChase. The majority of these are administered separately from the library's database account. Given the near impossibility of finding information about the volume of end-user searching, and with so many MEDLINE alternatives available, it is not possible to determine exact levels of MEDLINE use at Columbia. Estimates have been drawn by sampling users and by examining university accounting records, and are summarized in Section 3.9.

Environment: University of Washington Health Sciences Library and Information Center

The library is open to the public and is located in the Warren G. Magnusen Health Sciences Center building, along with the schools and institutions it serves. Its primary user groups include the schools of medicine, dentistry, pharmacy, public health, and nursing, the University Hospital, and related health care, instruction, and research programs. It is also heavily used by the campus at large, and by the general public as well. The Health Sciences Center is on the southern edge of the University of Washington campus.

As at Columbia, it is extremely difficult to quantify total MEDLINE use at the University of Washington. The library provides mediated MEDLINE searches on a cost-recovery basis. In addition, the library provides access to MEDLINE on compact disc in its End-User Searching Area, in which a microcomputer dedicated to PaperChase is also located along with NurseSearch and Micro-Medex stations. Subscriptions to many printed indexes, including *Index Medicus*, are maintained in addition to online and CD services. Many end-users maintain individual accounts with BRS, NLM, DIALOG, and PaperChase, and most of these are administered separately from the library's accounts.

Section 2. Methods

The data presented in this report were gathered in several separate data collection efforts designed to elicit information about different forms of MEDLINE at different locations. These various efforts are summarized in Table 2.1. The overall goal of each of the data collection efforts - to better understand the user response to MEDLINE - was the same, but the methods and the specific questions varied with the circumstances as described below.

Columbia University, the University of Washington, and Tufts University were chosen by NLM as test sites for the compact disc version of MEDLINE produced by Cambridge Scientific Abstracts. Each agreed to evaluate the system, and Columbia further agreed to coordinate parallel evaluations at the three sites. The primary means of data collection for this evaluation was an automated questionnaire designed by Columbia, modified slightly for Tufts and Washington, and incorporated in the Cambridge software so that it was automatically presented to each user at the end of a search. The questions included in the survey are shown in Appendix A.

Table 2.1 Summary of Data Collection Instruments

Questionnaire Name	Appendix Location	Sites	Dates	Number of Responses
Online #1	A	Columbia Univ. Library Univ. of Washington Library	December 1987- January 1988	120 103 223
Online #2	B	Columbia Univ. Library	April 1988	91
Paper - School of Nursing	C	Columbia Univer School of Nursing	September 1987- June 1988	23
Paper - Library	C	Columbia Univ. Library	August - November 1987	32
CLIO	D	Columbia Univ. Library	April 1988	70

The automated survey was installed at the three test sites on December 1, 1987 and maintained on the Cambridge system through January 31, 1988. Over this period of time, the questionnaire was completed by 120 users at Columbia and 103 users at Washington. Only two survey responses were collected at Tufts and these were, accordingly, not included in further analyses.

Not all system users completed the questionnaire; it was possible to skip particular questions or to exit the questionnaire at any point. To calculate response rate, we used the disc circulation records for the December-January time period at Columbia to determine that there had been 175 searches in total. Since we had 120 completed questionnaires for the same time period, the response rate was just under 70 percent.

The results of this first automated survey indicated that the patterns of use reported were very similar at Columbia and Washington. Some of the findings also suggested areas for further exploration - in particular, specifics about MEDLINE sources used and changes in searching behavior with the availability of Cambridge MEDLINE. We designed a second automated survey and, because of the similarity in first round responses, installed this questionnaire only on the Cambridge system at Columbia. The survey was carried out during April 1988, and 91 responses were received. Survey questions are shown in Appendix B.

At the same time as the NLM evaluation was being carried out, another CD-ROM evaluation study was taking place at Columbia University. Funds from a Pew grant were used to purchase a number of different CD-ROM systems and install them in libraries and other locations. The purposes of this effort were to study user response to CD systems and to investigate the effects of these systems on library services and budgets. Part of the evaluation effort involved determining which systems should be retained.

One of the systems which was acquired under Pew funding was a second Cambridge MEDLINE system, which was installed in the offices of the Columbia University School of Nursing in September 1987. Evaluation of the School of Nursing installation was carried out by observation and paper questionnaire, using the questionnaire shown in Appendix C. This report includes data collected from the School of Nursing over the period September - December 1987.

The questionnaire used in this effort was the predecessor of the first online Cambridge questionnaire, and so contains many of the same questions. It was used both in the School of Nursing and, for purposes of pretesting, with the Cambridge system when it was first installed in the Library. Results of 23 completed Cambridge questionnaires from the School of Nursing and 32 completed questionnaires from the Library are shown in Appendix C. and are combined, where appropriate, with other questionnaire responses in the tables and figures of this report.

The final data collection effort referenced in this report was a brief study of CLIO MEDLINE users conducted in April 1988. CLIO is the Columbia University Libraries' online catalog, and includes an 18 month subset of MEDLINE. It was introduced in December of 1987 as a part of our overall effort to investigate the costs and user response for different forms of MEDLINE. One part of our evaluation of CLIO MEDLINE was an interview survey conducted in April 1988. Library staff interviewed CLIO MEDLINE users using the interview guide shown in Appendix D; a total of 70 interviews were conducted. Again many of the questions were repeated from other MEDLINE evaluation efforts and so some comparative results are given in this report.

Most of the data presented in the body of this report reflect combined responses of Cambridge MEDLINE users from those surveys in which a particular topic was addressed. Where significant differences between subgroups were noted, for example between Washington and Columbia or between Columbia library and School of Nursing respondents, these are reported. Data on CLIO MEDLINE users are identified as such and are presented mainly for comparisons.

Section 3. Results

Cambridge MEDLINE was introduced in the NLM test sites in August 1987 and began to be used immediately. At both Columbia and Washington, the system is frequently in use and there are often individuals waiting to use it. There are, of course, variations in the level of use with the academic calendar. Levels of searching were lower at both schools during December, and lower at Columbia at the end of the spring term.

The number of searches (i.e., user interactions with the system) was estimated differently at the two test sites. At Columbia, we counted disc uses directly from the disc circulation cards, and the number of searches (a search may cover more than one disc) is estimated based on the number of disc uses per search during the first survey period. During this period, there were an average of 1.8 discs used by each searcher (see Table 3.8). The number of disc uses and searches per month at Columbia is shown in Figure 3.1 and Appendix E.

Over the ten months of Cambridge MEDLINE use in the Columbia Health Sciences Library, a total of 3,190 disc accesses or 1,772 searches were performed. Monthly figures (after the first month) ranged from 133 in December 1987 to 252 in March 1988, and there is a slight trend upward as well as the expected seasonal variation. Since the Cambridge system is made available for 236 one-hour time slots per month, the average utilization of 177 searches per month is about 75 percent of the available time.

The volume of searching of Cambridge MEDLINE at Washington was nearly twice as high as that of Columbia. During the same ten months period of August 1987 - May 1988, registration sheets indicate a total of 3,459 registered users performed searches at Washington. Monthly figures ranged from 104 in September 1987 to 584 in February 1988 with a significant upward trend. Until 15 September 1987, the Compact Cambridge system was made available for only an average of 320 half-hour time slots per month, when it was more than doubled (at user demand) to 656 half-hour time slots, averaging out to 597 slots per month for the ten month study. The average utilization of 346 searches per month is thus about 58 per cent of the available time.

Survey results reported here describe these searches in greater detail, focussing primarily on the individual users and their response to Cambridge

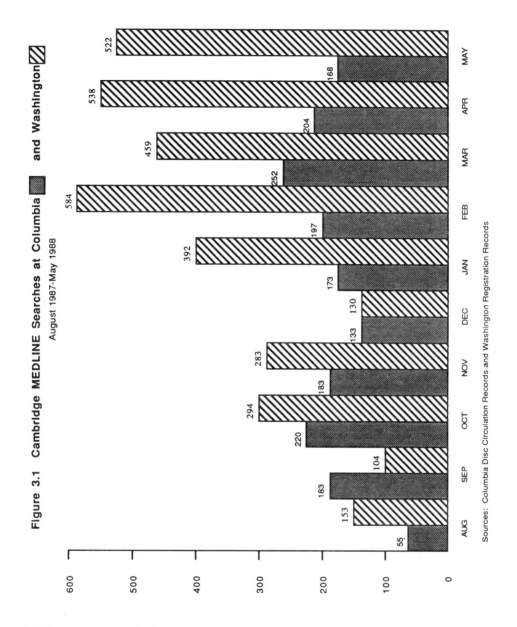

Figure 3.1 Cambridge MEDLINE Searches at Columbia and Washington

August 1987-May 1988

Sources: Columbia Disc Circulation Records and Washington Registration Records

MEDLINE. Sections below present survey results in terms of the key questions we attempted to answer.

3.1 Who Uses Cambridge? Are They New Users of Online Systems?

Table 3.1 looks at the affiliations of Cambridge MEDLINE users and the overall user population of both the University of Washington and Columbia

University. In both institutions, Medicine and Nursing make up a high proportion of the Cambridge user group, with Dentistry and the institutional hospitals accounting for a relatively small percentage of users. The School of

Table 3.1 Affiliations and the Overall User Population[2] of Cambridge MEDLINE Users[1] at Washington and Columbia

University of Washington

Affiliation[3]	Users		Population	
	Number	Percent	Number	Percent
Medicine	32	31	1,727	35
Dentistry	2	2	360	7
Nursing	14	14	825	17
Public Health	5	5	592	12
Hospital	7	7	534	11
Subtotal	60	60	4,038	82
Total	103	—	4,903	—

Columbia University

Affiliation[3]	Users		Population	
	Number	Percent	Number	Percent
Medicine	63	24	1,939	47
Dentistry	7	3	398	10
Nursing	38	14	520	12
Public Health	52	20	412	10
Hospital	4	2	551	13
Subtotal	164	62	3,820	92
Total	266	—	4,164	—

Sources: [1]Online Questionnaire #1,2; Paper Questionnaire.

[2]1986-87 Annual Statistics of Medical School Libraries in the United States and Canada.

[3]Not all departments are listed.

Public Health at Columbia also provided a relatively high proportion of Cambridge MEDLINE users. In both institutions, these five affiliations accounted for less than two-thirds of all Cambridge MEDLINE users, with the remaining coming from both other departments at the Health Sciences Centers and from outside.

Comparing the affiliations of Cambridge MEDLINE users with those of the total user population of each institution, we see (again in Table 3.1) that for the most part users are drawn representatively from all departments. Again, as noted above, there is a higher proportion of users from outside the listed departments than would be expected. At Columbia, the Schools of Public Health and Nursing accounted for more Cambridge users than would be expected proportionately. This pattern is similar to that for library use in general, that is, Public Health and Nursing students tend to be heavier users of the library.

In addition to affiliation we also looked at the profession of Cambridge users (See Table 3.2). As with affiliation, the user could indicate that he or she had more than one professional role, and many did. The four most frequently reported professions were student, researcher, physician, and nurse, in that order. Proportions of users with respect to profession was quite similar at Columbia and Washington. The majority of users in the School of Nursing, the departmental site at Columbia, gave nurse and educator as their professions.

Some of our hypotheses about Cambridge MEDLINE use had to do specifically with whether or not the user was a student. Students, it was felt, would be more likely to be in the library, would be more likely to use this "free" service than would funded faculty members, and would probably have different

Table 3.2 Profession of Cambridge MEDLINE Users at Washington and Columbia

Profession[2]	University of Washington		Columbia University	
	Number	Percent	Number	Percent
Student	38	37	67	38
Researcher	25	24	48	27
Physician	22	21	30	17
Nurse	15	14	27	15
N	103	—	175	—

Source: [1]Online Questionnaire #1, 2, Paper Questionnaire.

[2]Not all professional categories are listed. Multiple responses were allowed.

purposes for searching. Overall, as indicated in Table 3.2, students made up about 38 percent of all Cambridge MEDLINE users. Since they account for at least 50 percent of the overall user population at both schools, there is no reason to believe that students were more likely to use Cambridge. (They are, however, more likely to use CLIO; students make up 65 percent of the CLIO user population.) Other data presented later in this report show some differences in searching behavior between students and other groups.

Another study hypothesis was that Cambridge MEDLINE would attract a new group of users, users without previous experience with online searching or perhaps even bibliographic searching in general. To investigate this, we asked a number of questions about prior experience with both printed and online bibliographic tools.

The picture that emerged was of a small but significant proportion of new searchers. As shown in Table 3.3, about 13 percent of all the users questioned had never used any of the printed versions of MEDLINE (e.g. *Index Medicus,* the *International Nursing Index,* the *Index to Dental Literature,* or the *Hospital Literature Index*), and most of these had not been involved with an online MEDLINE search either. Almost a quarter of the users in all had no prior exper-

Table 3.3 Prior Search Experience of Cambridge MEDLINE Users at Washington and Columbia

	Users	
Printed Index Experience:	Number	Percent
Yes	228	81
No	36	13
Don't Know/No Answer	14	5

	Users	
Online Search Experience:	Number	Percent
Yes-Own Search	127	46
Yes-Librarian Search	100	36
No	64	23
Don't Know/No Answer	16	6
N	278	—

Source: Online Questionnaire #1, Paper Questionnaire

ience with an online search. When Cambridge was placed conveniently within the offices of the School of Nursing at Columbia, it attracted even more users without previous online experience.

We observed a similar pattern when looking at users of CLIO MEDLINE, our locally mounted MEDLINE subset. Again we expected that some users would have had no prior experience with other forms of MEDLINE. Our hypothesis was confirmed; survey results from CLIO MEDLINE users indicate that 20 percent of that group had no prior experience with either printed or online versions of MEDLINE.

3.2 How Much Is Cambridge MEDLINE Used? How Much Bibliographic Searching Is Done in General?

There are two components to the question of how much bibliographic searching, in total and on Cambridge, is done. One aspect of this is the number of people at the institution who search and the second is how many searches they do. Combining these two components gives a good picture of the volume of searching at the institution. We hypothesize that with a new form of MEDLINE available in an institution both the number of people who search and the number of searches that they do will increase.

Over the period that the Cambridge MEDLINE experiment was carried out, only a small proportion of the user populations of Columbia and the University of Washington used the system. At Columbia, for example, the size of the user population is over 4,000. Using circulation records, we estimate that the total number of Cambridge users is 150 - 200 or 4 - 5 percent of the total population. Clearly there are a large number of other individuals who do bibliographic searching in some other form. At the same time, however, as pointed out above, Cambridge did attract some users (students and others alike) who had previously not done any bibliographic searching. CLIO MEDLINE, which also attracts people who have not used bibliographic search tools previously, is used by a larger proportion of the Columbia population.

We asked Cambridge users both a general question about the amount of bibliographic searching they do and also specifically about their level of use of Cambridge. During the first survey period, when the Cambridge system had been available about four months, users reported their total use to date as:

Number of Uses	Users
1	33%
2	18%
3-5	23%
6 +	23%

187

At this point, then, the average number of uses was about 4. Projecting to a full year, we estimate a total of about 10-12 Cambridge searches per user per year, on the average. This includes, however, a few very heavy users and many occasional users.

Data on the total amount of bibliographic searching by Cambridge users suggest that, on the average, members of this group conduct about 50 searches a year. From the above, some of these will be done on Cambridge, while others will be done using any of the many other MEDLINE sources. The most likely alternative seems to be *Index Medicus* ; at Columbia, CLIO MEDLINE is also increasingly used.

Our first survey results and feedback from the reference staff suggested that some of the Cambridge searches were new searches, that is, searches that would not have been done were the Cambridge system not available. When the users were asked, for example, what they would have done had Cambridge not been available on this particular occasion (See Table 3.4), 87 percent said that they would have done a printed index or online search but the remaining 13 percent gave other answers that included asking a friend, browsing in the stacks, and even "nothing". Browsing was a more frequently identified alternative for users in the School of Nursing.

From these results we infer that the availability of additional MEDLINE alternatives like Cambridge will result in more bibliographic searching. To confirm this for both Cambridge and our local CLIO MEDLINE, we asked users of both how the availability of the system they used would affect their future

Table 3.4 User Alternatives to Cambridge MEDLINE for Current Search

| | Users | |
Alternative	Number	Percent
Use a Printed Index	101	57
Use an Online Search	53	30
Ask a Reference Librarian	37	21
Ask a Friend or Colleague	6	3
Browse Through the Stacks	25	14
Nothing	11	6
Other	9	5
N	177	—

Source: Online Questionnaire #1, Paper Questionnaire

searching for references to bibliographic journal articles. The response was clear - 80 percent of Cambridge users and 90 percent of CLIO MEDLINE users expected to search more frequently in the future. Among CLIO MEDLINE searchers, students are more likely than others to project more searching in the future.

3.3 Why Do Users Select Cambridge? What Other Information Sources Might They Use Instead?

Individuals at the test sites generally have access to a number of MEDLINE alternatives, including not only Cambridge but also printed indexes, librarian-mediated online searching, and direct online searching. Those who select Cambridge do so within the context of these other sources, at least those other sources with which they are familiar.

We asked Cambridge users both what source they would have used had Cambridge not been available and also what source they planned to use next time. Responses to the former were presented in Table 3.4; Table 3.5 shows users' future plans. In this context the choice of 83 percent of the users was to conduct their next search on Cambridge. About equal numbers planned to use printed indexes or to conduct an online search. We also learned here, as we did in other parts of our surveys, that some users would use several bibliographic sources in conducting their next search.

What are the features of Cambridge that caused users to select it? Responses to our first online survey suggested that there are a number of factors that are considered in making that choice, and that the decision is the result of some weighing of such factors as the cost of searching, the location of the source, how easy the source is to search, and the composition of the available MEDLINE file. In our second online survey we asked users to rank these four factors in terms of importance, obtaining the results shown in Figure 3.2.

Table 3.5 Intended Source for Next MEDLINE Search by Washington and Columbia Cambridge Users

Source	Number	Percent
Cambridge MEDLINE	230	83
Printed Index	34	12
Online Search	43	15
Another Source	24	9
N	278	—

Source: Online Questionnaire #1, Paper Questionnaire.

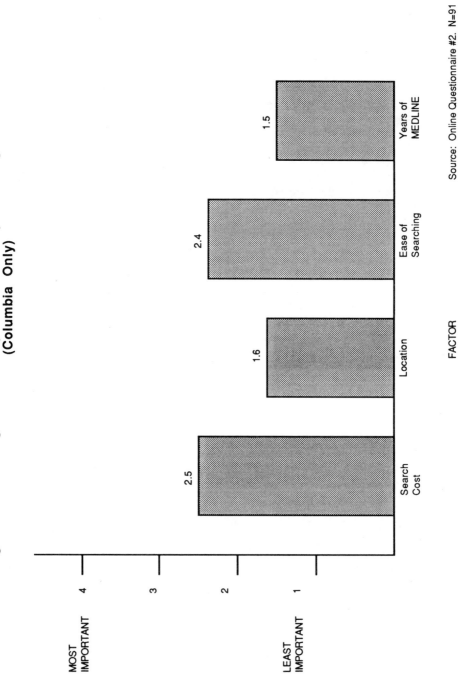

Figure 3.2   Ranking of Search System Factors by Cambridge MEDLINE Users
(Columbia Only)

Source: Online Questionnaire #2. N=91

190

As indicated, users rank cost and ease of searching as more important than the other two factors and about equal to each other. The location of the source and the number of years of MEDLINE references were also ranked about equally. We were surprised to find that students and non-students gave very similar rankings, in particular that non-students are as concerned as students about search costs. Interestingly, users with previous experience searching MEDLINE were more concerned with costs than new users of MEDLINE.

It is important to remember that these rankings were made by people who chose to use Cambridge. In this context, it seems reasonable that people who choose to use a free system consider cost to be an important factor. The high ranking that users give to ease of use seems to suggest that they find Cambridge relatively easy to use.

3.4 What Types of Questions Prompted Cambridge Use? Did the Users Find What They Were Looking For?

It will not come as a surprise to those who study bibliographic systems that the most frequent type of search of Cambridge MEDLINE was a subject search. This was the case for over 80 percent of all searches, sometimes in combination with other types of searches. About 20 percent of searches involved looking for a known author, and another 20 percent a known subject. Only 8 percent of searches overall involved a particular journal title.

Another aspect of a search that helps to characterize it is the way in which the information will be used. Table 3.6 shows the reported purposes for

Table 3.6 Purpose of Cambridge MEDLINE Search for Washington and Columbia Users

| | Searches | |
Purpose	Number	Percent
Patient Care	47	17
Paper or Report	85	31
Research Project	139	50
Keeping Current	42	15
Checking a Reference	18	6
Teaching/Planning a Course	21	8
Just Curious	15	5
Other	17	6
N	278	—

Source: Online Questionnaire #1, Paper Questionnaire

searching Cambridge MEDLINE, with some users reporting more than one purpose. As shown, half of the searches were for a research project and nearly a third were for a paper or report. More general purposes, such as keeping current and teaching or planning a course, were less often reported. Patient care was reported as the purpose for searching by 13 percent of the searchers; this figure reflects at least some use by the hospitals served by Columbia and Washington. In the School of Nursing departmental site, users reported a greater proportion of course planning searches and about the same proportion of patient care searches.

Users were asked directly whether or not they found what they were looking for. As shown in Figure 3.3, more than a third found what they were looking for and an additional 46 percent found some of what they needed. Six percent of searchers experienced the mixed blessing of finding more than they needed,

Figure 3.3 Cambridge MEDLINE Search Success at Washington and Columbia

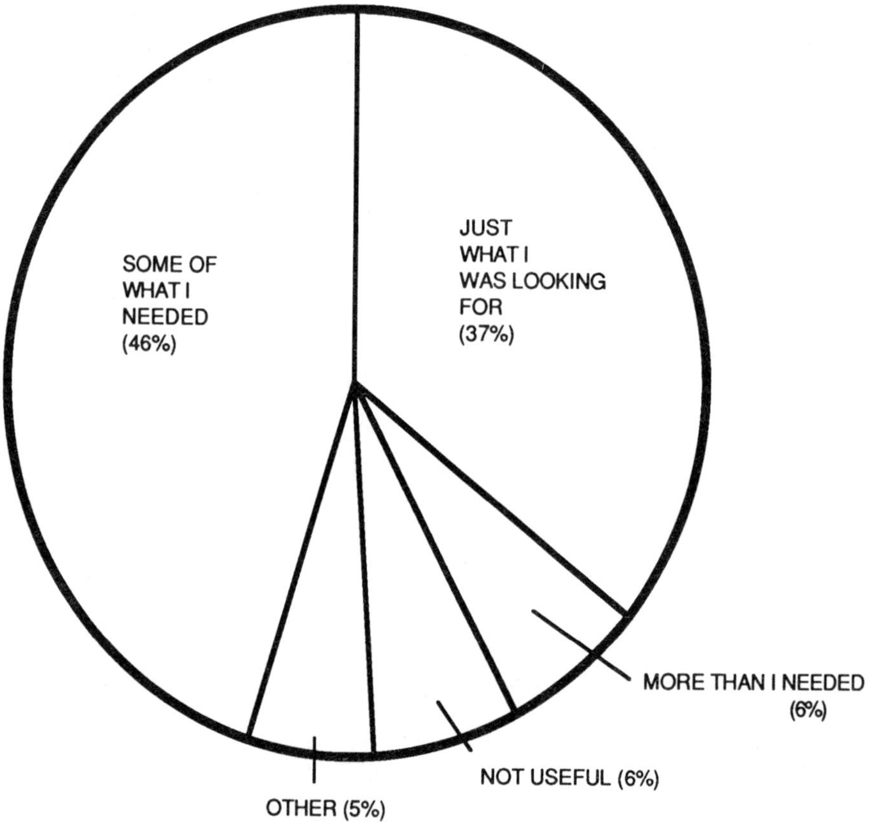

SOME OF
WHAT I
NEEDED
(46%)

JUST
WHAT I
WAS LOOKING
FOR
(37%)

MORE THAN I NEEDED
(6%)

NOT USEFUL (6%)

OTHER (5%)

Source: Online Questionnaire #1, Paper Questionnaire. N=278.

and only 6 percent found the search results not useful. The major area for concern here seems to be the nearly half of the searchers who found only some of what they needed. An even greater proportion of searchers in the School of Nursing site found only some of what they needed.

3.5 How Easy to Use Is Cambridge MEDLINE? How Do Users Compare It With Other MEDLINE Sources?

Our surveys took two different approaches to this question. We first asked users their opinions about specific features of the Cambridge system that we felt might be barriers to its successful use. This gave us a sense of the reaction to Cambridge as compared with similar, i.e., other compact disc, systems. We also asked users to compare Cambridge with other MEDLINE alternatives, including printed indexes and online searching. Since ease of use was found to be an important criterion in selecting a system, the comparative data give us at least some indication of the comparative ease of searching.

Questions about specific features of Cambridge involved a scale going from 1 for strongly agree to 5 for strongly disagree. Average ratings given by users were as follows:

Statement	Rating
Changing Cambridge MEDLINE discs is easy.	2.0
The rate at which the computer responds is satisfactory.	2.0
Instructions on Cambridge MEDLINE's screens were sufficient for my use.	2.2
The Cambridge manual helped me to use the system.	2.7

On the same scale, users gave an average rating of 1.9 to the statement "Overall, I found Cambridge MEDLINE easy to use."

These results are quite positive given that the questions addressed what were felt to be particularly negative features of the early Cambridge system. Feedback was provided to Cambridge and the manual, the feature that drew the most negative response, has since been considerably improved. Screen instructions, disc change procedures, and the response time have also been improved since these survey results were gathered.

On the general question of ease of use, Cambridge users were even more positive than they were about the particular features and generally agreed with the statement that the system is easy to use. When these ratings were calculated for different subgroups of users, we found that higher rankings were given by users who were successful and by users who had prior experience with other forms of MEDLINE. Ratings on the overall ease of use did not vary, however, with the type of search that was being performed or with the number of CD searches that a user had previously done.

To determine how users compare Cambridge MEDLINE with other sources of MEDLINE records, we asked those who have used other sources which they prefer. As indicated in Section 3.1, over 80 percent of the users of Cambridge have previously used printed indexes, 46 percent have done their own online searches, and 36 percent have obtained online searches from the library. Table 3.7 shows the preferences of each of these three groups.

Printed index users were asked which alternative they found easier to use, and nearly half of this group expressed a preference for Cambridge by indicating that they found printed indexes harder to use. About a third said that printed indexes are easier to use, and the remainder found the two comparable in terms of ease of use.

The question asked of users of online systems concerned which approach they preferred - Cambridge, their own online search, or an online search performed by the library. As indicated in Table 3.7, about half of those who have done their own online searches prefer this approach, and only 4 percent prefer Cambridge. Among those who have obtained librarian-mediated searches, about a third prefer this approach and about a quarter prefer Cambridge. Cambridge was preferred more often over library-mediated searches by the users in the School of Nursing with their own local CD station.

It is interesting to compare these data with those of Table 3.5, which show that 83 percent of Cambridge users intend to do their next MEDLINE search on Cambridge. Perhaps the implication is that users do not always follow the path that they prefer; other factors such as cost or convenience may intervene. It is also likely that, while 83 percent of users expect to use Cambridge next time, a smaller proportion actually do so.

Combining the results of these questions about preference, there is a suggestion that users who have experience with the variety of MEDLINE sources would generally rank them in this order (from most to least preferred): conduct an online search directly, search Cambridge MEDLINE, obtain an online search from the library, and use a printed index. There are, however, many individual exceptions to this ranking and many individuals who are not aware of all of the alternatives. More importantly, our observation of MEDLINE users suggests that users do not in fact select a single MEDLINE alternative for all searches but make their selection for each search depending upon the question and the circumstances.

3.6 What Is An Appropriate Content Mix?

The various compact disc systems and other MEDLINE alternatives provide different portions, or subsets, of the MEDLINE database. Subsets can be formed by using selective bibliographic elements, by using selective journal titles, or by limiting the time span covered. The rationale for limiting coverage is the restriction of storage space and costs - in the case of a compact disc,

Table 3.7 MEDLINE System Preferences of Washington and Columbia Cambridge MEDLINE Users

User Group: Printed Indexes

Preference	Number	Percent
Print easier	73	32
Print harder	111	49
Print and Cambridge about the same	29	13
Other	15	7
	228[1]	100

User Group: Own Online Search

Preference	Number	Percent
Prefer own search	62	49
Prefer librarian search	34	27
Prefer Cambridge search	6	4
Don't know/No answer	25	20
	127[1]	100

User Group: Librarian Online Search

Preference	Number	Percent
Prefer own search	19	19
Prefer librarian search	33	33
Prefer Cambridge search	24	24
Don't know/No answer	24	24
	100[1]	100

Source: Online Questionnaire #1, Paper Questionnaire

[1]Includes only users of the MEDLINE alternative indicated.

approximately one year of full bibliographic records for all MEDLINE titles requires one disc for storage.

Cambridge MEDLINE provides virtually the full MEDLINE record, including abstract. Users indicate that abstracts are useful in at least two ways; in screening citations prior to obtaining full text and, in some cases, as sources of the actual information that is needed. Some users have indicated that other fields in the record are not really necessary to them, particularly in the printed record.

Other subsets are selective in terms of journal titles, covering, for example, only English language titles or only titles held by the library. Cambridge MEDLINE includes all MEDLINE titles. This was felt to be particularly appropriate at Columbia and Washington, both libraries of which subscribe to a large proportion of the MEDLINE titles because of their large research populations.

As indicated, Cambridge MEDLINE uses one disc for each year of MEDLINE records. The first disc provided to the test sites was a 1987 disc, followed over a period of some months by 1986- 1982 discs. Columbia received an initial 1988 disc in June 1988 and Washington received theirs in May 1988. Updates to the current disc are provided quarterly.

Until the software release received in September 1988, when a user wished to search more than one year's records, he or she had to exit the system, remove the current disc, insert a new disc, restart the system, and rerun the search. At Columbia (and initially at Washington) this process was lengthened by the requirement that the user return the used disc to the reference desk and check out a new disc. It seems, under these circumstances, that the user who persevered and searched more than one year had a strong need for a multiple year search.

We analyzed the individual searches performed at Columbia in December and January to determine how often searchers were using multiple disks. During this period, four discs, covering 1984 - 1987, were available to searchers. Our results, which are shown in Table 3.8, indicate that almost half of all searches

Table 3.8. Cambridge CD-ROM Searches & Disc Use Dec. 1987 - Jan. 1988 (Columbia University Library)

Number of Searches   175

Discs Used	Number of Searches	Proportion of Searches
1	86	49%
2	52	30%
3	18	10%
4	19	11%

Average Number of Discs Used   1.8

Total Disc Uses   320

Source: Online Questionnaire #1

involved only one disc, i.e. one year. An additional 30 percent of searches involved two discs, 10 percent used three discs, and 11 percent used four discs. Nearly all cases of multiple disc use were of the most recent years. The implications of these data are that a two year file would have been sufficient for about 80 percent of the searches and a three year file would have met 90 percent of the needs.

At Washington, all discs have been available at the work station since January 1988. This was done to minimize difficulties in performing a multi-year search. Observation suggests that users generally search one or two discs, but this may in part be due to the short time slots (1/2 hour) allowed for searching Cambridge at Washington.

In addition to observing their behavior, Cambridge MEDLINE users were also asked their opinion about the time span covered by Cambridge. Measured on a 1 to 5 (strongly agree to strongly disagree) scale, the average user ranking of 1.9 indicates general satisfaction with the Cambridge time span. Given the evidence that many of them use a limited number of years, however, there may be a small marginal return for providing extensive backfiles.

3.7 Overall, Do Users Find Cambridge MEDLINE a Satisfactory Tool for Doing Their Own Searches?

Generally, Cambridge MEDLINE users do find the system a satisfactory tool for doing their own searches. Evidence of this, presented in earlier sections, includes the following:

- 83% of Cambridge users will use the system again for their next search;
- the average rating of Cambridge users indicates that they find the system easy to use.

In addition, nearly 80 percent of Cambridge MEDLINE users (and an even greater proportion of student users) indicated that they plan to use Cambridge MEDLINE regularly in the future.

These findings, however, should not be taken to suggest that Cambridge users will use only Cambridge. Most people at Columbia, for example, who use both Cambridge and CLIO, indicate that they will continue to use both. We believe that this can be generalized; that users will choose from the variety of systems that they know on the basis of the characteristics of the systems, system availability, and the nature of each particular question. What is perhaps more important, as documented by survey findings, is that awareness of the capabilities of Cambridge makes it more likely that users will formulate questions that Cambridge can be used to answer.

3.8 What Library Management Issues Arise in the Provision of Cambridge MEDLINE?

The effects of Cambridge MEDLINE (and other compact disc-based bibliographic information systems) on library management can be grouped into three general categories:

1. Budgetary issues

Although CD MEDLINE systems are bargains in their provision of bibliographic database searching for a fixed fee rather than on a pay-by-use basis, their expense can be significant. A library must first find money for equipment on which to install a system, and then must consider whether monetary resources are available to maintain an ongoing subscription to the system. Supplies such as printer ribbons and paper are also expenses to be taken into account. At the Columbia University Health Sciences Library's Cambridge workstation, for example, a box of 2,500 sheets of fan-fold computer paper can be consumed each month during high-use periods. Other costs are those associated with equipment maintenance and security.

2. Installation and maintenance issues

After deciding to install Cambridge MEDLINE, space must be found with electrical outlets and room for tables and chairs. Depending on the institutional environment, security may be a problem. Equipment may need to be bolted or cabled down, and discs may need to be kept in a secure area. The best locations for these systems are in areas of high visibility but which are out of direct traffic paths so users can concentrate on their work. The closer the system is to an information point the more likely the user will be to ask for help.

The procedures involved in initial system configuration and setup are theoretically simple, so that it should usually only take a few hours to install boards, assemble machinery, and load software. Problems occasionally arise, though, and efforts to resolve them can be extremely time-consuming. Initial installation of Cambridge MEDLINE at Columbia took several weeks.

Daily operation is also, theoretically, quite simple. The difficulties that arise stem from user inexperience or experimentation (when files are erased that shouldn't be, for example, or when a CD is inserted into a 5 1/4 inch floppy disk drive), heavy system use (compact discs can become smudged or scratched, disc player doors can break), and general equipment annoyances (such as loose cables and paper jams). Down time due to delays in delivery of supplies or repair of equipment can also be a problem.

3. Staffing Issues

Compact disc information systems in libraries bring changes to library staff workload. Mediated searches can be expected to decrease somewhat at sites where free CD systems are available. This trend is discussed further in Section 3.9.

While the availability of MEDLINE on CD has contributed, in part, to a decreased level of mediated searching at both the University of Washington and Columbia University, it is also partially responsible for a significant increase in reference desk traffic. Once again, because of counting differences, statistics should not be compared between institutions.

	Oct-Dec 1986	Oct-Dec 1987	% Increase
In-person reference and informational questions—			
University of Washington	6,802	7,153	5%
Columbia University	4,814	5,413	11%

Columbia University experienced an even greater change during January through March 1988, when a total of 5,960 reference and informational questions were answered, an increase of 51 percent over the volume of 3,935 during the same three months of 1987. Similarly, Washington's rate of questions increased by 13 percent the first quarter of 1988.

In both libraries, other end-user systems have been put in place as described earlier, so not all the increased activity at reference and information desks can be attributed to Cambridge MEDLINE. It has, however, been an important contributing factor.

In order to encourage use of CD systems, library staff can distribute publicity and conduct instructional sessions. Publicity must at present be designed in-house since little is supplied by CD vendors. Course development is very time-consuming. Although publicity and teaching can have severe impacts on staff workload, great benefits in public relations and user response can be realized. Both Columbia and Washington provide demonstration/training sessions for Cambridge MEDLINE to encourage use and reduce individual requests for assistance.

3.9 What Is the Impact of "Free" MEDLINE Use?

During the test period, the test libraries offered their patrons free use of the Cambridge MEDLINE system. At Columbia, CLIO MEDLINE is also made available without direct charge to the user. We were particularly interested in finding out how important cost was to users, and what effect the free availability of these MEDLINE sources had on other MEDLINE use.

We have already indicated (Section 3.3) that users reported the cost of searching as the most important factor in selecting a MEDLINE source. This is further confirmed by their response when asked specifically about the importance of cost in their decision to use Cambridge. These results were:

Level of Importance	Proportion of Users
very important	67%
somewhat important	13%
relatively unimportant	9%
other/no response	11%.

These data suggest that users have a strong preference for a "free" system over a system requiring out-of-pocket expenditures, but do not necessarily imply that with a free system there will be less use of alternatives that do cost money. An alternative hypothesis is that the free search systems are used to do searches that would not otherwise be done, and that even with the introduction of a free system in an institution the level of online searching will remain the same.

This is a difficult hypothesis to test, particularly because online statistics for an institution must be drawn from a number of sources. We did, however, look at two measures of online searching: the number of mediated searches conducted by the library and the estimated number of online searches conducted throughout the institution.

When looking at the number of mediated searches, statistics should not be compared between libraries because each institution counts its searches differently. However, both Columbia and Washington statistics, analyzed separately, show some decreases in the number of mediated searches during the test period. At the University of Washington, terminal use statistics of 283 MEDLINE searches for October through December 1986 and 275 for the same months of 1987 reveal a very slight decrease. At Columbia, paid mediated search counts (MEDLINE and other databases) were 333 for October through December 1986 and 268 for the same months of 1987, a decrease of 20 percent. These decreases can be accounted for in part by the availability of "free" MEDLINE searches but also by increases in the volume of searching done outside the library. Indications at both sites are that the complexity of mediated searches (as reflected in the search lengths) has increased as the number of searches has decreased.

At Columbia, we estimate that library-mediated searches make up about five percent or less of all the online searching that is done. Other searching is done through a large number of departmental and individual accounts with various vendors. By tracking some of the other major accounts, we have identified a pattern of continual increases in the level of online searching over the past few years, with no significant change in this pattern since the introduction of Cambridge MEDLINE and CLIO MEDLINE. Basically this says that searching outside the library is on the increase and is not affected by new in-library systems.

3.10   What Impact Will CD-ROM Systems Have on Library Services in the Future?

Up to this point in our analysis we have talked mainly about the effects of one specific CD-ROM system, Cambridge MEDLINE, on the users of the test site libraries. At this point, as we speculate about future use of MEDLINE alternatives, we must necessarily go beyond that specific system and try to visualize what will happen with the general availability of CD-ROM systems. We presume in this analysis that the library would choose the best CD-ROM system or systems available to it, just as it would also make choices among the various other types of MEDLINE sources.

What we conclude from the data presented in this report is that, from the user point of view, CD-ROM versions of MEDLINE such as Cambridge MEDLINE are a viable alternative to other MEDLINE sources. We have indications that the addition of a new and reasonable MEDLINE source to the array available to users will be used by some people for some questions, and that the availability of such a source is likely to result in increases in the number of bibliographic searches performed. To illustrate our point with specific numbers, consider the scenarios we at Columbia have developed to evaluate our future alternatives.

We began by identifying four configurations of MEDLINE that we might reasonably provide at Columbia. These four configurations and their estimated levels of demand are shown in Table 3.9.

- The remote configuration would have all MEDLINE access via remote hosts such as NLM, BRS, etc. There would be no local MEDLINE. Based on Columbia's recent levels of vendor searching, we predict an annual use level of 10,000 searches.

- The remote + CD configuration would retain vendor searching and add four CD stations distributed around the campus, including one in the library. We predict that this widespread availability of CD would cause a small drop in the volume of remote accesses. The figure of 8,000 searches for the CD systems is based on current usage of the Cambridge CD. Our predicted annual total is 16,000.

Table 3.9 Estimates of MEDLINE Use

Type of use	REMOTE	REMOTE+CDS	REMOTE+CLIO	REMOTE+CLIO2
Remote	10,000	8,000	10,000	2,000
Local (in library)	------	------	8,000	6,000
Local (other locations)	------	------	------	20,000
CD	------	8,000	------	------
TOTAL	10,000	16,000	18,000	28,000

- With the <u>remote + CLIO</u> configuration, CLIO MEDLINE, the locally mounted subset, would continue to be provided at no cost to users. Remote vendor searching would also continue. As was the case when it was originally introduced at Columbia, CLIO MEDLINE would only be available in the library. We predict, based on current CLIO MEDLINE use, about 8,000 CLIO MEDLINE searches a year. We predict that remote vendor searches would remain at a level of 10,000 since users would prefer the convenience of continuing to search from their office. Total searches is thus 18,000.

- The <u>remote + CLIO2</u> configuration again retains remote vendor searching but adds campus-wide availability of the free local MEDLINE subset, CLIO MEDLINE. With this configuration, we would expect remote searching and in-library CLIO search levels to drop. Based on the experiences other libraries have had with their local MEDLINE systems, we predict a very high level of use of CLIO MEDLINE on the network. The total predicted use with this configuration is 28,000 searches per year.

One point of these scenarios, with their quite conservative estimates of demand, is that levels of use will vary significantly depending upon the alternative, or combination of alternatives, that is provided. To some extent any new and reasonable alternative will create some additional demand, but more importantly, new alternatives with significant advantages in terms of cost, availability, ease of searching, and/or file composition will increase the overall level of searching. This was the case when online services were first introduced, and all indications are that there will be continued expansion with compact disc systems.

To this point we have not addressed the economic issues, yet these clearly will have an impact on the role of compact disc systems in the future. There are two broad levels of economic issues here, with the first concerned with selecting the most cost-efficient system from among similar alternatives, for example, from among the various compact disc systems. At this level, system characteristics may be a more important consideration than cost.

Once likely alternatives are identified, however, the question becomes the most cost-effective combination of these alternatives. The cost structures associated with the various alternatives are very different, with compact disc systems having relatively high fixed costs and online searching having high per-search costs. Also varying among types of systems is the level of library or institutional support required, and the cost of this. Institutional levels of demand, and the associated cost estimates, will be highly specific to the institution. Library choices will depend upon these economic analyses and upon internal priorities that determine the level of bibliographic searching that the institution is willing to support. The end result, it seems likely, will be that compact disc systems will remain a part of the array of MEDLINE alternatives, thus adding to the levels of bibliographic searching that are done.

Section 4. Conclusions

The user response to Cambridge MEDLINE in the test site institutions was generally positive. Users appreciated having "free" access to MEDLINE in a convenient location, felt that the database was generally sufficient for their needs, and found the search system relatively easy to use. When comparing Cambridge with other MEDLINE sources available to them, they suggested that Cambridge was sufficiently attractive to be used again, probably in combination with these other alternatives.

Cambridge attracted some users who had not previously used other MEDLINE sources, either printed indexes or online vendor searching. Thus the availability of Cambridge resulted in a group of new bibliographic searchers. Users also reported that, with Cambridge, they would now be likely to do more searching. Thus we have indications that not only the number of people searching but also the number of searches each performed increased with Cambridge MEDLINE. The Cambridge system was used, however, by a relatively small percentage of the total medical center populations to which it was made available. Use was restricted not only by lack of awareness of the system but also because it is available at only one location and to only a single user at a time.

The provision of Cambridge MEDLINE without cost to the user was a significant factor in its use. Those who chose to use Cambridge were were very clear about the importance of free availability, and few would be willing to pay for use.

Users had questions about the Cambridge search system, and relied heavily upon library reference staff for assistance in answering these questions. The original user's manual provided with Cambridge was not very helpful; instructions on the screens were more so. Staff effort required to introduce patrons to the system, to answer user questions, and to provide system support were considerable.

Users responded positively to the Cambridge database, which contains all MEDLINE records, with abstracts, and goes back to 1982. Most felt that this time span was satisfactory. When actual use was monitored, there was relatively little use of the discs covering earlier years.

Some of our findings can be generalized to all compact disc systems. The advantages of compact disc versions of MEDLINE, in general, are in their ease of searching and in their local availability. Because an individual system will serve a relatively small user group, the selection of system can be tailored to the particular needs of that group. The disadvantages of compact disc are, at least to date, the relatively limited data that can be accessed at once and the inability to provide compact disc services over a network. Compact disc systems provide most of the search and database features of online systems. The user response suggests that compact disc systems will attract new users and increase the level of bibliographic searching within the institution.

**A. Cambridge Online Questionnaire #1
(Columbia University and
University of Washington Health Sciences Libraries)**

December 1987 - January 1988

n=120+103=223

Question	Columbia University Response averages	University of Washington Response averages
1. My primary affiliation is:		
a. Medicine	23%	31%
b. Dentistry	3%	2%
c. Nursing	4%	14%
d. Pharmacy	in other	in other
e. Public Health	17%	5%
f. Rehabilitation	in other	in other
g. Presbyterian Hospital (Columbia)/ University Hospital (Washington)	2%	7%
h. Harborview Medical Center		
i. Other	28%	31%
Physical Therapy	8%	
Psychiatric Institute	5%	

Enter ONE only--->

	Columbia University Response averages	University of Washington Response averages
2. My profession is:		
a. physician	15%	21%
b. nurse	7%	15%
c. dentist	2%	1%
d. other health care professional	7%	3%
e. educator	6%	5%
f. scientist/researcher	33%	24%
g. student	43%	37%
h. librarian	5%	6%
i. other	5%	7%

Enter ALL that apply--->

	Combined average
3. I was looking for articles:	
a. by an author	21%
b. under a title	17%
c. on a subject	79%
d. in a journal	8%
e. other	5%

Enter ALL that apply--->

4. I needed the information for:

a.	patient care	18%
b.	a paper or report	30%
c.	a research project	52%
d.	keeping current	13%
e.	to check a reference	6%
f.	teaching/planning a course	6%
g.	not needed, just curious	6%
h.	other	6%

    Enter ALL that apply--->

5. The information I found was:

a.	what I was looking for	36%
b.	more than I needed	6%
c.	some of what I needed	43%
d.	not useful	7%
e.	other	6%

    Enter ONE only--->

6. Have you used any of the printed publications produced from the MEDLINE system
    (e.g. *Index Medicus*, the *International Nursing Index*, the *Index to Dental
    Literature*, or the *Hospital Literature Index*)?

a.	yes	84%
b.	no	12%
c.	don't know	4%

    Enter ONE only--->

7. If yes, you've used printed versions, how do they compare to Cambridge
    MEDLINE?

a.	easier to use	31%
b.	harder to use	51%
c.	about the same to use	12%
d.	other	6%

    Enter ONE only--->

8. Have you used an online version of MEDLINE (either yourself or by having
    a librarian process a search for you)?

a.	yes, by myself	50%
b.	yes, librarian search	30%
c.	no	18%
d.	don't know	6%

    Enter ALL that apply--->

9. If yes, you've used online MEDLINE, which system do you prefer?

	own	librarian
a. online, own search	42%	18%
b. Cambridge MEDLINE	5%	15%
c. online, librarian search	30%	36%
d. don't know	21%	27%

Enter ONE only--->

10. If Cambridge MEDLINE had not been available today, what would you have done?

a. used a printed version	62%
b. used an online version	16%
c. asked a library staff member	18%
d. asked a friend or colleague	3%
e. browsed through the stacks	14%
f. nothing	6%
g. other	6%

Enter ALL that apply--->

11. Next time you need this sort of information, what will you do?

a. try Cambridge MEDLINE	84%
b. try a printed version	14%
c. try an online version	17%
d. try another source	11%

Enter ALL that apply--->

12. Cambridge MEDLINE is provided free of charge to library users. How important a consideration was this in your decision to use this system, instead of an online version of MEDLINE?

a. very important	70%
b. somewhat important	15%
c. relatively unimportant	8%
d. would not have used an online version of MEDLINE	3%

Enter ONE only--->

13. How often have you used Cambridge MEDLINE?

a. first time	33%
b. once before	18%
c. 3-5 times	23%
d. 6 or more times	23%

Enter ONE only--->

Appendix A-4

SCALE:

	1	2	3	4	5
	Strongly Agree	Agree	Neutral	Disagree	Strongly Disagree

14. Instructions on Cambridge MEDLINE screens were sufficient for my use.

   AVERAGE RESPONSE: 2.2

15. The rate at which the computer responds is satisfactory.

   AVERAGE RESPONSE: 2.0

16. The time span covered by Cambridge MEDLINE was sufficient for my needs.

   AVERAGE RESPONSE: 2.6

17. Overall, I found Cambridge MEDLINE easy to use.

   AVERAGE RESPONSE: 1.9

18. Changing Cambridge MEDLINE discs is easy.

   AVERAGE RESPONSE: 2.2

19. The Cambridge MEDLINE manual helped me to learn the system.

   AVERAGE RESPONSE: 2.7

B. Cambridge Online Questionnaire #2 (Columbia only)

April 1988

n=91

<u>Question</u>

Columbia
University
<u>Response averages</u>

1. What is your primary affiliation?

a.	Medicine	25%
b.	Dentistry	4%
c.	Nursing	10%
d.	Public Health	26%
e.	Occupational/Physical Therapy	2%
f.	Presbyterian Hospital	2%
g.	Psychiatric Institute	2%
h.	Other	27%

    Enter ONE only--->

2. Are you a student?

a.	yes	66%
b.	no	33%

    Enter ONE only--->

3. How often do you search for references to biomedical journal articles?

a.	daily	10%
b.	approximately once a week	41%
c.	approximately once a month	29%
d.	rarely	18%
e.	never	3%

    Enter ONE only--->

4. Do you plan to use Cambridge MEDLINE regularly?

a.	yes	78%
b.	no	10%
c.	don't know	12%

    Enter ONE only--->

5. How do expect that the availability of Cambridge MEDLINE will affect your searches for references to biomedical journal articles?

a.	plan to search more frequently	80%
b.	do not expect a change	14%
c.	other (please specify)	5%

    Enter ONE only--->

6. Which of these other MEDLINE sources do you use regularly?

a.	*Index Medicus*	60% (44% IM only, 16% w/ others)
b.	BRS Colleague	9%
c.	Dialog Medical Connection	1%
d.	PaperChase	3%
e.	Reference librarian conducting a MEDLINE search	12%
f.	none	21%
g.	other (please specify)	8%

Enter ALL that apply--->

7. How do you expect that the availability of Cambridge MEDLINE will affect your choice of sources for searching?

a.	will continue to use the same sources	27%
b.	will use the same sources PLUS Cambridge	58%
c.	will discontinue use of one or more sources	
	(please specify which)	5% (IM)
	NO RESPONSE	10%

Enter ONE only--->

8. Have you ever used CLIO MEDLINE?

a.	yes	69%
b.	no	26%

Enter ONE only--->

9. Which system do you prefer?

a.	Cambridge MEDLINE	82%
b.	CLIO MEDLINE	7%
c.	It depends (please explain)	12%

Enter ONE only--->

10. Various aspects of the different sources of MEDLINE my affect which you choose to use. Please rank the following factors in terms of their importance to you, starting with the most important:

a.	the cost of searching (1)	(192)
b.	the location of the source (3)	(118)
c.	how easy the source is to search (2)	(179)
d.	the number of years of MEDLINE references available (4)	(111)

Enter 4 or 5 letters, in order of preference--->

C. Paper Questionnaire,
Columbia University Health Sciences Library and School of Nursing
n=32+23=55

Question	Library Responses	School of Nursing Responses
1. My primary affiliation is: (Circle **one** only)		
a. Medicine	41%	--
b. Dentistry	--	--
c. Nursing	6%	96%
d. Public Health	22%	4%
e. Occupational/Physical Therapy	--	--
f. Presbyterian Hospital	--	--
g. Psychiatric Institute	13%	--
h. Other (please specify):	13%	--
2. My profession is: (Circle **all** that apply)		
a. physician	38%	--
b. nurse	3%	78%
c. dentist	--	--
d. other health care professional	3%	--
e. educator	--	52%
f. scientist/researcher	16%	13%
g. student	38%	17%
h. librarian	--	--
i. other (please specify):	6%	9%

Question	Library/School of Nursing Responses
3. I was looking for articles: (Circle **all** that apply)	
a. by an author	15%
b. under a title	22%
c. on a subject	87%
d. in a journal	5%
e. other (please explain):	--
4. I needed the information for: (Circle **all** that apply)	
a. patient care	13%
b. a paper or report	33%
c. a research project	42%
d. keeping current	24%
e. to check a reference	9%
f. teaching/planning a course	15%
g. not needed, just curious	4%
h. other (please explain):	7%

Question	Library/School of Nursing Responses

5. The information I found was:
(Circle **one** only)

a.	what I was looking for	42%
b.	more than I needed	7%
c.	some of what I needed	58%
d.	not useful	--
e.	other (please explain):	--

6. Have you used any of the printed
publications produced from the
MEDLINE system (e.g., **Index Medicus**,
the **International Nursing Index**,
the **Index to Dental Literature**,
or the **Hospital Literature Index**)?
(Circle **one** only)

a.	yes	82%
b.	no	16%
c.	don't know	2%

If yes, how do the printed versions
compare to **Cambridge MEDLINE**?
(Circle **one** only)

a.	easier to use	38%
b.	harder to use	38%
c.	about the same to use	16%
d.	other (please explain):	4%

7. Have you used an online version of
MEDLINE (either yourself or by
having a librarian process a search
for you?
(Circle **all** that apply)

a.	yes, by myself	27%
b.	yes, librarian search	60%
c.	no	41%
d.	don't know	4%

If yes, which system do you prefer?
(Circle **one** only)

a.	online, own search	34%
b.	**Cambridge MEDLINE**	32%
c.	online, librarian search	20%
d.	don't know	14%

Appendix C-3

<u>Question</u>	Library /School of Nursing <u>Responses</u>

8. If **Cambridge MEDLINE**
    had not been available, what
    would you have done?
    (Circle **all** that apply)

a.	used a printed version	45%
b.	used an online version	11%
c.	asked a library staff member	27%
d.	asked a friend or colleague	4%
e.	browsed through the stacks	15%
f.	nothing	7%
g.	other (please explain):	4%

9. **Cambridge MEDLINE** is provided
    free of charge to library users.
    How important a consideration
    was this in your decision today
    to use this system, instead of an
    online version of MEDLINE?
    (Circle **one** only)

a.	very important	56%
b.	somewhat important	13%
c.	relatively unimportant	4%
d.	would not have used an online version of MEDLINE	2%
	NO RESPONSE	22%

10. If you obtained results from using
    Cambridge MEDLINE, did you:
    (Circle **all** that apply)

a.	use printer	75%
b.	download results	2%
c.	copy needed information by hand	11%
d.	other (please explain):	--
	NO RESPONSE	13%

11. Next time you need this sort of
    information, what will you do?
    (Circle **all** that apply)

a.	try **Cambridge MEDLINE**	76%
b.	try a printed version	5%
c.	try an online version	11%
d.	try another source	--
e.	other (please explain):	--

12. Please check the appropriate spaces below:

	1 Strongly agree	2 Agree	3 Neither agree nor disagree	4 Disagree	5 Strongly disagree
Instructions on **Cambridge MEDLINE**'s screens were sufficient for my use.	____	____	____	____	____

Library/School of Nursing average: 2.4

The **Cambridge MEDLINE** manual helped me to use the system.	____	____	____	____	____

Library/School of Nursing average: 2.8

The rate at which the computer responds is satisfactory.	____	____	____	____	____

Library/School of Nursing average: 1.9

Changing **Cambridge MEDLINE** discs is easy.	____	____	____	____	____

Library/School of Nursing average: 1.7

To use **Cambridge MEDLINE**, I would be willing to pay $5 for half an hour.	____	____	____	____	____

Library/School of Nursing average: 3.6

The time span covered by **Cambridge MEDLINE** was sufficient for my needs.	____	____	____	____	____

Library/School of Nursing average: 2.6

Overall, I found **Cambridge MEDLINE** easy to use.	____	____	____	____	____

Library/School of Nursing average: 1.7

13. How much time did you spend working with this system? _____

Library/School of nursing average: 58 minutes

14. Comments:

Appendix D

D. CLIO MEDLINE Interviews

April 1988

		Yes	No
1.	What is your affiliation? Are you a student?	65%	35%
2.	Have you searched CLIO MEDLINE before?	74%	26%
3.	Did you find what you were looking for today?	90%	3%
4.	Do you plan to use CLIO MEDLINE again?	97%	3%

If yes, how often?   Daily: 6%   Weekly: 47%   Monthly: 29%   Other: 18%

5.   (If yes to 4) With CLIO MEDLINE available,
do you/will you search for journal article
references more frequently?   90%   10%

6.   Which of these other MEDLINE sources have you used regularly?
(If yes, will you continue to use it?)

	Have used	Will continue
Index Medicus (30% only IM)	71%	63%
BRS Colleague	7%	50%
Dialog Medical Connection	1%	---
PaperChase	3%	---
Reference librarian search	22%	50%
Cambridge CD-ROM	28%	100%
None	20%	

7.   (If user of Cambridge) Do you prefer CLIO or Cambridge? Why? (n=21)

CLIO	Cambridge	Both
5%	76%	19%

8.   Do you have any comments about CLIO MEDLINE?

Appendix E

E. Number of Cambridge Cd-ROM Disc Uses and Searches, August-December 1987

(Columbia University Library)

	Aug.	Sep.	Oct.	Nov.	Dec.	Jan.	Feb.	Mar.	Apr.	May
Discs Used										
1987	36	91	117	133	105	131	154	182	158	124
1986	33	139	132	99	76	83	87	98	81	63
1985	18	59	86	57	37	47	50	69	49	44
1984	12	41	62	41	26	31	27	47	31	26
1983						10	18	33	26	24
1982						9	18	25	23	22
Total Disc Uses	99	330	397	330	244	311	354	454	368	303
Estimated Searches	55	183	220	183	133	173	197	252	204	168

3190/10
/1.8=177

Source: Count of signout cards

215

DIALOG OnDisc
MEDLINE

AT THE NEW YORK ACADEMY OF MEDICINE

By *Claudia A. Perry*

New York Academy of Medicine
2 East 103rd Street
New York, New York 10029

* The author would like to acknowledge the assistance of Anjannette McCullough in compiling statistical data and preparing the appendices. The study would not have been possible without the cooperation of the professional staff of the Academy Library, particularly the CD-ROM Project Working Group: John Balkema, Richard Clare, Arthur Downing and Donald Potts.

DIALOG OnDisc MEDLINE
At The New York
Academy Of Medicine

DIALOG OnDisc MEDLINE has been available to staff and users of the New York Academy of Medicine (NYAM) Library since mid-April 1988 as part of the National Library of Medicine's (NLM) nationwide evaluation of MEDLINE CD-ROM products. Hardware, software and CD-ROM discs were provided by DIALOG Information Services, Inc. to be used in testing the system through September 1988. As part of the agreement to participate, the Academy adapted a generic questionnaire designed by the NLM for use in the evaluation process. Users of the system were required, insofar as was possible, to fill out the questionnaire each time a CD-ROM search session was conducted. The analysis which follows is based upon the questionnaire results, observations of system use from initial training of staff in March 1988 through mid-September 1988, and interviews with all staff working in public reference points who assisted Library users with DIALOG OnDisc.

CD-ROM Project Working Group

A five person working group was organized to coordinate the DIALOG OnDisc project. The group included department heads representing both technical and public services areas, most with a fairly strong background in microcomputers, and was chaired by the head of the Reference Department. The group adapted the generic questionnaire provided by NLM, discussed security and training issues and procedures, and decided on the location of the system for public access. A subset of the group set up the equipment, installed the software, and conducted training of other staff members. The coordination of the project by a group representing a cross-section of the Library staff did much to facilitate the acceptance of the system, while the varied experience of the members of the group was helpful in the anticipation of possible problems with the implementation process.

The Study Site

The New York Academy of Medicine (NYAM) Library is both a sizable research library and the only major medical library open to the public in the New York City Metropolitan area. Individuals with medical questions are referred to NYAM from the New York Public Library, as well as from many other public, school and academic libraries in the area. The Library is also an important resource for corporate users. It attracts a varied clientele, ranging from high school students doing term papers or concerned parents reading about the illness of a family member, to foreign visitors conducting research for publication in scholarly papers. Over two-thirds of Library reference queries originate with this varied public. Telephone questions outnumber in-person requests by nearly two to one, but on-site use is substantial. An average of 55 individuals requested materials from the Library's closed stacks each day in April 1988, the month DIALOG OnDisc was introduced to the public. This does not include on-site users able to meet their needs from materials located on open shelves in the reading room areas. Fellows of the Academy and clients who pay for subscriptions to the Library (Subscribers) are accorded priority service at the exhaustive level, while members of the general public are given guidance in using the Library but are expected to conduct their own research. Most research assistance provided for primary users is handled over the telephone and by mail or messenger, although a number of representatives of subscribing firms are regular users of the Library's mediated photocopy service as well. Mediated computerized literature searches are provided to all users for a fee, but searches from the general public must be submitted in writing rather than over the telephone, and may not be completed for several days. It was anticipated that the availability of MEDLINE on CD-ROM would be of particular benefit to these individuals.

The Library is an interesting mixture of the old and the new. An online public access catalog (OPAC) system provides rapid access to materials obtained since 1976, but users must wait for books to be retrieved from over fourteen floors of closed stacks, a time-consuming process many do not anticipate. Books are classed not only according to the familiar NLM or Library of Congress classification systems, but also the Academy's own classification scheme. Orienting a variety of users in such a setting can be a challenge.

Staff Training for the CD-ROM Evaluation Project

The public Reference Desk is staffed 36 hours per week (28 in summer) by professional staff from all departments in the Library. Reference staff are on call at other hours the Library is open. Professional staff vary in degree of experience with computer systems, and in familiarity with Medical Subject Headings (MeSH) and the conceptual aspects of online searching. Nearly all have attended training in the fundamentals of searching MEDLINE, but for many training has not been recent.

Orientation sessions were conducted by two members of the CD-ROM project working group. Groups of three or four staff were shown how to turn on each piece of equipment, call up the software, and select appropriate terms from an annotated *MeSH*. The trainer then demonstrated a sample search incorporating most basic functions, while the group followed along with individual copies of the search printed directly from sample screens. Venn diagrams were used selectively to illustrate Boolean logic, and to explain what a particular menu choice was accomplishing if this was unclear. Each staff member then took turns searching and printing, with assistance from the trainer, as needed. Interest expressed in the CD-ROM system was so substantial that after orientations for professional staff, demonstrations were arranged for support staff as well. The CD-ROM system was made available for staff to practice on their own for two weeks before being moved to the public area, and could be used by staff whenever it was free thereafter.

Written instructions for booting the system were posted at the Circulation and Reference Desks, and were included with the sample search displayed next to the computer. The DIALOG OnDisc manual was also located nearby, but was rarely used. Initially, the system was loaded only with the 1987 MEDLINE disc. The cumulated *Index Medicus (IM)* had not yet been received for that year, so use of DIALOG OnDisc was suggested to users as an alternative to poring through twelve monthly issues of *IM*. As more discs were received and staff grew more accustomed to using CD-ROM, additional training was provided to small groups or to individual staff members on how to change discs and restart the search process. Members of the project working group were available for one-on-one assistance with staff throughout the duration of the evaluation project, and were responsible for changing paper and checking ink cartridges on the printer as needed.

Problems with Staff Training

By June, nearly all professional staff assisting with reference desk coverage felt fairly comfortable with the basics of using the system and assisting Library users. Most had not used the more sophisticated features of the system, and sought assistance from a member of the project working group whenever there was some difficulty with hardware or software. A frequent software problem which resulted in a "Fatal Error" message when the most recent disc was changed caused some consternation among those who were less familiar with computers. (This problem was corrected with a later version of the search software.)

Professional staff varied in their reactions to the way in which training was handled. Half preferred to have had more detailed, individualized instruction, and expressed a need for a better manual as well as simple written guidelines to get one started, and then to lead the user to more sophisticated features. One stated that the training received was "terrible" and that it was awkward to have to try the system for the first time while others stood around watching. Others, generally those with more automation experience, believed that the best way to learn how to use the system was simply to practice on their own, and to ask for assistance from others when it was needed. Yet another staff member particularly enjoyed practicing with two other inexperienced colleagues. This individual regularly referred users to the sample search ("the blue typed instruction sheets"), and felt this had helped them (and himself) to get started.

Two professional staff suggested that a workbook might be a useful way to introduce different functions and system capabilities. Others felt they would not have read documentation even if better written materials had been available. While the DIALOG OnDisc manual was clearly inadequate, since it was designed for a completely different product (DIALOG OnDisc ERIC; the MEDLINE manual is still forthcoming), this writer can attest to the difficulty of developing easy-to-follow written instructions given the multiplicity of routes which can be taken from each menu. A member of the project working group suggested that the idea of menus and windows is still foreign to many users, particularly those used to communicating with computers by typing in commands. As the icono-graphic approach to computer software becomes more widespread, it is possible that many difficulties presently associated with training on this system will diminish.

Several members of the project working group felt that many training problems were related as much to a lack of computer literacy among the staff as to difficulties with use of DIALOG OnDisc itself. Individuals with a minimal exposure to online searching had more difficulty constructing search strategy and choosing the appropriate Medical Subject Heading (MeSH) than those who search MEDLINE regularly. Those who had never worked with microcomputers had difficulty remembering how to log on to the system or how to deal with a software or printer problem. One might therefore expect fewer problems training reference librarians whose responsibilities include online searching and microcomputer use than individuals who lack such experience. It should be emphasized that no matter what the levels of experience of the user population or the ease of use of a system, differences in individual learning preferences indicate the need to allow for flexibility and a variety of approaches to training. But despite occasional criticisms, nearly all staff interviewed agreed that the system is "really easy to learn", and were almost unanimous in their conviction that it would be great if DIALOG OnDisc became a permanent feature in the Library.

Publicity

DIALOG OnDisc MEDLINE was set up in the Library Lobby April 17, 1988, sandwiched between the Circulation Desk and a row of four Online Public Access Catalog terminals (OPACs), and in clear sight of the public Reference Desk. Availability of the system was announced in the Academy newsletter, which is mailed to all Fellows, in a Library newsletter distributed to Subscribers, other libraries, and selected others, and by a sign greeting all visitors as they entered the Library. Staff stationed at the Reference Desk and answering the Reference Department telephones selectively suggested to those seeking assistance that DIALOG OnDisc might help them to meet their information needs. For the first weeks after the system was introduced, colored handouts were left by the computer and alongside other Library guides describing the pilot project (Appendix A) and directions for use (Appendix B). Finally, Library users learned of the system by word of mouth, and by observing others using the CD-ROM.

Patron Training in the Use of DIALOG OnDisc

Library users were encouraged, though not required, to sign up in advance for half-hour search sessions. In practice, the half-hour limit was only enforced if others were waiting to use the system, and patrons would frequently remain at the CD-ROM station for several hours. Use of the system took some time to build, and initial use was not as heavy as expected.

Each user asking for assistance or observed using the system by a librarian at the reference desk was given a questionnaire attached to the one page "Directions for Use" sheet. This sheet specifically directed the user to start with the *Medical Subject Headings (MeSH),* since use of *MeSH* is already stressed in orienting patrons to the OPACs and *Index Medicus,* and the working group believed that better results would be obtained by working with established headings rather than simply key words. Users were requested to fill out a questionnaire after every search session, even if they had used the system previously.

The procedures used by staff assisting with reference desk coverage to orient CD-ROM users varied from reader to reader and from staff member to staff member. Nearly all librarians began by trying to identify an appropriate MeSH term with which to search. Many staff members encouraged the patron to use the keyboard from the very start, and provided verbal instructions on how to proceed, feeling that more effective learning takes place by doing than by observing. Others demonstrated a sample search, and then encouraged users to continue on their own. If it appeared that a patron needed just a few good references on a topic and was likely not to be a regular visitor to the Library, several librarians conducted a quick search for the patron, instructed them in displaying and printing citations, and left them to peruse the results at their leisure, in the belief that this was a more effective use of their time and the patron's time than trying to instruct the individual in the use of the system. This was particularly appropriate for those who were unfamiliar with library and computer use in general. The various approaches demonstrate some philosophical differences in the concept of reference service, as well as differences in the ways in which dissimilar library users may need to be handled in different settings. Appropriate orientation in an academic setting may be quite different than assistance in a public or special library. Within any institution it is increasingly likely that these issues will need to be discussed and clarified, so that the degree of assistance provided is not subject to mere chance.

Time spent with individual users ranged from less than five minutes to a case where one aggressive patron working with a particular staff member demanded well over an hour of attention. Efforts by certain patrons to monopolize staff, or attempts to pressure a librarian to conduct extensive searches for them, point up the need for an explicit policy, clearly understood by all staff working at this service point, as to the extent of instruction and assistance which can and should be provided, and under what circumstances. While such a policy is recommended in any reference setting, it is particularly important with a new technology, where patrons may feel anxious and may not understand what the system is providing them. Librarians commented that patrons frequently did not realize that citations corresponding to only one year of MEDLINE were available at one time. Many also did not understand that it was possible to switch discs, once this option was made available to users, despite the presence of a sign on the computer indicating which years were available and directing the user to ask a librarian if they needed to change discs. Questionnaire comments indicated occasional lack of understanding of the means to refine search results. It is thus important that staff provide sufficient assistance so that misunderstandings do not occur. At the same time, alleged lack of understanding can be used by patrons in attempts to monopolize a librarian or to avoid doing the actual work themselves. Clear guidelines could help less assertive staff to deal with such manipulative behavior.

Most librarians felt that the amount of time needed to orient users to the CD-ROM was only slightly more than that needed to teach individuals how to use *Index Medicus* or the OPAC, and that results were far better than if the patron had used a printed index. In some cases, the availability of DIALOG OnDisc was merely a convenience; in others, particularly when searching by keyword if a relevant MeSH heading was unavailable, information could not have been easily obtained in any other way. Despite occasional misunderstandings of what the system was capable of providing, most librarians felt that the availability of DIALOG OnDisc made it easier for them to assist patrons in meeting their needs.

Questionnaire Administration and Analysis

Questionnaires were distributed to all observed users of the CD-ROM system from the time when it was first made available to the public April 17 through the end of August 1988. The major analysis of responses was conducted on 122 completed questionnaires received by June 30. At that time, the Library had not advertised the availability of discs with earlier bibliographic data, so respondents were working only with the 1987 or 1988 MEDLINE disc. Discs containing citations for the years 1984 through 1986 were received from the vendor throughout the Spring, but were not made publicly available until June to give staff and users an opportunity to become familiar with the basic functioning of DIALOG OnDisc. Questionnaires received after June 30 were analyzed separately in order to examine the impact of the availability of a larger MEDLINE data set (1984-1988) on responses. Seasonal variations in the responses were also of interest since far fewer students use the Library during the summer months, and students are a large proportion of the Library's user population during the academic year. Most of the analysis which follows deals with the spring survey results. A separate section then compares the spring and summer survey responses.

Questionnaire Return Rate—Spring Survey

A total of 150 questionnaires were distributed during the survey period from April 17 - June 30. Fifty-four forms were handed out during the pretest phase and 96 following a minor revision of the questionnaire. Forty-three pretest questionnaires and 79 revised questionnaires were completed, or a total of 122 out of 150. This yielded a return rate of 81.33%. All returns were included in the final tally due to the relative similarity of the two versions. (Appendix C)

After examining initial returns in the context of observed behavior, the working group was concerned that individuals receiving a great deal of staff assistance were overestimating the degree to which they could have used the system without orientation from a librarian (see question II-6 in Appendix C). A question (I-14) was therefore added to indicate what was used to get started using the system (orientation with a librarian, help screen, or written instructions), in order to clarify the responses made in section II of the questionnaire. There was also some confusion as to whether respondents had really used the DIALOG OnDisc Manual. Staff had found it singularly unhelpful, yet 37% of initial respondents agreed or strongly agreed that the manual helped them to use the system (question II-3). When a question was added concerning reactions to the "blue typed instruction sheets" (question II-4), positive reactions to question II-3 fell to only 15% of new responses. Moreover, responses to the new question I-14 indicated that only 6 of 79 respondents (7.59%) had used the black bound manual, as compared to 17.72% of respondents who reported using the blue instruction sheets. It is thus likely that the positive reaction to the manual provided by the vendor is overstated by the questionnaire, and that some of these positive reactions may have referred to the instruction sheets developed in-house.

Following receipt of a questionnaire in which a high school student stated that his or her primary affiliation was medicine, two initial questions concerning affiliation/profession were collapsed into one for the revised questionnaire (and the presentation of results in Appendix C). The number of total responses varied from question to question because of these changes, and due to the fact that not all respondents answered all questions. Whenever possible, the number of actual responses to a question was used as the denominator in computing a percentage of responses in the analysis of results. In cases where more than one answer was permitted, the denominator used was the maximum number of possible responses (e.g. n=79 for question I-14).

While efforts were made to encourage all users to fill out a questionnaire, there were undoubtedly a fair number of individuals who tried the system without an appointment, who were not assisted or noticed by a librarian, and who did not receive a questionnaire. Librarians staffing the Reference Desk were asked to distribute a questionnaire and provide assistance, if needed, to all those using the system, or to suggest its use to patrons when appropriate. Nonetheless, at busy periods individuals could readily use the machine without receiving this attention. Interviews revealed that repeat users often did not realize that completion of a questionnaire was requested after each use. Thus, the survey may under-represent those who used the system numerous times. Others who failed to fill out a questionnaire may have used the CD-ROM only briefly and abandoned their efforts after a short time either because they were disinterested, frustrated, or intimidated. The CD-ROM system was located next to a row of Online Public Access Catalog terminals (OPACs), so some individuals may have been unsure of what the system really could do, confusing it with the OPAC terminals or viewing it as a public access microcomputer. (Some students, for example, inquired as to what games were available for the system.) Others appear to have tried the CD-ROM out of curiosity, while waiting for library materials to be retrieved from the stacks, or waiting for an available OPAC terminal.

Yet another group who may be under-represented by the survey are those who learned to use the system either without assistance, or with the assistance of another library patron, rather than a librarian. One staff member observed that CD-ROM users are far more likely to assist one another in the system's use than are OPAC users, perhaps because there is only one CD-ROM system, which all have to share. One might expect that individuals who did not receive or fill out questionnaires were therefore relatively comfortable with its use, not seriously interested in the system, or quite uncomfortable and unwilling to ask for help.

It should also be noted that the respondents to the questionnaire were to a large extent a self-selected group, who may be somewhat more likely to be computer-oriented than the average user of the Academy Library. OPAC terminals have been available in the Library for over 15 months, but the card catalog has not been closed and many patrons continue to use printed sources to check Library holdings. Staff used their own judgment in suggesting to patrons that they might wish to try the CD-ROM system, based on the nature of the patron's questions, their sense of the patron's capabilities, and the availability of the machine. While this may have encouraged use from some individuals who would not have tried the system on their own, other patrons flatly refused to use it, even though the CD-ROM might have saved them time. The fact that the Academy Library is the only sizable medical library open to the public in the Greater Metropolitan New York City area means that it attracts a varied clientele, some of whom have never used a research library, not to mention a computer. At the same time, the profile obtained of CD-ROM users did not differ greatly from an informal survey of Library users conducted in late 1983. While the categories and the methods of data collection and analysis of the two surveys are not strictly comparable, they do provide some basis for evaluating the representativeness of the response to the CD-ROM questionnaire.

In the discussion which follows, "CD-ROM users" will be used to refer to the 122 respondents to this questionnaire during the spring survey period. It is understood that this group may not be fully representative of the total CD-ROM user population in this setting, but as there does not appear to be systematic bias among nonrespondents, the survey results will be used in conjunction with observations by staff to present a portrait of CD-ROM use at this particular library.

Profile of CD-ROM User—Spring Survey

The largest single category of CD-ROM users were students, constituting 30% of those filling out questionnaires during the period from April through June (see question 1 of Appendix C). College students were the most numerous, followed by high school, graduate school and medical school students. Similarly, approximately 37% of weekend users and 23% of weekday users identified themselves as students in the 1983 survey.

When all health professionals were grouped together they totaled nearly 20% of CD-ROM respondents, with physicians approximately 8% of the user population. In 1983, health professionals constituted one quarter of Saturday users and nearly 9% of weekday users. Scientist/researchers and attorney/-paralegals numbered 18% and 13% respectively in the current survey, while over 25% of weekday users in 1983 were from the law field. The most obvious discrepancy between the two profiles is the relative absence of scientist/-researchers in the earlier period. Only about 4% of users in 1983 identified themselves as "medical researchers," and there was no category for scientists. Other users in the current study included educators (8%) and those involved in publishing (6.56%). Of the nearly 14% who did not fit any predefined category, respondents included several professional writers, a computer scientist, an actuary, a mechanical equipment manager, a mother, and an individual involved in corporate film and video (see Appendix D). Other health care professionals included a clinical psychologist, a medical anthropologist, a chiropractor and a health advocate.

Comparison with Requesters of Mediated Computer Searches

There were 174 mediated searches conducted for a fee during the survey period from April through June 1988. Over 70% of these searches were conducted for Academy Fellows and Subscribers to the Library, who are permitted to submit requests by telephone and who receive priority service. Appendix E presents data on the affiliations of requesters of mediated searches during this time. More than double the percentage of requests for mediated searches originated with physicians, as compared with CD-ROM searches conducted by physicians. This is not surprising given that Fellows, as primary clientele of the Library, are charged one-half the regular rate for computer searches, and receive priority service. A substantial number of requests for mediated searches were received from law firms and advertising firms, many of whom are Subcribers to the Library. No requests originated with students, who are likely to be on a limited budget, or to have access to less expensive search services through their schools. The percentage of requests for mediated searches from "others" is nearly the same as in the CD-ROM user profile (13%), but two-thirds of these fee-for-service requests came from commercial enterprises: several consultants, a chemical company, and an insurance company. Four requests for mediated searches appear to be from patients.

Clearly, corporate firms seem to need comprehensive mediated searches, and seem more willing to pay for them than they are interested in sending representatives to the Library to use a free CD-ROM system. Students, scientists, researchers, educators, nurses, dentists and librarians appear willing to spend time using a free CD-ROM system on their own rather than paying the costs of a mediated search. The relatively low number of responses by physicians to the CD-ROM questionnaire may reflect the tendency of most Fellows of the Academy to request their services by telephone, rather than by visiting the Library in person. The CD-ROM questionnaire did not inquire if a respondent was affiliated with the Library, so there is no way of determining if physicians using CD-ROM were Fellows or if they were unaffiliated users.

Willingness to Pay for CD-ROM Searches — Spring Survey

While one can hardly assume that all individuals expressing an opinion on the maximum charge they would be willing to pay for a CD-ROM search would, in fact, pay such a fee, it is still useful to note that over 70% were willing to pay something. Although only slightly more than 16% would pay more than $15.00, well over half the individuals responding to this question appeared willing to consider a charge of $5 to $10 reasonable. As stated previously, at the time most of the questionnaires were completed, the Library had not advertised the availability of discs with earlier bibliographic data, so respondents were working only with the 1987 or 1988 MEDLINE disc. The results from the summer survey, when discs were available for the years 1984 through 1988, are discussed below.

The Impact of the Availability of CD-ROM on Fee-based Search Requests

Over the last several years, the number of search requests at the Academy has been dropping, by 8% from 1986 to 1987, and by 18% from 1985 to 1986. The monthly average in the first half of 1988 was 60, as compared to 65 in 1987, and 74 in 1986. Given this trend, the slight decrease in the number of searches performed in April-June of 1988 (182 as compared to 200 in the same period in the previous year) did not appear to be unusual. It was therefore assumed that the availability of a CD-ROM system during that period was having little impact on the Academy's mediated search service.

An analysis of the distribution of requests from April 17 through June 30 presents a slightly different picture of one of the possible effects of the CD-ROM system. There were only slight decreases in the numbers of mediated searches conducted for Fellows of the Academy, and a 36% increase in numbers of searches performed for Subscribers to the Library. No searches were conducted for staff during this quarter, as compared to twenty-three for the same period during 1987. Demand for searches for staff members may have decreased in 1988 (there were only two searches conducted for staff in the first quarter of

1988, as compared to fifteen in 1987). It is also true that staff could easily use the CD-ROM system to meet their needs for information from MEDLINE, particularly at less hectic times of the day when the system was not in use by the public. Many commented that it was easy to use the CD-ROM to scan for the availability of information on a topic, to conduct a preliminary search before doing a full-fledged search online, or to find answers to questions of a personal concern. This may account in part for the reduction in the number of searches conducted for staff in 1988 as compared to previous periods. While using the system to practice or to answer work-related questions, staff did not fill out a questionnaire.

Reduction in the Number of Requests from the General Public

While the total number of requests for mediated searches in the second quarter of 1988 dropped by only 18 searches as compared to the previous year, there were eleven fewer requests from "others", or a drop of more than 25%. Nearly 20% of questionnaire respondents during the spring indicated they would have requested an online search or conducted their own online search if the CD-ROM system had been unavailable, but it is difficult to tell how many of these searches would have resulted in a request from the Academy's search service. Since nearly 35% of respondents report having conducted their own searches, it is likely that at least some of these individuals would have searched for themselves. Approximately 16% of those who reported having used online MEDLINE claimed to prefer conducting their own searches online. Nearly 42% preferred DIALOG OnDisc MEDLINE, while close to 13% preferred requesting a search from a librarian (see questions 7-9 in Appendix C). But for most individuals (55.74%), if a MEDLINE CD-ROM system had not been available, they would have relied instead on a printed source such as *Index Medicus*.

Purposes for Which Information Was Sought

When asked for what purposes they needed information, spring respondents were most likely to select a research project (41.8%) or a paper or report (31.15%). This corresponds well with the needs one might expect to be expressed by students and researchers, the two single largest groups in the spring survey population. Respondents were directed to circle all relevant responses, which may account for the choice of more than 17% who reported investigating a personal concern. It is likely that respondents may have searched more than one topic in a single session. Nearly 14% were conducting research for an employer, consistent with the presence of a sizable number of representatives from the fields of law and publishing.

As noted earlier the Academy is a closed stack library which, by its very nature, is better suited to the pace of scholarly research than to finding quick answers to clinical questions. It is hardly surprising that respondents reported that only 4% of CD-ROM use was concerned with patient care. It would appear that most physicians requiring clinical information meet their needs from a source other than the Academy Library.

Types of Searches and Success Rates—Spring Survey

The vast majority of respondents (95.08%) reported looking for articles on a subject. Author searches were conducted by slightly more than 16%, and title searches (presumably citation verifications) by only 10.66%. Almost 42% reported finding what they were looking for while 45% found some of what they sought. (Respondents to this question, I-4, were directed to choose all choices which applied.) Only 9% found no useful information. More than 12% were faced with more information than was needed, possibly indicating a problem of information overload. Some respondents appear not to have fully comprehended the capabilities of the system to refine search results. One commented that he or she was forced to review over 800 citations, a possible indication of lack of awareness of the ability to limit results by crossing with another concept.

A far more successful incident was recounted by a Fellow of the Academy, a self-described computer neophyte who nonetheless feels comfortable searching MEDLINE online using GRATEFUL MED. This physician had been unable to identify any relevant citations using GRATEFUL MED, but found 24 excellent references on his topic with DIALOG OnDisc MEDLINE. While hardly good news for proponents of GRATEFUL MED, this is an encouraging anecdote for beginning users of CD-ROM.

Experience Levels of Spring CD-ROM Users

Nearly one third of spring users were unfamiliar with the print counterparts to MEDLINE. Of the 61% who had previously used *Index Medicus* or a similar source, there was a nearly even split between those who felt the print indexes are easier to use (40.79%) and those who felt they are harder to use (45.74%). Nonetheless, nearly 75% of respondents were ready to try DIALOG OnDisc MEDLINE the next time they needed similar information, with another 17% willing to try CD-ROM, a print index, an online version of MEDLINE, as well as other sources (i.e. all choices listed).

As has been mentioned earlier, it is likely that patrons using DIALOG OnDisc multiple times did not always fill out a questionnaire. Data indicate that almost 83% of respondents were first time users, with only 13.67% of questionnaires being returned by those using the system three or more times. It may be more accurate to interpret the questionnaire results as an indicator of what most spring users thought on their initial experiences with the system than as a sign that few returned to use the system more than twice.

Interest in Retrospective Searching—Spring Users

Rather than present users with predefined time frames, the questionnaire included an open-ended query as to how far back individuals would be interested in searching. Of the 85 responses to question I-13 in the spring survey period, 44.7% specified five years, and an additional 17.64% indicated one to three years. Only four respondents were interested in searching back more than 30 years. It would seem that for most users, the present range of availability of MEDLINE on CD-ROM is adequate.

Ease of Use and System Problems—Spring Survey

Although only 20% of spring respondents indicated that they felt they would have been unable to use the system without the aid of a librarian, approximately three-quarters of those responding reported that they had received an orientation with a staff member. Librarians helping users felt that in numerous cases, no matter what the patron may have replied on the questionnaire, the individual would have had some difficulty using the system without any orientation. Written comments on the questionnaire also tended to stress the need for assistance (see Appendix H). Among particular problems was the occasional mistaken selection of the DIALOG search mode from the menu instead of the "Easy menu" choice. Users possessing no knowledge of DIALOG command structure were then unable to extricate themselves from this mode. Several librarians and users felt that better explanations were needed to steer neophytes away from this particular choice, even though written instructions clearly indicated that the user should select the "Easy Menu".

Some individuals found it confusing that after selecting a particular highlighted selection, the item was no longer highlighted. Others appeared not to grasp the conceptual aspects of Boolean logic. In some people's view, the biggest system problem was the inability to save search strategy from one disc to another. There were numerous complaints about the speed of the printer (a Hewlett Packard Thinkjet), although some admitted grudgingly that at least it was quiet.

Despite these criticisms, over 80% of spring respondents found the system easy to use overall, and nearly 85% considered the response rate satisfactory. Users were particularly delighted with the availability of abstracts, and staff considered the presence of the system a good public relations tool, which often made it easier to assist patrons. Despite minor reservations by two librarians interviewed, all professional staff working with the system considered it important for the Library to consider one or more CD-ROM installations on a permanent basis, and most were enthusiastic about such a prospect.

Comparison of Spring and Summer Survey Results

As anticipated, the summer user group included far fewer students, but also a much lower proportion of scientist/researchers (4.41% as compared to 18.03%

in the spring). Proportions of corporate representatives (29%, including attorneys), physicians (13.24%) and "others" increased in summer (see Appendix C-G). More respondents identified themselves as a relative of a patient than in the earlier period. Not surprisingly, given this shift in the user group, more users reported that they needed information for patient care (10.29%) or a personal concern (25%) and fewer for a paper or report (17.65%, down from 31.15% in the spring). A slightly higher proportion (45% as compared to 41%) indicated during the summer that information was needed for a research project, which may reflect the needs of corporate users.

With a larger data set available (1984-1988), respondents were more likely to report that they found what they were looking for (57% as compared to 41.8% in spring) and less likely to indicate that what they found was not useful (2.94% in summer, 9% in spring). More summer users thought that the printed indexes were harder to use than DIALOG OnDisc MEDLINE (56.09%, compared with 44.7%) and more (82.35% compared to 74.59%) indicated that they would try the system again the next time they needed this type of information. The summer responses included a higher proportion of repeat users, but this probably reflects greater vigilance on the part of library staff in encouraging users to fill out a questionnaire than it does a major change in use patterns.

Summer users also indicated a greater willingness to pay for a DIALOG OnDisc search. Over 78% were willing to pay something, compared with 70% in spring, and nearly 30% of summer users were willing to pay more than $15 to use the system. Only 16.24% of spring users held this view. This may reflect the availability of more years of bibliographic data, or the financial standing of the summer user population.   Finally, summer users were far more likely to have received an orientation with a librarian (88.24%) than spring users (74.59%), possibly due to the less hectic pace of the Library during July and August. It may also be that since users did not usually have to wait to use the system, they were less likely to have watched or received assistance from the user preceding them.

Impact on In-Person Reference Service

Despite the fact that staff feel that the availability of DIALOG OnDisc MEDLINE frequently makes it easier to assist patrons, it also has an undeniable impact on patterns of user assistance. Reference staff at the Academy continue to switch discs for users rather than allow them to do so for themselves, primarily for security reasons. As one librarian commented, readers manage to misplace large reference books on a regular basis; CD-ROM discs could all too easily be lost. While discs may be more secure if staff retain control, this approach has its drawbacks. A user conducting an author search may need to have discs switched every five minutes or so. Staff may find they are spending a great deal of time with one user, or users may need to wait until a librarian is free to bring them a new disc. The availability of multiple disc readers, while a more expensive option than single disc readers, would cut down substantially on the amount of disc-switching assistance required from staff.

While a CD-ROM system may facilitate the provision of better service, it may also demand more instructional time. Between 10-13% of reference questions logged during July and August dealt with CD-ROM use. CD-ROM orientations are usually more time-consuming than other categories of questions, except for in-depth reference questions and instructions on the use of OPAC terminals. Orientations to *Index Medicus* typically are shorter than orientations to CD-ROM because a CD-ROM session involves multiple steps. If the user lacks typing skills and is unfamiliar with computers, the CD-ROM instruction session can be even longer.

The degree of assistance expected is also related to physical setting. *Index Medicus* is located in a separate room at the Academy, and it may not be readily apparent to staff when a reader is having trouble with its use. For their part, *Index Medicus* users must get up and walk to the Reference Desk to request help. The CD-ROM, however, is sandwiched between two public services points: the Circulation and Reference desks. Close physical proximity makes it difficult for staff to avoid eye contact with frustrated CD-ROM users, particularly if beeps emanating from the system signal that a user is having trouble. The answer is not, of course, to move a CD-ROM system to the far reaches of the Library. It should be well-understood, however, that the addition of a CD-ROM system to the library is likely to result in an increase in the demand for reference assistance.

Long Range Results of the Evaluation Program

The availability of DIALOG OnDisc MEDLINE has been an undeniable success thus far, achieving a degree of acceptance, particularly among staff not accustomed to microcomputers, that was unanticipated. The Library has, in fact, decided to make DIALOG OnDisc a permanent fixture, and to provide access without charge at least for the foreseeable future. We are pleased that this has been possible, but recognize that other institutions may need to recoup some of the costs involved with a similar subscription. Most vendors will make their products available for a free trial of thirty days, which can be helpful in the comparison of alternative products. Potential subscribers would be wise to try such a free evaluation period, but they may wish to closely ponder the pros and cons of providing the service free to users if it is anticipated that there will be fees once CD-ROM is permanently available.

The presence of DIALOG OnDisc MEDLINE, or any similar product, on a trial basis without charge may create subsequent difficulties with changing the arrangement. In the current fiscal climate, it was considered unlikely that a CD-ROM installation would be possible at this site without some minimal level of cost-recovery. Several staff commented that charging for availability could alter expectations and cause users to be far more demanding. Thus far there has been relatively little problem with regulating the length of time an individual may use the system. If others are waiting, users are asked to restrict their use to approximately 30 minutes. But if searches were fee-based, length of a search session could become a monitoring problem which the Library is presently ill-equipped to handle. (Alternative arrangements for collecting fees would need to be investigated if cost-recovery was adopted for this service.) Paying patrons might also expect a higher level of assistance and training on the system, and hold the Library accountable for their results. While on the surface there seems to be no quarrel with the desirability of subscribing to CD-ROM, administrative questions abound.

Although the Academy Library relies solely on income from fees for service, gifts, grants, contracts and its endowment for funding, it is frequently mistakenly perceived as a tax-supported institution because it is open to the public. Library users who already complain about charges for photocopies ($0.25 per page) may react negatively to the imposition of fees for access to a previously free service. As one respondent wrote: "Why should this service cost, and all other library services be free? It will jeopardize the concept of free library services!" Regardless of the fact that all other library services are *not* free in this setting, many library patrons may be negatively impressed by a fee for self-service searching, particularly one that was originally offered at no charge. While it is important for the Academy and similar organizations to seriously consider the availability of CD-ROM in their libraries, there are also major problems and implications associated with such a step that cannot be overlooked or minimized. Consideration of CD-ROM necessitates a close scrutiny of costs and benefits, for its availability is likely to come only at the expense of other library functions or services.

Appendix A

```
                    DIALOG OnDisc MEDLINE
                       Pilot Project


    This compact disk version of the MEDLINE database is being tested
by the New York Academy of Medicine (NYAM) through September 1988 as
part of the National Library of Medicine's nation-wide evaluation of
MEDLINE CD ROM products.  The MEDLINE database corresponds to the
printed Cumulated Index Medicus, International Nursing Index, and
Index to Dental Literature.  MEDLINE provides citations to the journal
literature of biomedicine and allows you to find and print out
references on a topic of your choice.  One can search DIALOG OnDisc by
subject, author, or keyword, and can limit retrieval to human studies
or articles in English.  Approximately 60% of the citations contain
abstracts.  For the purposes of the pilot project only those citations
indexed in 1987 can be searched on the system.

    The NYAM Library does not own all the journals indexed on the
disk.  Please consult a reference librarian for assistance in locating
these journals, or refer to the pink guide entitled  "Locating Journals
in the New York Academy of Medicine Library".

    If you wish to try the system please ask the Reference
Librarian for the "Directions for Use" and then fill out the
Questionnaire upon completion of your search.


                      Guidelines for Use

1.  Please sign up for a search session at the Lobby Reference Desk
    between the hours of 10:00 a.m. and 4:00 p.m.  After 4:00 or before
    10:00 sign up sheets will be available in the Reference office.

2.  Each daily appointment is limited to a maximum of 30 minutes per
    person.  Specific permission is required for all exceptions.

3.  Signups may be made up to one week in advance.  All signups
    must be made in person with the exception of Fellows and
    Subscribers, who may call for an appointment.

4.  All users must fill out a questionnaire following each search
    session.
```

Appendix B

```
                    DIALOG OnDisc MEDLINE


                      Directions for Use


1.  Before beginning your search session please consult the Medical
    Subject Headings (MESH) or Permuted Medical Subject Headings to
    identify the appropriate search terms under which to search.  Try
    to select the most specific terms possible (e.g. "Arteriosclerosis"
    rather than "Cardiovascular Diseases").  You may cross a number
    of terms, such as "Arteriosclerosis" and "Cholesterol" to
    retrieve articles dealing with both concepts.

2.  At the initial menu, highlight "Easy Menu Search" and press
    carriage return.  Follow the menu directions on succeeding
    screens to conduct your search.  Choices on each screen may be
    selected by pressing the appropriate highlighted letter.
    Alternatively, you may use the arrows on the keypad to
    highlight your choice, then  press the carriage return.  A
    sample search is available near the computer for your review.

3.  If you make a mistake and wish to begin again press the "F9"
    key to start over.

4.  You can limit your retrieval to articles in English or human
    studies by selecting the appropriate choices.  Citations can be
    printed at the attached printer.

5.  For additional assistance, please consult a Reference Librarian or
    the DIALOG OnDisc user manual.

6.  At the conclusion of your search session please complete the
    Questionnaire and hand it to the Reference Librarian at the
    Lobby Reference Desk.
```

```
            DIALOG OnDisc MEDLINE EVALUATION QUESTIONNAIRE
                          (Spring 1988)
                      (Analysis of Responses)
```

Instructions

I. This MEDLINE DIALOG OnDisc system is being tested by the New York
Academy of Medicine. We would like you to fill out this questionnaire
in order to help us find out who is using the system, and how useful it
is to you. If you need assistance in using the system please ask at
the Reference Desk. After completing your search please return the
questionnaire to the Lobby Reference Desk. Thank you!

Please circle the correct response.

1. My primary affiliation/profession is:

    (Circle ONE only)

    a. physician   i. advertising (public relations)
        (10/122) = 8.19%   (0)
    b. dentist   j. publishing
        (2/122) = 1.64%   (8/122) = 6.56%
    c. scientist/researcher   k. nurse
        (22/122) = 18.03%   (4/122) = 3.28%
    d. attorney/paralegal   l. educator
        (16/122) = 13.11%   (10/122) = 8.19%
    e. public health   m. librarian
        (1/122) = 0.82%   (5/122) = 4.10%
    f. pharmaceutical company   n. other (See appendix D)
                                             please specify
        (0)   (17/122) = 13.93%
    g. other health care professional (See appendix E)
                                         please specify
        (7/122) = 5.74%
    h. student   1.high school (10)   4.medical school (3)
                       2.college (16)   5.graduate school (7)
                       3.nursing (0)   6.other health care
                                               field (1)

        total students = (37/122) = 30.32%

2. I was looking for articles:

    (Circle ALL that apply)

    a. on a subject (116/122) = 95.08%

    b. under a title (13/122) = 10.66%

    c. by an author (20/122) = 16.39%

    d. in a particular journal (9/122) = 7.37%

    e. other (2/122) = 1.64%
```
```

Appendix C-2

3. I needed the information for:

    (Circle ALL that apply)

    a. personal concern   g. not needed, just curious
        (21/122) = 17.21%   (5/122) = 4.09%
    b. a paper or report   h. patient care
        (38/122) = 31.15%   (5/122) = 4.09%
    c. a research project   i. drug research
        (51/122) = 41.8%   (13/122) = 10.66%
    d. keeping current   j. legal matters
        (5/122) = 4.09%   (14/122) = 11.48%
    e. to check a reference   k. work for employer
        (6/122) = 4.92%   (17/122) = 13.94%
    f. teaching/planning a course   l. other
        (5/122) = 4.09%   (5/122) = 4.09%

4. The information I found was:

    (Circle ALL that apply)

    a. what I was looking for (51/122) = 41.80%

    b. more than I needed (15/122) = 12.30%

    c. some of what I needed (55/122) = 45.08%

    d. not useful (11/122) = 9.01%

    e. for someone else (3/122) = 2.46%

    f. other (2/122) = 1.64%

5. Have you ever used any of the printed publications produced
    from the MEDLINE system (e.g. INDEX MEDICUS, the INTERNATIONAL
    NURSING INDEX, the INDEX TO DENTAL LITERATURE, or the HOSPITAL
    LITERATURE INDEX)? (Circle ONE only)

    a. yes   b. no   c. don't know
    (75/122) =   (40/122) =   (7/122) =
    61.48%   32.79%   5.74%

6. If yes, you've used printed versions, how do they compare to
    the DIALOG OnDisc MEDLINE you have just used?

    (Circle ONE only)

    a. easier to use (31/76) = 40.79%

    b. harder to use (34/76) = 44.74%

    c. about the same to use (7/76) = 9.21%

    d. other (4/76) = 5.26%

7. Have you used an online version of MEDLINE (either yourself or by having a librarian process a search for you)?

   (Circle ALL that apply)

   a. yes, by myself (42/122) = 34.43%

   b. yes, librarian search (35/122) = 28.69%

   c. no (53/122) = 43.44%

   d. don't know (5/122) = 4.09%

8. If yes, you've used online MEDLINE, which system do you prefer?

   a. online, own search (e.g. Grateful Med., BRS Colleague, Paper Chase)   (which one?) (10/62) = 16.13%

   b. DIALOG OnDisc MEDLINE (26/62) = 41.94%

   c. online, librarian search (8/62) = 12.90%

   d. don't know (18/62) = 29.03%

9. If this MEDLINE CD-ROM system had not been available today, what would you have done?

   (Circle ALL that apply)

   a. used a printed version (e.g. Index Medicus)
      (68/122) = 55.74%
   b. requested an online search or conducted own online search
      (24/122) = 19.67%
   c. asked a library staff member
      (47/122) = 38.52%
   d. asked a friend or colleague
      (3/122) = 2.46%
   e. used online or card catalog
      (30/122) = 24.59%
   f. nothing
      (7/122) = 5.74%
   g. other
      (3/122) = 2.46%

10. Next time you need this sort of information, what will you
    do?

    (Circle ALL that apply)

    a. try DIALOG OnDisc MEDLINE (91/122) = 74.59%

    b. try a printed version (Index Medicus etc.)
        (20/122) = 16.39%
    c. try an online version (30/122) = 24.59%

    d. try another source (10/122) = 8.20%

    e. all of the above (21/122) = 17.21%

11. During this test, DIALOG OnDisc MEDLINE is provided free of
    charge to library users.

    What is the maximum amount you would be willing to pay per
    search to use this system?

    (Check the highest amount that applies)

    a. nothing   d. $15.00 - 20.00
    (35/117) = 29.91%   (10/11) = 8.55%
    b. $5.00   e. $25.00 - 35.00
    (44/117) = 36.07%   (5/117) = 4.10%
    c. $10.00   f. $40.00 - 50.00
    (19/117) = 15.57%   (4/117) = 3.42%

12. How often have you used DIALOG OnDisc MEDLINE

    a. first time (97/117) = 82.91%

    b. once before (9/117) = 7.70%

    c. 3-5 times (7/117) = 5.98%

    d. 6 or more times (4/117) = 3.42%

13. How many years back would you be interested in searching?
    1-3 yrs. - (14),   5 yrs. - (38),   10 yrs. - (9)
    15-20 yrs. - (10),   21-30 yrs. - (10),   >30 yrs. - (4)

14. To get started using DIALOG OnDisc, I used the following sources:

(Circle ALL that apply)

a. orientation with a librarian (59/79) = 74.68%

b. blue typed instruction sheets (14/79) = 17.72%

c. black bound DIALOG OnDisc manual (6/79) = 7.59%

d. DIALOG OnDisc menus and help screen (27/79) = 34.18%

II. Enter one response only (on the following 5 point scale) for each of the questions 1 through 5.

SCALE:	A Strongly Agree	B Agree	C Neutral	D Disagree	E Strongly Disagree

_____1. Instructions on DIALOG OnDisc MEDLINE screens were sufficient for my use.

A	B	C	D	E
27/105	47/105	19/105	12/105	-
25.71%	44.76%	18.10%	11.43%	

_____2. The rate at which the computer responds is satisfactory.

A	B	C	D	E
52/113	44/113	15/113	1/113	1/113
46.01%	38.94%	13.27%	0.88%	0.88%

_____3. The black bound DIALOG OnDisc manual helped me to use the system.

A	B	C	D	E
6/88	22/88	48/88	9/88	3/88
6.82%	25%	54.55%	10.23%	3.41%

_____4. The DIALOG OnDisc blue typed instruction sheets helped me to use the system.

A	B	C	D	E
3/53	18/53	25/53	4/53	3/53
5.66%	33.96%	47.17%	7.55%	5.66%

_____5. Overall, I found DIALOG OnDisc MEDLINE easy to use.

A	B	C	D	E
36/109	52/109	10/109	10/109	1/109
33.03%	47.71%	9.17%	9.17%	0.92%

_____6. I could use the system without assistance from a librarian.

A	B	C	D	E
25/103	38/103	19/103	13/103	8/103
24.27%	36.90%	18.45%	12.62%	7.77%

Comments
        In what ways could the system be improved? Other comments?

(see Appendix H)

Your cooperation in responding to this questionnaire is very much
appreciated. Please give the completed questionnaire to the librarian
at the Lobby Reference Desk.

Appendix D

Respondent Affiliations--Spring Survey

Question 1N: "Others":

1 Actuary
1 Analyst
7 Chemical Company Representative
1 Computer Science
5 Consultant
1 Corporate Communication Company
1 Corporate Video/Film
1 Design Company
5 Editor/Writer
3 Insurance
1 Mechanical Equipment Manufacturer
1 Parent
4 Patient

Question 1G: Other Health Care Professional:

2 Chiropractor
1 Clinical Psychologist
1 Health Advocate
1 Medical Anthropologist
1 Psychologist
2 Psychotherapist

Appendix E

Mediated Computerized Literature Search Requests
(April 17 - June 30,1988)

Primary affiliation/profession of search requesters:

a. physician
    (33/174) = 18.96%

i. advertising (public relations)
    (48/174) = 27.59%

b. dentist
    (0)

j. publishing
    (8/174) = 4.60%

c. scientist/researcher
    (2/174) = 1.15%

k. nurse
    (0)

d. attorney/paralegal
    (55/174) = 31.61%

l. educator
    (0)

e. public health
    (0)

m. librarian
    (0)

f. pharmaceutical company

    (1/174) = 0.57%

n. other _____
              please specify
    (23/174) = 13.22%

g. other health care professional _____

    (4/174) = 2.30%

                                   please specify

h. student   1.high school   4.medical school
    (0)   2.college   5.graduate school
                 3.nursing   6.other health care
                                      field

Appendix F-1

DIALOG OnDisc MEDLINE EVALUATION QUESTIONNAIRE
(Summer 1988)
[Analysis of Responses]

Instructions

I. This MEDLINE DIALOG OnDisc system is being tested by the New York
Academy of Medicine. We would like you to fill out this questionnaire
in order to help us find out who is using the system, and how useful it
is to you. If you need assistance in using the system please ask at
the Reference Desk. After completing your search please return the
questionnaire to the Lobby Reference Desk. Thank you!

Please circle the correct response.

1. My primary affiliation/profession is:

(Circle ONE only)

a. physician   i. advertising (public relations)
    (9/68) = 13.24%   (2/68) = 2.94%
b. dentist   j. publishing
                                          (6/68) = 8.82%
c. scientist/researcher   k. nurse
    (3/68) = 4.41%   (1/68) = 1.47%
d. attorney/paralegal   l. educator
    (7/68) = 10.29%   (4/68) = 5.88%
e. public health   m. librarian
    (2/68) = 2.94%
f. pharmaceutical company   n. other (12/68) = 17.64%
    (5/68) = 7.35%
g. other health care professional (3/68) = 4.41%

h. student   1.high school   4.medical school (2)
                   2.college (2)   5.graduate school (8)
                   3.nursing   6.other health care
                                         field (1)

    total students = (13/68) = 19.12%

2. I was looking for articles:

(Circle ALL that apply)

a. on a subject (64/68) = 94.11%

b. under a title (1/68) = 1.48%

c. by an author (9/68) = 13.24%

d. in a particular journal (3/68) = 4.4%

244

e. other

3. I needed the information for:

    (Circle ALL that apply)

    a. personal concern   g. not needed, just curious
        (17/68) = 25%   (2/68) = 2.94%
    b. a paper or report   h. patient care
        (12/68) = 17.65%   (7/68) = 10.29%
    c. a research project   i. drug research
        (31/68) = 45.59%   (7/68) = 10.29%
    d. keeping current   j. legal matters
        (4/68) = 5.88%   (9/68) = 13.24%
    e. to check a reference   k. work for employer
        (2/68) = 2.94%   (9/68) = 13.24%
    f. teaching/planning a course l. other
        (2/68) = 2.94%   (4/68) = 5.89%

4. The information I found was:

    (Circle ALL that apply)

    a. what I was looking for (39/68) = 57.35%

    b. more than I needed (4/68) = 5.88%

    c. some of what I needed (26/68) = 38.24%

    d. not useful (2/68) = 2.94%

    e. for someone else (5/68) = 7.35%

    f. other (2/68) = 2.94%

5. Have you ever used any of the printed publications produced
    from the MEDLINE system (e.g. INDEX MEDICUS, the INTERNATIONAL
    NURSING INDEX, the INDEX TO DENTAL LITERATURE, or the HOSPITAL
    LITERATURE INDEX)? (Circle ONE only)

    a. yes   b. no   c. don't know
    (44/68) =   (22/68) =   (2/68) =
    64.47%   32.35%   2.94%

6. If yes, you've used printed versions, how do they compare to
    the DIALOG OnDisc MEDLINE you have just used?

    (Circle ONE only)

    a. easier to use (11/41) = 26.83%

    b. harder to use (23/41) = 56.09%

c. about the same to use (7/41) = 17.07%

d. other

7. Have you used an online version of MEDLINE (either yourself or by having a librarian process a search for you)?

(Circle ALL that apply)

a. yes, by myself (25/68) = 36.76%

b. yes, librarian search (17/68) = 25%

c. no (32/68) = 47.06%

d. don't know

8. If yes, you've used online MEDLINE, which system do you prefer?

a. online, own search (e.g. Grateful Med., BRS Colleague, Paper Chase) (which one?) (9/42) = 21.43%

b. DIALOG OnDisc MEDLINE (21/42) = 5%

c. online, librarian search (1/42) = 2.38%

d. don't know (8/42) = 19.05%

9. If this MEDLINE CD-ROM system had not been available today, what would you have done?

(Circle ALL that apply)

a. used a printed version (e.g. Index Medicus)
   (42/68) = 61.76%
b. requested an online search or conducted own online search
   (23/68) = 33.82%
c. asked a library staff member
   (25/68) = 36.76%
d. asked a friend or colleague
   (5/68) = 7.35%
e. used online or card catalog
   (13/68) = 19.11%
f. nothing
   (2/68) = 2.94%
g. other
   (6/68) = 8.82%

10. Next time you need this sort of information, what will you do?

    (Circle ALL that apply)

    a.   try DIALOG OnDisc MEDLINE   (56/68) = 82.35%

    b.   try a printed version (Index Medicus etc.)
         (15/68) = 22.06)
    c.   try an online version   (10/68) = 14.71%

    d.   try another source   (6/68) = 8.82%

    e.   all of the above   (13/68) = 19.12%

11. During this test, DIALOG OnDisc MEDLINE is provided free of charge to library users.

    What is the maximum amount you would be willing to pay per search to use this system?

    (Check the highest amount that applies)

    a. nothing   d. $15.00 - 20.00
    (10/57) = 17.54%   (7/57) = 12.28%

    b. $5.00   e. $25.00 - 35.00
    (15/57) = 26.32%   (3/57) = 5.26%

    c. $10.00   f. $40.00 - 50.00
    (15/57) = 26.32%   (7/57) = 12.28%

12. How often have you used DIALOG OnDisc MEDLINE

    a.   first time   (47/68) = 69.11%

    b.   once before   (12/68) = 17.65%

    c.   3-5 times   (4/68) = 5.88%

    d.   6 or more times   (5/68) = 7.35%

13. How many years back would you be interested in searching?
    1-3 yrs. - (9),   5 yrs. - (24),   10 yrs. - (11)
    15-20 yrs. - (7),   21-30 yrs. - (1),   >30 yrs. - (1)

14. To get started using DIALOG OnDisc, I used the following sources:

   (Circle ALL that apply)

   a. orientation with a librarian (60/68) = 88.24%

   b. blue typed instruction sheets (16/68) = 23.53%

   c. black bound DIALOG OnDisc manual (7/68) = 10.29%

   d. DIALOG OnDisc menus and help screen (26/68) = 38.24%

II. Enter one response only (on the following 5 point scale) for
   each of the questions 1 through 5.

SCALE:	A Strongly Agree	B Agree	C Neutral	D Disagree	E Strongly Disagree

_____1. Instructions on DIALOG OnDisc MEDLINE screens were
       sufficient for my use.

A	B	C	D	E
18/65	32/65	6/65	7/65	2/65
27.69%	49.23%	9.23%	10.77%	3.08%

_____2. The rate at which the computer responds is satisfactory.

A	B	C	D	E
34/64	23/64	6/64	1/64	-
53.13%	35.94%	9.38%	1.56%	

_____3. The black bound DIALOG OnDisc manual helped me to use
       the system.

A	B	C	D	E
5/52	8/52	34/52	3/52	2/52
9.62%	15.38%	65.38%	5.77%	3.85%

_____4. The DIALOG OnDisc blue typed instruction sheets helped
       me to use the system.

A	B	C	D	E
4/56	18/56	25/56	7/56	2/56
7.14%	32.14%	44.64%	12.5%	3.57%

_____5. Overall, I found DIALOG OnDisc MEDLINE easy to use.

	A	B	C	D	E
	29/63	30/63	1/63	2/63	1/63
	46.03%	47.62%	1.59%	3.17%	1.59%

_____6. I could use the system without assistance from a librarian.

	A	B	C	D	E
	22/59	17/59	8/59	5/59	7/59
	37.29%	28.81%	13.56%	8.47%	11.86%

Comments
       In what ways could the system be improved? Other comments?

(see Appendix H)

Your cooperation in responding to this questionnaire is very much
appreciated. Please give the completed questionnaire to the librarian
at the Lobby Reference Desk.

Appendix G

Respondent Affiliations--Summer-Survey

Question <u>1N</u>: "Others":

1 Journalist
1 Layperson
1 NYS Assemblyman
1 Photo-researcher
1 Producer on neurological disorders
1 Programmer
3 Relative of ill patient
1 Research consultant
1 Theological
1 Writer

Question <u>1G</u>: <u>Other</u> <u>Health</u> <u>Care</u> <u>Professional</u>:

1 Chiropractor
1 Medical Assistant
1 Psychoanalyst

QUESTIONNAIRE COMMENTS--SPRING 1988

[9000 series numbers refer to the Pretest responses.]

#9005 - More instructions/explanations in BLUE CHARTS on screen. For instance, parenthesis explanations while still in blue phase. The constant switching back and forth is confusing and the red instructions are confusing and too wordy. (Educator)

#9906 - In trial session choosing a non-available option (ex. DIALOG or on-line) search caused software lock-up causing need to reboot. (Health Care Professional)

#9009 - Need manual for user & hand-holding first time used.

#9010 - Being able to use more selects--instead, in my scan, I needed to review over 800 items.

#9017 - The rate was excellent, but the instructions and orientation were not easy to understand or use. The system is beautiful but needs a lot of work. (Graduate student)

#9027 - A one page simple outline with minimum amount of information--how to get into computer and what to do. Each page would be titled--SUBJECT SEARCH, NAME SEARCH etc. (College student)

#9028 - More listings going back 20 years or more. (Medical Anthropology)

#9032 - While printing out titles non-recoverable error on CD-ROM (after 7th title). (Financial Communication System)

#9038 - The availability of the printed copy really is helpful. The Reference Librarian was extremely helpful as well.

#9044 - Sort by item # in a search file would help. To print #s 1, 2, 7, 10, 15 of 30. Should be able to limit by 'non-human' also. (Scientist)

#9046 - Some fairly complicated searches can be set up by easy menu. It is a big disadvantage that they cannot be saved from disc to disc. (Physician)

#9054 - Faster computer and faster printer, directions card. (Physician)

* * * * *

#109 - Name of journal should be indicated more clearly (hold for type, perhaps. (Scientist/researcher)

#112 - Darker printing/display function. (Physician)

#114 - Faster printer. (Corporate Comm. Co.)

#122 - Have instruction sheet and book by the machine. (Actuary)

#126 - More years, more speed. (Scientist/researcher)

#133 - Dialogue does not have sufficient ways to modify searches online. (Writer/editor)

#135 - Don't understand why you need to highlight a topic and also F10 it also should be able to narrow search yourself (similar to BRS). (Publishing)

#140 - Without the direct assistance of a very cooperative Librarian, I would not have been able to use the system. (Physician)

#142 - More keywords! (Publishing)

#143 - The author index, in the few minutes I had, retrieved papers by someone else - possible first names or some other more particular means of specifying authors, would help. (Scientist/researcher)

#159 - Did not have material under topic of "harmful psychotherapy" that is, negative effects caused by therapist factors. (Researcher)

#167 - It would be helpful to be able to go back at least five-ten years. Otherwise, its a terrific service to have. (Publishing)

#178 - Cleaner & more complete screen printouts. (Scientist/researcher)

Appendix H-3

#210 - The system is fairly simple but, I found that the orientation with the reference Librarian was necessary. Even going back to use the system again, I may have additional questions as I become more comfortable and want to branch out. Thus, I may need to ask the Librarian for assistance after the initial 1/2 hr. orientation. (Educator)

#211 - NO STRUCTURE! I want to key in (Laser)(Printers) (Toxic or Adverse) in any order & get results. I do not want to have to select Lasers after I select Laser. Tedious. (Computer Programmer)

#212 - "Free" search - help with key words not on system, e.g., type in key words & system should refer you to online correct (accepted) terms. (Research)

#216 - Help screen first would be helpful. Otherwise, I'm aware of the vast amount of data stored on each disk - I am very impressed. (Grad. School student)

#222 - There are separate discs for each year, 1988-1984. Completed years will undoubtedly be put on one hard disc, accessable to one search. (Attorney/paralegal)

#227 - As a complete amateur I was very pleasantly pleased that with only brief instruction I could proceed. The librarian, however was critical when I made a fatal mistake. (Physician)

#236 - With my lack of computer know-how it was very easy to use. The abstracts & printing them were very convient. (Research/ intern)

#238 - One screen indicating the exact sequence (keys) for processing the search. (Physician)

#244 - Put more years together (5 years at a time) or get more Librarians. (Medical Assistant)

#263 - Printed Chart of what functions keys are for. (Attorney/paralegal)

#270 - Great system - but it won't replace print version search for many things. (Scientist/researcher)

#274 - Less keystrokes (Publishing)

#275 - Easier to follow instructions (Public Health)

EVALUATION AT

UNIVERSITY OF TEXAS SOUTHWESTERN

MEDICAL CENTER AT DALLAS LIBRARY

DIALOG MEDLINE
ONDISC

By *Helen Mayo*
    Leslie Dworkin
    Glenn Bunton

University of Texas Southwestern
Medical Center at Dallas Library
5323 Harry Hines Blvd.
Dallas, TX 75235

EVALUATION AT UNIVERSITY OF TEXAS SOUTHWESTERN MEDICAL CENTER AT DALLAS LIBRARY DIALOG MEDLINE ONDISC

Introduction

The University of Texas Southwestern Medical Center at Dallas Library participated in the National Library of Medicine's evaluation of MEDLINE CD-ROM products, testing DIALOG MEDLINE OnDisc. The following describes our experiences with the equipment and software and presents the results of the data collected from surveys of users between April and May 1988.

The computer, CD-ROM player, and printer were set up near the Information Desk in the Library. By having the equipment in close proximity to the Information Desk we were able to monitor use of the equipment, inform clients about the system, suggest its use when appropriate, and assist clients with any questions that arose (either of a mechanical or search strategy nature). The discs were kept at the Information Desk. This allowed us to ask the client to fill out a questionnaire at the same time that we handed out the discs. Our clients were generally very cooperative in filling out the evaluation forms. However, some of our repeat users, knowing the location of the discs, "helped themselves" and were missed from the data collection process. In addition, during the first week of the evaluation, we did not emphasize filling out the forms to our clients. Because of this we do not know the actual number of users on the system during the evaluation period.

The decision to assist clients not only with equipment and software questions, but also with formulation of search strategies using DIALOG MEDLINE OnDisc was deliberate. We have a policy of assisting our clients with other computer-based information sources which we have available (such as PaperChase and Micromedex on CD-ROM) and felt that our clients deserved the same assistance with the use of this test product.

We also made the decision to allow any library user access to this product. This is in contrast to the current library policies described below regarding intermediated searches and use of the PaperChase terminals.

The computer-assisted reference service unit (CARS) in our Library performs intermediated online searches for a select group of library clients defined as follows:

> students, staff, faculty, fellows, and residents associated with our

institution or 2 locally-affiliated hospitals (primary clientele); local area health care professionals, the lay public, and direct patient care product or services businesses (secondary clientele)

We do not perform online searches for students from other academic institutions, attorneys, or businesses (unless they meet the criteria previously stated).

PaperChase use is restricted to our primary clientele.

Results

The results of our evaluation are based on 132 questionnaires completed and returned during the test period. (Appendix A) The original questionnaire received from NLM was revised to fit our particular information environment. The changes made to the evaluation form reflect our specific interests and information that we felt would be useful for future planning and for provision of services and resources for our clients.

Of 113 responses to question number 1, thirty represented students affiliated with this institution (these include medical students, undergraduate and graduate students in allied health programs, and graduate students in the biological sciences) [Figure 1]. The next largest single group was students from other institutions which is not surprising since they frequently request online searches, and we always refer this user group back to their home institutions for

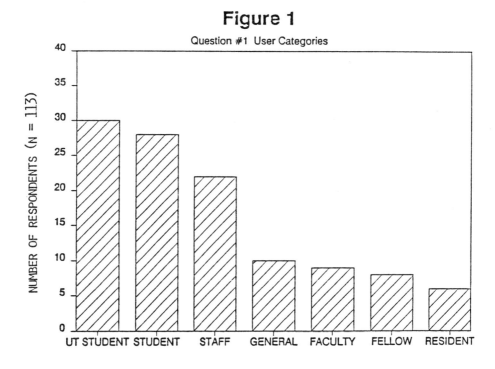

Figure 1

Question #1 User Categories

intermediated searches. During the test period we routinely recommended the DIALOG MEDLINE OnDisc to these students which may account for the large size of this group.

Users of MEDLINE CD-ROM did not always follow the user patterns established by PaperChase searchers in our Library. Approximately 30% of our PaperChase users are our students, and 26.5% of the CD-ROM users were students at this institution. Whereas faculty comprise 30% of our PaperChase users, they accounted for only 8% of DIALOG CD-ROM users. In fact, approximately 35% fewer faculty, fellows, and residents used the CD-ROM product than use PaperChase in our Library. This may be due in part to their not being aware that DIALOG MEDLINE OnDisc was available since we did not advertise this fact. It could also have been a result of PaperChase's broader time coverage (1966-1988). There may be a certain product loyalty, in this case to PaperChase. Some PaperChase users may also have decided not to learn a new system for such short-term use.

The majority of those responding on the evaluation form were familiar with MEDLINE (#8)**. Whereas 31.9% of those who responded said that they had previously only searched MEDLINE online themselves, 17.7% had previously requested an intermediated search, and 28.3% had done both. But 22.1% answered that they had not used MEDLINE in any way; students from other institutions comprised by far the largest percentage in this category.

From our observations all clients used the Easy Menu Mode. Of 112 persons responding to the question on DIALOG MEDLINE OnDisc use, 77 were first-time users at the time they completed the evaluation form (#12). But 35 persons returning the form had previously used DIALOG MEDLINE OnDisc one or more times before [Figure 2]. Unfortunately, we have no way of comparing the same individual's responses following his or her initial use of the MEDLINE CD product and after subsequent uses. It would have been informative to see how clients' responses on questions did or did not change after more use of and greater familiarity with the system.

Our results demonstrated that when cost differences were ignored a majority of users preferred this CD-ROM product over printed indexes, PaperChase or BRS Colleague, and intermediated searches. Exactly one-half of the respondents said that the cost factor (i.e. free during the evaluation period) was very important and 30.6% that it was somewhat important in their decision to use the CD product rather than request an online search (#10). Only 12% replied that the cost factor was unimportant. Of the total responding, 7.4% would not have done an online search if DIALOG MEDLINE OnDisc was not available [Figure 3]. A total of 57.7% would have used a printed index if DIALOG MEDLINE OnDisc had not been available. Even though the majority of that group would have been eligible for an online search they still would have preferred to use a printed index. Thirty-six percent would have used another end-user system or asked library staff to perform the search (#13). Significantly,

**number in parentheses refers to question on the evaluation

Figure 2

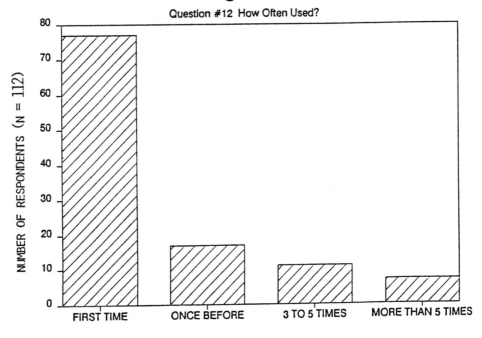

Question #12 How Often Used?

Figure 3

Question #10 Cost Importance

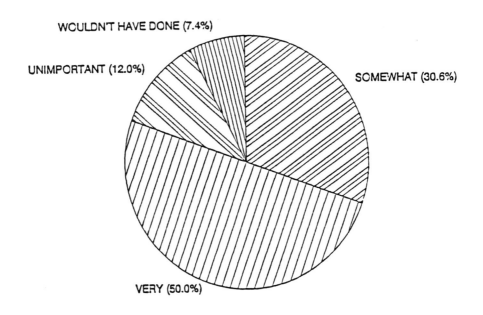

62.7% of the responses indicated that ignoring cost factors they preferred DIALOG MEDLINE OnDisc to either an end-user system (i.e. PaperChase or BRS Colleague) or intermediated searching (#9) [Figure 4]. However, we have no way of ascertaining when regular users of PaperChase and BRS Colleague, with a bias toward these systems, tried DIALOG MEDLINE OnDisc. For 20.6% the preferred mode of database searching varied depending on their topic. Although most clients knew MEDLINE existed, it appears that DIALOG MEDLINE CD-ROM attracted those clients who would frequently choose to do their searches using printed indexes.

The greatest number of our clients, 50 out of 132, used DIALOG MEDLINE OnDisc to get information for a report or paper, and 44 clients used it for a research project (#4) [Figure 5]. It is interesting to note that 9 out of 132 respondents or 6.8% said that they used this product for patient care information. Subject searches comprised 80.3% of the searches, but only 13.9% were by author (#3). While 37.7% said that the references they found were "just what I needed," only 0.8% replied that the information was "not useful" (#5) [Figure 6]. There was no relationship between the access point with which the users searched or for what purpose they needed the information (i.e. for patient care or research) and the satisfaction level response in question number 5.

Figure 4

Question #9 Preferred Method

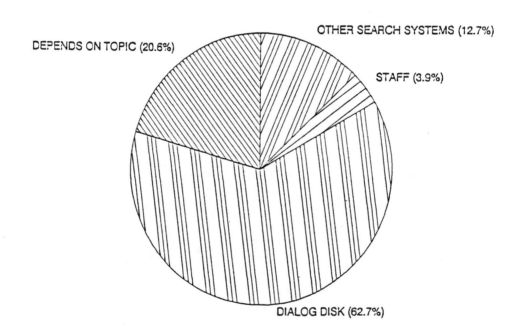

OTHER SEARCH SYSTEMS (12.7%)

DEPENDS ON TOPIC (20.6%)

STAFF (3.9%)

DIALOG DISK (62.7%)

Figure 5

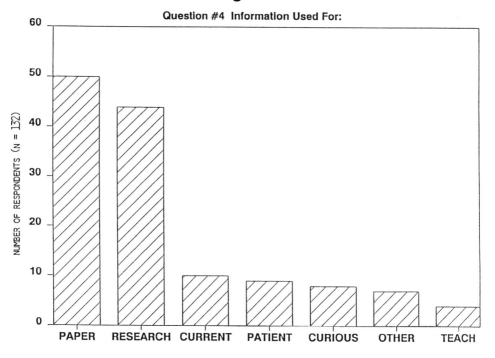

Question #4 Information Used For:

Figure 6

Question #5 Information Retrieved

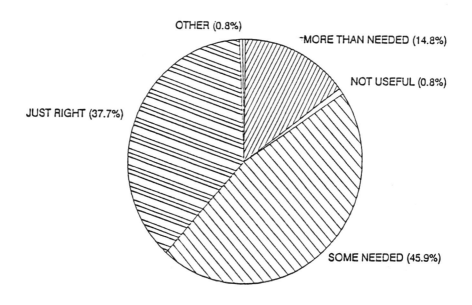

The majority of responses regarding ease of use of DIALOG MEDLINE OnDisc were very favorable. As seen from question number seven, 55 out of 90 respondents who had previously used indexes (*Index Medicus, International Nursing Index, Index to Dental Literature,* or *Hospital Literature Index*) stated that this CD-ROM product was easier to use than the printed indexes [Figure 7]. In our general experience we have observed that most of our clients tend to respond favorably to machines, so it is not surprising that 21.1% felt that printed indexes are less fun to use (#7). Seventy-eight percent of those who found references that were "just what I needed" felt that the printed indexes were harder to use while only 49% of those who found "some that I needed" responded in the same manner. In fact, twenty percent of this second group responded that the printed indexes are easier to use or about the same as this CD product.

Overall, 105 of 111 persons responding found DIALOG MEDLINE OnDisc easy to use (#21) [Figure 8]. A majority of users (85.6%) agreed or agreed strongly that the response rate of the system was satisfactory (#18). Also 80.4% said that changing discs during a search was easy (#19).

One surprising result was that 58.2% of the users would have been satisfied to search 4 or 5 years back while only 23.5% would have preferred to search more than 5 years (#11) [Figure 9]. When asked whether the current time span covered (1986-1988) is sufficient, 47.7% responded favorably (agree or strongly

Figure 7

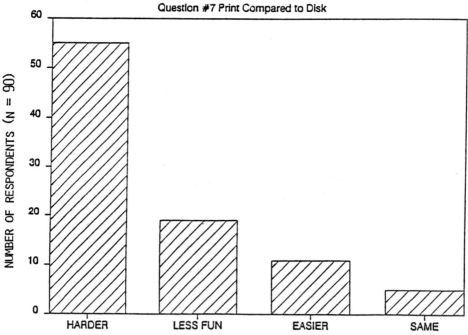

Question #7 Print Compared to Disk

Figure 8

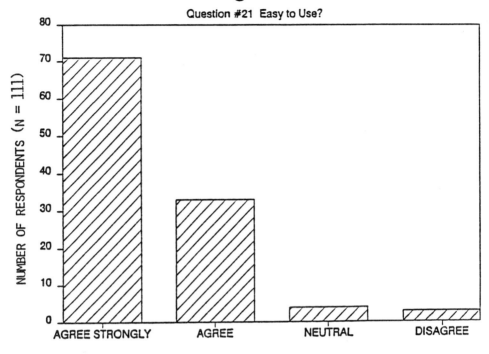

Question #21 Easy to Use?

Figure 9

Question #11 Preferred Time Coverage

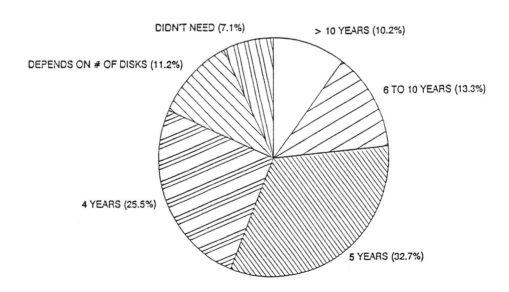

agree), 18% were neutral, 20.7% disagreed, and 13.6% disagreed strongly (#20). These are interesting statistics considering that 29.1% of our users used one disc, 42.7% used two discs, and 28.2% reported that they used three discs going back to 1986 (#14).

Conclusions and Observations

The impact of CD-ROM technology and other new technologies on information retrieval and library services is already being felt at our institution. Many of our clients now do MEDLINE searching themselves and are accessing MEDLINE through various vendors from computers in their offices or using the PaperChase terminals in the Library. Our own in-house CL-MEDLINE system will soon be available for access from three terminals in the Library and, shortly, from offices on campus.

The CD-ROM technology will allow users to access databases previously available only online. How will charges be assessed or will the Library assume the costs? What will the role of the librarian be in a CD-ROM environment? We have already seen a change in our role from one of strictly search intermediaries to instructors for end-user searching.

It appears from this evaluation that DIALOG MEDLINE OnDisc was generally easy for the users to operate and provided the majority of those responding to our questionnaire with satisfactory search results. However, we would have liked the opportunity to evaluate other MEDLINE CD-ROM products to compare and contrast strengths and weaknesses of each system. Some of the problems which we noticed in our personal use of DIALOG MEDLINE OnDisc which may have escaped the notice of our clients were:

1) In the index, subject terms with subheadings followed alpha-betically after subject headings with commas, leading to incomplete and ineffective searches.

2) Inability to explode and lack of tree structures

3) Inability to save a search and execute with subsequent discs (several of our clients mentioned this)

4) Occurrence of Fatal error #7 - inconsistent occurrences of system crashing. Unable to determine any common pattern for this.

5) Vocabulary inconsistent with other systems - e.g. use of the term "include" to indicate the Boolean "and" caused confusion for clients

6) This is not a system that all can intuitively use, but must be explained in some detail to the first-time user. As an example, most users never "discovered" the "Other Search Options Screen."

Some additional positive aspects which we noted include:

1) Excellent sort capability

2) Ease of use after initial explanation

3) Librarians enjoyed the fast response and ease of input in the Command Mode.

DIALOG CD-ROM was very popular with clients and librarians alike. While most of the design flaws noted above by our staff are not serious, they did impede quick orientation to the system and, in some cases, hindered access to the information sought. In addition, a hardware problem which caused the screen to fade was not only disconcerting to the user, but rendered the screen nearly impossible to read. If these deficiencies are corrected in future versions, this system would likely be most welcome in many libraries.

CD-ROM EVALUATION DATA

1. Please circle the category that best applies to you

a.	Staff	22	19.5%
b.	Faculty	8	7.1%
c.	Clinical Faculty	1	.9%
d.	Fellow	8	7.1%
e.	Resident	6	5.3%
f.	UT Southwestern Student	30	26.5%
g.	Other student	28	24.8%
h.	general public	10	8.8%
		113	100%

2. For categories a-e, please write the name of your primary department

3. Did you search by:

a.	Author name	17	13.9%
b.	Article title	2	1.6%
c.	Subject of article	98	80.3%
d.	Journal title	1	.8%
e.	Other	4	3.4%
		122	100%

4. I needed the information for:

a.	patient care	9	6.8%
b.	paper or report	50	37.9%
c.	research project	44	33.3%
d.	keeping current	10	7.6%
e.	verify reference	1	.8%
f.	teaching	4	3.0%
g.	just trying the system	8	6.1%
h.	other	6	4.5%
		132	100%

5. The references I found were:

a.	just what I needed	46	37.7%
b.	more than I needed	18	14.8%
c.	not useful	1	.8%
d.	some that I needed	56	45.9%
e.	other	1	.8%
		122	100%

6. Have you used any of the following printed indexes: (Index Medicus, Intl. Nursing Index, Index to Dental Lit, Hosp Lit Index?)

a. yes	87	77.7%
b. no	25	22.3%
c. don't remember	0	
	112	100%

7. If you have used any of the above, how do they compare to this Dialog-On-Disc?

a. printed index easier	11	12.2%
b. about the same	5	5.6%
c. printed index harder	55	61.1%
d. printed index less fun	19	21.1%
	90	100%

8. Have you searched Medline online yourself (Paperchase or BRS Colleague) or ordered an online search from the library?

a. searched myself	36	31.9%
b. library staff searched	20	17.7%
c. both a. and b.	32	28.3%
d. no	25	22.1%
e. don't remember	0	
	113	100%

9. Ignoring cost factors, which do you prefer?

a. Paperchase/Brs Colleague	13	12.7%
b. this Dialog-On-Disc	64	62.7%
c. Having Library staff do	4	3.9%
d. depends on topic	21	20.6%
	102	99.9%

10. Dialog-On-Disc is free during this evaluation period. How important was this factor in deciding to use it instead of doing an online search today?

a. very important	54	50.0%
b. somewhat important	33	30.6%
c. unimportant	13	12.0%
d. wouldn't have done	8	7.4%
	108	100%

11. About how far back in years would you have preferred to search
    on this topic if Dialog-On-Disc covered years before 1986?

    a. 4 years   25   25.5%
    b. 5 years   32   32.7%
    c. 6-10 years   13   13.3%
    d. >10 years   10   10.2%
    e. depends on # of discs   11   11.2%
    f. didn't need   7   7.1%

                                        ___   ____
                                        98   100%

12. How often have you used Dialog-On-Disc before?

    a. first time   77   68.8%
    b. once before   17   15.2%
    c. 3-5 times   11   10.0%
    d. >5 times   7   6.0%

                                        ___   ____
                                        112   100%

13. If Dialog-On-Disc weren't available today, what would you have
    done to locate information?

    a. used printed index   64   57.7%
    b. used Paperchase/BRS Colleague   18   16.2%
    c. asked a friend   0
    d. as library staff   22   19.8%
    e. something else   2   1.8%
    f. nothing today   5   4.5%

                                        ___   ____
                                        111   100%

14. Dialog-On-Disc covers the years 1986 through 1988 on separate
    discs. How many discs did you use today?

    a. one   32   29.1%
    b. two   47   42.7%
    c. three   31   28.2%

                                        ___   ____
                                        110   100%

15. About how many citations did you print today?

    a. 0   8   7.4%
    b. <10   40   37.0%
    c. 10-29   39   36.1%
    d. 30-50   17   15.7%
    e. >50   4   3.8%

                                        ___   ____
                                        108   100%

16. Did you print any abstracts today?

a. yes	69	62.7%
b. no	41	37.3%
	110	100%

17. Did you select any subject terms from the Medical Subject Headings list before you started searching?

a. yes	71	64.5%
b. no	39	35.5%
	110	100%

18. Response rate of the system is satisfactory

a. agree strongly	61	55.0%
b. agree	34	30.6%
c. neutral	6	5.4%
d. disagree	9	8.1%
e. disagree strongly	1	.9%
	111	100%

19. Changing discs during a search is easy

a. agree strongly	47	43.9%
b. agree	39	36.5%
c. neutral	14	13.1%
d. disagree	6	5.6%
e. disagree strongly	1	.9%
	107	100%

20. Time span covered is sufficient

a. agree strongly	33	29.7%
b. agree	20	18.0%
c. neutral	20	18.0%
d. disagree	23	20.7%
e. disagree strongly	15	13.6%
	111	100%

21. Overall, I found Dialog-On-Disc easy to use

a. agree strongly	72	64.9%
b. agree	33	29.7%
c. neutral	4	3.6%
d. disagree	2	1.8%
e. disagree strongly	0	
	111	100%

EVALUATION OF

MEDLINE
DIALOG ONDISC

AT UNIVERSITY OF NEBRASKA
MEDICAL CENTER

A Field Study and a Comparative Test of Five Systems

By *Nancy N. Woelfl*
Claire Gadzikowski
Suzanne Kehm
Audrey Powderly Newcomer
Marie A. Reidelbach

The McGoogan Library of Medicine
University of Nebraska Medical Center
42nd St. and Dewey Ave.,
Omaha, NE 68105

EVALUATION OF
MEDLINE DIALOG ONDISC
AT UNIVERSITY OF NEBRASKA
MEDICAL CENTER

Introduction

Once the exclusive domain of librarians, information and computer specialists, the National Library of Medicine's (NLM) ELHILL system and its MEDLINE database are now routinely used by a new and originally unanticipated class of users. Dubbed end users, these individuals perform for themselves many of the online database searches that librarians and information specialists once performed for them. Sales of MEDLINE subsets on magnetic tape and of Grateful Med (TM), NLM's user friendly interface to the MEDLINE database, indicate that end user searching is continuing to rise: by December, 1987, NLM had sold 11,399 copies of Grateful Med's three successive versions to end users and to institutions.

Many factors have stimulated the growth of end user searching including advances in computing equipment, telecommunications technology, and increasing levels of computer literacy. Lingering questions over the quality and effectiveness of mediated searches have led some to believe that physicians and biomedical scientists can master search protocols and mechanics as well as intermediaries or that they can compensate for lack of procedural skills by virtue of their superior subject knowledge and technical vocabularies. Convenience factors have also stimulated end user searching. Having personal access to relevant databases from one's home or office saves users a call or trip to the library. They no longer need to articulate the search topic to an intermediary or wait for search results. Finally, rising expectations have also played a role. Today's physicians are expected to search machine readable indexes as readily as they once searched the printed versions.

During the 1970's, access to the ELHILL system and the MEDLINE database was largely limited to institutions and individuals that could afford the cost of accessing mainframe computers located at the National Library of Medicine or commercial database vendors. By the early 1980's, some academic health sciences libraries had begun to purchase their own MEDLINE subsets, but the costs associated with this form of access also restricted its use to a fairly limited group of larger institutions. Optical disc technology which offered the potential to provide the MEDLINE database to smaller organizations began to mature in the 1980's and finally came of age as a viable storage and distribution medium late in the decade. Given the rapid proliferation of such databases, the National Library of Medicine decided to conduct a comprehensive evaluation of MEDLINE products on compact disc during Spring, 1988, to assess the impact of the technology on end users and institutions.

To collect representative data on all of the compact disc products available, NLM invited 21 health sciences libraries to participate in the study. The McGoogan Library of Medicine, a large academic health sciences library at the University of Nebraska Medical Center (UNMC), was invited to test Dialog OnDisc, Version 2.11, of the MEDLINE database.

The McGoogan Library of Medicine has an active end user search population. Early in 1987 the Library installed an integrated library system using the LIS software developed at Georgetown University. In addition to the basic acquisition, cataloging, serial, and bibliographic utility modules, the library also installed a miniMEDLINE (TM) subset containing 12 month's references from 550 English language titles currently acquired by the library. Originally available from sixteen hardwired terminals in the library, the system later became available 24 hours a day on a dial-up basis to authorized Medical Center faculty, staff, and students. Because UNMC's miniMEDLINE system had been well received, the library had no plans to acquire a compact version of the MEDLINE database. However, the staff had followed the development of CD-ROM databases with interest and looked upon the invitation to participate in the study as an opportunity to learn about the new technology.

The evaluation team had many questions about compact disc retrieval systems but given that there was neither time nor resources to answer them all, decided to concentrate on comparing actual to perceived ease of use.

Given that the UNMC study involved two somewhat different evaluative components, it required the use of two separate methods. To gather data on perceived ease of use, the library surveyed users for subjective reactions to Dialog OnDisc, version 2.11, in effect, asking them how well they liked this particular compact disc database. Determining actual ease of use required a more objective method. To collect this data, the library conducted a controlled comparative test of the Dialog OnDisc and four other database interfaces.

Field Study Method

To collect data on perceived ease of use, the library conducted an unobtrusive field test designed to focus on user reactions to the Dialog OnDisc version of the MEDLINE database. Dialog OnDisc, Version 2.11, was installed on a dedicated microcomputer in the reference area and made available to end-users on a first-come, first-served basis during normal library hours. Walk-in users who tried the system were asked to complete a brief questionnaire describing themselves and their experience with Dialog OnDisc (Appendix A).

Individuals who tried the system pursued their own unique search topics. Although users were asked the purpose of the search, they were not required to divulge the subject. Time limits were not imposed, nor were sign up sheets required to use the workstation. The Dialog OnDisc quick reference card and user manual were available at the workstation. In addition, the Reference staff provided personal assistance if needed.

The questionnaire shown in Appendix A was formulated to collect information about participants and factors that could affect their ability to use the system. These factors included previous microcomputing experience, exposure to NLM indexes and databases, and their purpose in trying out the system.

Prior to the field test, both components of the evaluation project were promoted extensively using the campus newsletter, individual letters, and a poster designed to emphasize the study theme, "User Friendly? YOU Be the Judge!"

Controlled Test Method

UNMC's controlled test was designed to focus on measurable behaviors and required little subjective input on the part of participants. The controlled study attempted to compare actual ease of use for five different compact disc interfaces to the MEDLINE database.

The controlled test presented a number of design and logistic problems. The primary design problem involved insuring enough observations of each interface to allow for valid comparisons and conclusions. The study team elected to use a single measures design in which each participant performed only one trial of one product. This was done to prevent learning or practice results from obscuring product differences and making it difficult to tell whether interface characteristics or practice by the subjects were actually responsible for good performance. Although appropriate, obtaining large enough samples is always a challenge when using single measures designs. The study team set a goal of 250 observations to permit fifty on each of the five compact disc versions of MEDLINE being tested, but only obtained 129.

To allow for a fair test of the products involved, it was also necessary to place some constraints on user behavior. Information retrieval system users come to systems with many different information needs and problems, some more difficult than others. In order to prevent question characteristics from influencing study results, participants were asked to perform a preformulated search rather than one of their own. The preformulated search, referred to as a benchmark search, retrieved a single reference and was neither excessively difficult nor excessively easy to perform. However, it could be performed more efficiently if the participant had previous end user search experience and was familiar with Boolean operators.

The benchmark search was developed by searching for a common author name such as Smith or Brown for which it was assumed there would be a large set of postings, a set too awkward to review item by item. This effort produced the following reference:

The use of a single daily theophylline dose and metered-dose albuterol in asthma treatment

BUSSE WW; SMITH A; RUSH RK
J Allergy Clin Immunol
Oct 1986
78 (4 Pt 1) p577-82

The comparative study also placed another restriction on user behavior. To prevent some subjects from succeeding simply because they devoted unlimited time to the task, participants were allowed no more than 15 minutes to find and print the target reference.

To conduct the comparative study, the BRS, Compact Cambridge, Dialog, Ebsco Electronic Information and SilverPlatter versions of MEDLINE on compact disc, were mounted on identical equipment configurations and installed in one of the library's seminar rooms. A project assistant was hired to distribute and collect testing materials, time the participants, and generally monitor the testing room. The project assistant was specifically instructed not to answer questions or help subjects until their fifteen minute testing time had elapsed.

As each participant arrived in the testing room, he was logged in, asked to complete a brief questionnaire (Appendix B), and randomly assigned to one of the five workstations in the room in such a way that equal numbers of subjects were assigned to each workstation.

Although no effort was made to obscure the identity of the products being tested, the study team avoided visible labelling of the workstations. Instead, each compact disc system and the testing materials associated with it were color coded, allowing the project assistant to direct participants to the blue system, the green system, and so on.

Field Test Results

The field test was conducted from May through July, 1988. Ninety-four questionnaires were collected, forming the basis for this analysis. Actual usage of the Dialog OnDisc workstation was considerably higher given that many persons who participated in the field test chose not to fill out a questionnaire because they were not required to do so. For results, see Appendix A.

Participants

The majority of individuals that tested Dialog OnDisc described themselves as students or faculty at the University of Nebraska Medical Center. (Question 1) Clinicians—physicians, nurses, and other health professionals—

constituted the second largest group, representing slightly more than one-third of the users that responded. Although 25% indicated they had used Dialog OnDisc before, the majority (70/94) had not, suggesting that most were walk-in traffic to the library and therefore typical of users in an academic health sciences library. Approximately 10% of the respondents indicated they tried the workstation because they were "just curious" about it.

In terms of familiarity with the workstation hardware, 89 participants (95%) indicated they had previous experience with microcomputers and 63% characterized themselves as regular microcomputer users. Only five respondents had never used a microcomputer before. (Question 2)

Many had also had some exposure to NLM indexes and databases. (Question 6) Eighty percent had used the printed Index Medicus and somewhat more than half (54/94) had searched the UNMC subset for themselves. Another 18 were regular or occasional consumers of mediated searches. Forty of the 94 participants (43%) had never used UNMC's local miniMEDLINE (TM) subset, and approximately 19 appeared to be completely naive when it came to NLM indexes and databases (Question 8). Given that the local UNMC MEDLINE subset is free to authorized faculty, staff, and students, and is available on a dial-in basis, it was surprising that such a sizable group had not used it.

When asked about the purpose of their search, more than half the participants replied they were working on a research project. In fact, searching for references on research in progress out-numbered the next most frequent use, searching for information on patient care, by an almost four-to-one margin. Presentations and reports accounted for nearly equal numbers of use, and as noted earlier, a fair number of participants tried Dialog OnDisc simply because they were curious about it. (Question 4)

Search Characteristics

Most of the individuals that participated in the field test used Dialog OnDisc to search the database for articles on a specific subject. Although a few author, title, and journal searches were reported, the vast majority of participants (84%) did not attempt other approaches to the literature. (Question 3)

Only thirteen of the 94 participants pursued a search across three or more discs. Six participants pursued searches across all four. The total set of searches was divided almost evenly between those that required a single disc (45/93) and those that required removing one disc from the player and inserting another (48/93). Thus, almost half the persons who participated in the field test did not try to change discs. (Question 13)

Search Results

By and large, most field test participants indicated they were satisfied with Dialog OnDisc using a number of self-report measures. One of these was repeated usage, with one quarter of the participants reporting two or more searches and some as many as ten. Most users found what they were looking for in the database. Of the 94 recorded searches, 84% of the users indicated they found at least some or all of what they were seeking. Six percent reported finding more than they expected. Only six individuals replied that the information they retrieved was not useful. (Question 5)

Although one could assume that previous experience with NLM databases and indexes would contribute to search success, when viewed in relation to other variables, previous exposure to NLM indexes and databases appeared to have little effect on search results. Previous microcomputer experience is the one variable that did. By a 2-1 margin regular microcomputer users appeared to be more successful in finding what they wanted.

Perhaps the best measure of satisfaction with Dialog Ondisc is the fact that when asked which system they would use for their next bibliographic search, participants chose Dialog OnDisc by a four-to- one margin over all other forms of access combined, including the local subset. Having tried Dialog OnDisc, very few respondents— only fifteen indicated the would select another form of access.

Although most agreed that response time was adequate, there was less agreement about database coverage. When the study began, UNMC had only two discs covering the time period from January, 1986 through December, 1987. However, two additional discs were received before the field study was completed. Thus some respondents based their response to this question on partial database and others on the full database. Fifty-four percent found the coverage was adequate; twenty percent did not. The remaining 30% expressed no opinion, most probably because they satisfied their information needs with a single disc.

Perceived Ease of Use

The last seven questions of the survey form consisted of a rating scale that allowed users to comment on other aspects of the Dialog OnDisc package. Of the five questions that referred specifically to ease of use, 80 participants expressed very strong agreement with the statement that "Dialog OnDisc is very easy to use." Only six indicated they found the system difficult to use.

Although only half the respondents initiated a search that required changing discs, those who tried it (52/94) agreed it was easy to do, in part perhaps because the library had posted clear directions on the workstations after several mishaps. Only one respondent encountered difficulties changing discs.

Many participants (44/94) felt they needed little help in using the system. Of those who referred to the manual, 27 found it adequate; sixteen did not. Many apparently did not try to use the manual at all since 33 respondents gave neutral replies and 18 did not reply at all. Replies to the question about the help screens indicate that more participants referred to the help screens than printed aids.

Controlled Test Results

One hundred twenty-nine UNMC faculty, staff, and students participated in the controlled test, which was conducted from April 1 through April 29, 1988. Twenty-seven individuals were assigned to test the BRS retrieval system, 27 to Dialog OnDisc, 27 to Ebsco, and 28 to SilverPlatter. Only 20 observations were recorded using the Compact Cambridge system which malfunctioned during the third week of the study and could not be restored.

Participants

The 129 individuals that participated in the study classified themselves primarily as students and library staff in response to the question, "What is your profession?" Faculty members and nonhealth professionals constituted the next most sizable groups. (See question 1 on questionnaire in Appendix B.)

Participants were asked to report previous experience with microcomputers using a three-point nominal scale that differentiated between regular microcomputer users, occasional users, and individuals who had never used a microcomputer before. By an almost two-to-one margin, most of the participants in this study (80/129) described themselves as regular microcomputer users. Forty described themselves as occasional users, and nine had never used a microcomputer at all before attempting the benchmark search. (Question 2)

With respect to previous end-user search experience it was assumed that many study participants would already have had exposure to a machine readable version of the MEDLINE database, since the University of Nebraska Medical Center leases a MEDLINE subset. However, less than half the participants (62/129) had conducted an end-user search using the local subset. Twenty of the participants indicated they requested mediated searches, and 47 had never used the MEDLINE database at all before participating in the study. (Question 3)

A fair number of respondents (51/129) had both considerable microcomputer and end-user experience found by correlating question 2 and 3 of questionnaire. Table 1 shows the relationship between microcomputing and previous MEDLINE experience among the sample. It was assumed that these individuals would have some degree of success with the bench mark search given their familiarity with the keyboard and function keys, grasp of boolean operators, and familiarity with the MEDLINE database.

Search Results

As noted earlier, the objective of the controlled study was to determine whether users could find and print a target reference within 15 minutes regardless of which retrieval system they used to search the MEDLINE database. Less than half the study participants (60/129) were actually able to do so. Sixty-nine individual tried but failed to complete the benchmark search.

TABLE 1
MICROCOMPUTING AND END USE EXPERIENCE
OF CONTROLLED TEST PARTICIPANTS

Use of Microcomputing Equipment

PREVIOUS EXPOSURE TO MEDLINE	Regular	Occasional	None	Total
End-User	51	10	1	62
Mediated Use	8	11	2	21
No Reported Use	21	198	6	46
TOTAL	80	40	9	129

In attempting to determine why some users could not complete the benchmark search, the possible effect of user characteristics on search results was considered. As noted, it was assumed that previous experience with MEDLINE would have a positive effect on ability to complete the benchmark search. However such an effect was not visible (Table 3).

TABLE 2
EFFECT OF MICROCOMPUTING EXPERIENCE
ON BENCHMARK SEARCH RESULTS

| | COMPLETED SEARCH | | |
	YES	NO	TOTAL
PREVIOUS MICROCOMPUTING EXPERIENCE			
Regular User	46	34	80
Occasional User	12	28	40
No Previous Experience	2	7	9
TOTAL	60	69	129

TABLE 3

EFFECT OF MEDLINE EXPERIENCE ON
BENCHMARK SEARCH RESULTS

SEARCH COMPLETED?

PREVIOUS MEDLINE USE	YES	NO	Total
Own Search	33	29	62
Mediated Search	10	10	20
Never Searched	17	30	47
Total	60	69	129

As shown in Table 2, microcomputing experience did seem to account for some of the differences in search results.

In summary, by a small margin, regular microcomputer users appeared more likely than occasional or naive users to succeed in completing the benchmark search. Occasional users were twice as likely to fail as to succeed, and those who had no previous microcomputing experience failed by a three-to-one ratio. Looking at this table, it appears that the level of success did rise among participants that had previous microcomputing or MEDLINE experience, although previous microcomputing experience was no guarantee of success.

The combined effect of these variables is examined in Table 4. This table shows the respective distributions of success and failure for users with varying degrees of microcomputing and MEDLINE end-user experience. Had these variables had an additive effect, the cell frequency for successful regular end-users would have been much higher. In studying these distributions, it is obvious that for every experienced end-user that tried the benchmark search and succeeded, another failed.

Interface Characteristics

Only after the possible effect of user characteristics on search results had been examined was the interface difference considered. Table 5 shows the distribution of success and failures by compact disc product.

TABLE 4

EFFECT OF MICROCOMPUTING
AND MEDLINE EXPERIENCE ON SEARCH RESULTS

A. ABLE TO COMPLETE BENCHMARK SEARCH

Previous Microcomputing Experience

	Regular	Occasional	None	Total
End User	29	4	0	33
Mediated Use	5	4	1	10
No Reported Use	13	3	1	17
Total	47	11	2	60

B. UNABLE TO COMPLETE BENCHMARK SEARCH

Use of Microcomputing Equipment

	Regular	Occasional	None	Total
End User	22	6	1	29
Mediated Use	3	6	1	10
No Reported Use	9	16	5	30
Total	34	28	7	69

TABLE 5

RELATIONSHIP BETWEEN PRODUCT
INTERFACE AND BENCHMARK SEARCH RESULTS

SEARCH COMPLETED?

SYSTEM	YES	NO*	TOTAL
BRS	19	8	27
Compact Cambridge	13	7	20
Dialog	12	15	27
Ebsco	9	8	27
SilverPlatter	7	21	28
TOTAL	60	69	129

* On all systems these negative results were often affected by the
difficulties encountered in *printing* the reference after retrieving it.
(See comments in *Discussion* section of this paper.)

More BRS and Compact Cambridge users were successful in searching than were unsuccessful. For every participant that searched Dialog successfully, one tried it and failed. For every user that searched Ebsco successfully, two failed; and for every user that successfully searched SilverPlatter, three others failed.

As previously noted, the results suggest that previous microcomputing and MEDLINE end-user experience were not good predictors of search results. The distribution of users by type was also checked. (Table 6). With few exceptions, the distribution appeared to be random. The fact that no nurse was assigned to test Compact Cambridge appears to be a function of small sample size. Nurses who did participate were for the most part evenly assigned to other systems. There was some clustering of Other Health Professionals to Dialog and BRS. None of this subgroup tested SilverPlatter.

Librarians clustered to BRS and were highly successful in using this product.

TABLE 6

DISTRIBUTION OF CONTROLLED TEST PARTICIPANTS
TO PRODUCT INTERFACES

SYSTEM NAME

USER TYPE	SILVER PLATTER	EBSCO	DIALOG	BRS	COMPACT CAMBRIDGE	TOTAL
Nurse	2	2	2	1	0	7
Physician	3	1	2	1	1	8
Other Health Prof.	0	1	4	4	1	10
Faculty	4	4	2	1	6	17
Librarian	6	7	6	10	2	31
Student	9	10	6	7	7	39
Other	4	2	5	3	3	17
TOTAL	28	27	27	27	20	129

Discussion

Based on this evaluation, the field test indicates that perceived ease of use for MEDLINE on compact disc is high. The University of Nebraska Medical Center began its study of Dialog OnDisc with one loaned workstation and quickly purchased another of its own despite the fact that it leases and operates a local MEDLINE subset. Both compact disc workstations and the local subset terminals received constant use. Among researchers, who constituted the most frequent compact disc user group at University of Nebraska Medical Center, the large Dialog OnDisc database proved to be an attraction. The Dialog OnDisc database contained almost five years worth of references from all indexed Index Medicus titles as opposed to the local subset's approximately 12 months of references from 550 titles purchased by the library.

The results of UNMC's comparative study suggest that many of the existing CD interfaces to the MEDLINE database do not facilitate successful searches especially for first time users. Slightly more than half the controlled study participants could not complete a simple search and print the retrieved reference.

One of the most common problems involved changing the compact discs. This problem can be solved in several ways, one of which is to post clear and simple instructions listing sequence of actions to be taken in several visible places near the workstation. Most users do not consult manuals for this information, but guess or experiment, sometimes with unfortunate results. As multiple disc drives become more available, changing discs will become less of a problem.

The comparative test revealed one inherent design flaw that was common to all the compact disc systems tested. With few exceptions users found print instructions confusing whether they were menu or function key driven. For all of the products tested during this study, some participants were able to locate the target reference but unable to print it. Many specifically commented on this interface feature afterwards, suggesting that compact disc distributors may need to devote more attention to this aspect of their interfaces.

The evaluation test identified several product specific problems unique to Dialog OnDisc, version 2.11. Both evaluative methods indicated that some users did not understand the Easy Menu instruction "F10 when done," which creates sets of postings and activates Boolean operators. After it was explained to them, they seldom found it a problem. The instruction may need to be rephrased.

During both tests, a number of participants selected the Dialog command search mode, either inadvertently or deliberately and did not know how to exit or escape from it. This was one of the most identifiable causes of failure during the controlled study. While it is not a problem that should discourage any institution from purchasing Dialog OnDisc, any library that does buy Dialog OnDisc should be sure that every staff member recognizes the Dialog command search prompt (?) and knows how to enter the LOGOFF command. This is especially important in public service areas where one frustrated user can walk away and leave the terminal "locked up" for others.

The University of Nebraska Medical Center also experienced other terminal lock ups that were not associated with the command search mode. These tended to occur while Easy Menu users were reviewing search results and produced a "Fatal Error No. 7" message. Most users had no idea how to free up the terminal and the only thing the staff could often do was reboot the workstation, losing the search in the process. Dialog Information Services has corrected this problem in later versions of the interface.

Conclusion

Although the UNMC study has some limitations, it did accomplish what it was designed to do — compare actual to perceived ease of use of compact

MEDLINE databases in an objective way. In retrospect, the study design could have been improved in a number of ways.

With respect to the field test, the participant questionnaire could be revised to differentiate more clearly between classes or types of users. Although many users at an academic health sciences center fill multiple roles, determining a primary responsibility is important. Some categories were not mutually exclusive and did not allow us to differentiate sufficiently between types of users.

The field test questionnaire should also have given users more of an opportunity to explain in their own words what they liked and did not like about Dialog OnDisc. The study design was almost too objective in this sense.

The comparative study accomplished only half of what it was hoped it would do. It did not provide specific diagnostic information identifying why products were difficult to use. An effort to record search transcripts, which would have allowed the study team to reconstruct this information, had to be abandoned for lack of time and resources.

Based on the results of the field study, MEDLINE on compact disc does provide a cost-effective alternative for any library considering an end user search system. Many end users enjoy being able to search for themselves and found Dialog OnDisc's extensive database—five years' coverage of all indexed titles—a real attraction. Quite frankly, University of Nebraska Medical Center was not prepared for the enthusiastic reception Dialog OnDisc received on campus.

The fact that nearly fifty percent of the controlled test participants succeeded in completing the benchmark search should be considered encouraging. Most users will become better searchers with experience and familiarity, so it is important not to generalize the findings of the controlled study too far.

Finally, any library that is considering a compact disc retrieval system is well advised to compare the available products before making a decision. It is important to develop several local benchmark searches and try them consistently on each product that is being considered for purchase. This type of informal evaluation will allow a realistic comparison of product features and help insure that the library selects a product that is well suited to its own user clientele.

DIALOG ON-DISC EVALUATION

Instructions

This MEDLINE CD-ROM Dialog OnDisc system is being tested by the McGoogan Library of Medicine. We would like you to fill out this questionnaire in order to help us find out who is using the system, and how useful it is for you. Thank you!

1. What is your profession: (Check all that apply) n=94

    __20__ Physician   21%

    __6__   Nurse   6%

    __8__   Other Health Professional   9%

    __14__ Faculty   15%

    __1__   Computing Services   1%

    __2__   Librarian/Information Specialist   2%

    __34__ Student   36%

    __9__   Other   10%

2. Have you had previous experience with microcomputers: n=94
    (Check one)

    __59__ Use regularly   63%

    __30__ Slight experience   32%

    __5__   No experience   5%

3. I was looking for articles: (Check one) n=94

    __8__   by an author   9%

    __5__   under a title   5%

    __79__ on a subject   84%

    __1__   in a journal   1%

    __1__   other   1%

4. I needed the information for: (Check one) n=94

   12   patient care   13%

   7   a paper or report   7%

   49   a research project   52%

   3   keeping current   3%

   4   to check a reference   4%

   1   teaching/planning a course   1%

   8   a presentation   9%

   8   not needed, just curious   9%

   2   no response   2%

5. The information I found was: (Check one) n=94

   50   what I was looking for   54%

   6   more than I needed   6%

   25   some of what I needed   27%

   6   not useful   6%

   3   other   3%

   4   no response   4%

6. Have you used any other printed publications produced from the MEDLINE system (e.g. Index Medicus, the International Nursing Index, and the Index to Dental Literature)? (Check one) n=94

   75   yes   14   no   3   don't know   2   no response

7. If you answered yes to question 6, how do they compare to Dialog OnDisc MEDLINE? (Check one) n=75

   15   easier to use   20%

   40   harder to use   53%

   17   about the same to use   23%

   2   other   3%

   1   no response   1%

8. Have you used an online version of MEDLINE (either running the search yourself or by having a librarian process a search for you)? (Check all that apply) n=94

    __54__ yes, by myself using the LEON MiniMEDLINE system   57%

    __18__ yes, librarian search   19%

    __20__ no   21%

    __1__ don't know   1%

    1 no response   1%

9. If you answered yes to question 9 which system do you prefer? n=72

    __13__ online, own search using the LEON MiniMEDLINE system   18%

    __49__ Dialog OnDisc MEDLINE   68%

    __4__ online, librarian search   6%

    __4__ don't know   6%

    2 no response   2%

10. Next time you want to do a search from the library what will you do? (Check one) n=94

    __76__ try Dialog OnDisc MEDLINE   82%

    __2__ try a printed version   2%

    __6__ use the LEON MiniMEDLINE system   6%

    __4__ try an online version   4%

    __3__ try another source   3%

    3 no response   3%

11. Dialog OnDisc MEDLINE is provided free of charge to library users. How important a consideration was this in your decision to use this system instead of an online version of MEDLINE. (Check one only) n=94

    __54__ very important   58%

    __21__ somewhat important   22%

    __10__ relatively important   11%

    __5__ would not have used an online version of MEDLINE   5%

    4 no response   4%

12. How often have you used Dialog OnDisc MEDLINE? n=94

   __70__ first time   __10__ 3 - 5 times   11%

   __3__ once before   __10__ 6 or more times   11%
                           1   no response   1%

13. Dialog OnDisc MEDLINE contains material on two discs covering two years. How many discs did you use today? n=94

   __45__ 1 disc   __35__ 2 discs   _7_ 3 discs _6_ 4 discs   1 no resp.=1%

Using the 5 point scale, answer the following questions using only one number.

SCALE: 1   2   3   4   5
           Strongly   Agree   Neutral   Disagree   Strongly
            Agree   Disagree

14. Dialog OnDisc is very easy to use. _____

15. The rate at which the computer responds is satisfactory. ___

16. The Dialog OnDisc manual helped me use the system. _____

17. Changing MEDLINE discs was easy. _____

18. The time span covered by Dialog OnDisc MEDLINE was sufficient for my needs. _____

19. The online help screens were very helpful. _____

20. A new user needs additional help beyond the manual to search Dialog OnDisc MEDLINE. _____

Appendix B

CD-ROM COMPARATIVE TESTING QUESTIONNAIRE

These MEDLINE on CD-ROM programs are being tested by the McGoogan Library of Medicine. We would like you to fill out the following questionnaire before completing the assigned search. Thank you!!

1. What is your profession: (Check one) n=129

__8__	Physician	6%
__7__	Nurse	5%
__10__	Other Health Professional	8%
__17__	Faculty	13%
__0__	Computing Services	
__31__	Librarian/Information Specialist	24%
__40__	Student	31%
__16__	Other	13%

2. Have you had previous experience with microcomputers: n=129 (Check one)

__80__	Use regularly	62%
__40__	Slight experience	31%
__9__	No experience	7%

3. Have you used an online version of MEDLINE (either running the search yourself or by having a librarian process a search for you)? (Check all that apply) n=129

__62__	yes, by myself	48%
__20__	yes, librarian search	16%
__47__	no	36%
__0__	don't know	

4. How many computer searches did you do last week?

__82__	None	64%
__34__	1 - 5	26%
__5__	5 - 10	4%
__8__	More than 10	6%

LM-31 (3/88)

290

EVALUATION REPORTS OF

BiblioMed AND
CAMBRIDGE
CD-ROM

AT OREGON HEALTH SCIENCES
UNIVERSITY LIBRARY

By Millard F. Johnson Jr.
Leslie Wykoff
Derrin Arnett

Oregon Health Sciences
University Library
3181 S. W. Sam Jackson Park Road
Portland, Oregon 97201

EVALUATION REPORTS OF BIBLIOMED AND CAMBRIDGE CD-ROM AT OREGON HEALTH SCIENCES UNIVERSITY LIBRARY

Introduction

Between March 14, 1988 and June 1, 1988 the Oregon Health Sciences University Library conducted a formal evaluation of the BiblioMed CD-ROM MEDLINE retrieval system.

The OHSU Library had the advantage that it had previously conducted a formal but less rigorous evaluation of the Compact Cambridge CD-MEDLINE system. We modified NLM's suggested survey instrument based on our earlier study and our conception of the role we expect the CD-MEDLINE system to play.

In our earlier evaluation we tested whether a CD-MEDLINE system could be used by students, faculty and staff without a training program and without intervention by staff. Because our earlier results had been positive we assumed that the system could be used without training and we focused our study on determining user satisfaction and system performance.

This research was performed at the request of, and with the support of the National Library of Medicine. Our objective in evaluating was to assess the utility of the BiblioMed CD-MEDLINE system at the Oregon Health Sciences University (OHSU) Library. The OHSU Library is a medium-sized health sciences library subscribing to approximately 2400 periodicals. It serves graduate schools of Medicine and Nursing and is part of a larger health sciences center complex that includes a teaching hospital, a VA medical center, and a School of Dentistry. A branch library serving the School of Dentistry is removed from the main library.

BiblioMed Evaluation

The BiblioMed CD-ROM work station was located in a small "end-user" room off of the lobby of the library but near the reference department, the circulation department and the printed literature indexes. A person working in the end-user room is not visible to librarians working in the reference department. The CD-MEDLINE work station was equipped with a Televideo computer, dot matrix printer, single drive CD player, and three years of the BiblioMed MEDLINE subset. A poster above the computer advised users that the system contained only a 1985-87 subset of 500 clinical journals indexed in MEDLINE and asked patrons to inquire at the reference desk if they had any questions. Librarians would "drop in" occasionally during searches and would provide assistance when asked, but essentially the system was available "self-service" and without training during all of the hours the library was open.

We advertised the availability of the system by flyers around campus, several notices in CampusGram, (a weekly institutional newsletter), an announcement on INFONET (the campus electronic mail system), a large poster beside the circulation desk, and a personal letter to department heads and key faculty members.

The survey itself and the survey tally are shown in Appendix A. The survey instrument is based on our earlier study and on the sample questionnaire prepared by NLM and it was pretested before the beginning of the investigation.

Our earlier experience had indicated that many users would not complete a questionnaire unless someone were "standing over" the work station. To circumvent this problem we elected to passively collect some data from every user, as part of the logon process but to carefully administer the full formal survey only on 11 selected days. On these sample days the user was required to enter a password before gaining access to the system. To learn the password, the user had to go to the circulation desk and get a survey with the password written on it. The password was different on each sample day. (See Appendix B for report on Log of Use from Menu Program.)

Results

(Please refer to Appendix A for the raw scores from which this discussion is drawn.)

The Users

More than 50% of the sample set of users cited MEDICINE as their primary affiliation. Thirty percent listed OTHER. Comments indicated that the other were from Pharmacology, graduate department of biochemistry, patient and other populations. About three-fourths of all sample users were about equally divided among the professional affiliations of physician, scientist/researcher and students.

Nature of Activity

About 75% of all searches were by subject with author searching being the only other significant searching at 17% of the total. Nearly 40% of the subjects indicated they would use the results of the MEDLINE search in relation to their research. The remainder was distributed between educational and clinical uses. Sixteen percent of the uses were for patient care and another 16% intended to use the results in preparation of a paper or report.

Several questions were designed to test whether the search was effective or not. One question asked whether the subject found what they were looking for. Only 18% indicated that the information was either not useful or they could not find what was needed. Forty percent said that they found some of what they needed and another 42% indicated that they found either what they were looking for or more than they needed.

In a question on the OHSU survey that was not suggested by the NLM, subjects were asked how many citations their search retrieved and how many of these were relevant. Seventy-three percent of searches reported were successful in that they produced some output but less than 100 citations. In those reports where both the number of citations retrieved and the number relevant were reported (n=28), the mean number of citations retrieved was 29.61 and the mean number relevant was 12.89. Therefore 43.55% of the citations retrieved were relevant.

Searching Experience

The sample subjects were fairly experienced in using the index products produced by the NLM. Almost 90% of them had used the print-based products of the NLM. More than 50% had had MEDLINE searches done by their librarian and nearly 35% had done their own MEDLINE searching. Better than 69% of these users were either uncertain (25%), or preferred BiblioMed to any other search option. Significantly, fewer people prefer to do their own MEDLINE searching than have experience doing it. Apparently some people who search MEDLINE directly, through BRS or by using GRATEFUL MED prefer the CD-ROM access. Also significantly, less than 6% of searchers prefer to have the library do their MEDLINE searching for them even though more than 50% have had the library do MEDLINE searching for them in the past.

The favorable assessment of BiblioMed is due in part to its performance and in part to the quality and accessibility of alternatives. If BiblioMed were not available, 50% would have done a manual search and another 30% would have paid to do the search online themselves or had a librarian do it for them.

Price seems to have been a major factor in this assessment. The OHSU Library charges its clients the full "out of pocket" costs. Persons who are not primary clientele of the library are charged an additional surcharge to cover part of the overhead of conducting searches. More than 87% indicated that price (free) was either somewhat or very important in their choice of Biblio-Med. For whatever reason BiblioMed CD-ROM is remarkably satisfactory to users and more than 66% of subjects report that the next time they need information they would choose BiblioMed over the printed version (8%), online access (library and self) 20% and all other sources (6%).

BiblioMed Interface

Six questions attempted to ascertain the subjects' perception of the quality of BiblioMed as an information product. The subjects were asked to rate the quality of instructions on the BiblioMed screens, response time, instruction manual, and size and coverage of the database. The last question inquired into the overall ease of use of BiblioMed.

The relatively small size of the sample (n=50) and the scatter of responses among the three mid-range ranking (agree, neutral, and disagree) make it difficult to come to any firm conclusions. This probably reflects very different levels of experience on the part of the subject population but the lack of a bulge at either extreme (strongly agree and strongly disagree) probably reflects our intuitive feeling that users see BiblioMed as very good but could be better still.

Only 15% of our subjects felt that BiblioMed screens were insufficient. Another 22% felt that the response time was unsatisfactory while 62% felt it was satisfactory. More than 50% of the subjects felt that the 3 year time span was insufficient but more than 50% felt that the database consisting of only 500 journals was sufficient.

Finally, only 15% of our sample subjects would disagree with the statement that "Overall, you found BiblioMed easy to use."

Conclusion

BiblioMed would be an effective tool in a medium-sized health sciences library in a university setting. It is useful for patient care, research, education and current awareness. It can be used by all classes of users without significant instruction. We feel that the characteristics of the MEDLINE subset covered by BiblioMed suggest that it is a better tool for clinical than research applications. It also lacks significant nursing journals. Perhaps the greatest benefit of BiblioMed in the health sciences center environment, which is not obvious, is that it will relieve the reference staff of the burden of conducting simple searches, thus allowing them to concentrate on personalized services and more difficult reference transactions.

Our one fear is that patrons finding some information by using the BiblioMed system will make the false assumption that they have conducted a thorough and exhaustive search of the biomedical literature. This suggests that an educational effort directed at the library's clients to instruct them, not in how to use the system, but in when to use BiblioMed and when to use other, more appropriate tools, is imperative.

Compact Cambridge Evaluation

The Oregon Health Sciences University Medical Library conducted a one-month test of Cambridge Scientific Abstracts Compact MEDLINE system during the month of December 1987.

We were interested to know whether the system could be used successfully by medical school students, faculty and staff without a training program and without intervention by library staff.

System availability was announced in the campus newspaper, on posters around campus, over the campus electronic mail network and by letter to department heads. The system was set up in an "end-user searching" room near, but not visible from the reference office.

Only one station was available and it was equipped with an IBM XT computer, dot matrix printer, CD-drive and one year of the English language MEDLINE subset. A poster above the computer advised users that the system contained only one year of the data base and asked patrons to go to the reference office for a complete search. Librarians would "drop in" occasionally during searches and would provide assistance when asked, but essentially the system was available "self-service" and without training during all of the hours the library was open.

We began the test with a work station consisting of hardware, CD-ROM database, and a single copy of the product description provided by Cambridge. Due to demand for better "help" we tore apart the product announcement and stapled it to a thick poster board with the major sections shingled and highlighted as our printed help aid. We also made available a complete set of the MeSH subject headings from the National Library of Medicine.

A number of copies of an evaluation form and a collection box for completed forms was placed on the table that held hardware, MeSH and documentation.

Results

An evaluation form consisting of six questions was available next to the CD work station. Ninety questionnaires were analyzed. The form was not pretested so the data shown should be taken as indicative only. The following cautions should be remembered.

Question 1.

Forty-five persons claimed to have some experience doing their own MEDLINE searching. It may be that, for some users, "doing your own MEDLINE search" is interpreted as asking a reference librarian to do a search for them. In any case, over one-half of the users have no end-user searching experience.

Question 2.

For more than three-fourths of the users of the system this was their first searching experience with the Cambridge CD system. Only 6 users used the system more than twice and only one user used it more than 3 times.

The respondents were, then, relatively novice searchers.

Question 3.

About 25% of all searches were conducted in less than 20 minutes. All but about 5% of searches were conducted in an hour or less. While we have no solid evidence to this effect, we observe that most of the short searches were done by curious browsers while content-producing searches by novice users are closer to the hour figure.

Question 4.

Figures show that almost 40 of 90 users needed some help. This figure is misleading. Comments in the margin of the evaluation form about needing help occasionally say - "Yes, a little at first" or "Someone already using the system got me started". While a few a people faulted the lack of help and some help aid is clearly needed, most people got on quite well with surprisingly little assistance.

Question 5.

About 90% of the people who used the system were able to find useful information. Considering the time invested in training and searching this is really remarkably good performance.

Question 6.

Sixty-one of 90 users gave the system the highest possible rating on a 1 to 10 scale. This rating would have been even higher except that the form was improperly designed with 1 being the highest rating. Even though the meanings of the rating scale were clearly stated (1=MUST HAVE and 10=NOT IMPORTANT) some users obviously did not read the rating labels and assumed that 10 was high. Where this was obvious from context (eg., a user rates the system 10 and comments "This is a great system.") we substituted the superlative score, but some of the '8' scores at the negative end of the scale should probably have been at the superlative end of the scale.

Conclusion

Clearly, end-users love this system. It is so much better than thumbing through bound volumes of *Index Medicus* and is viewed as a remarkable advancement. There are, however, some things that can be done immediately to improve it. These are (in our perceived order of priority):

1. Produce good, brief printed help.

We suspect that there is a different set of help needs for experienced users but for novice users simple printed directions are badly needed.

2. Include more years of the database on a single search station. We did not tell users that they could swap discs and we believe that if the data base must spill over to different discs it is better to have multiple stations than to have users swapping discs.

3. Redesign the software as it relates to searching the MeSH major subject heading and "anding" current and previously done searches.

4. Provide print spooling

5. More flexibility in printing specific citations

Recommendations

Based on our observations and the comments of test users, the Cambridge Scientific Abstracts MEDLINE CD search system can be highly recommended. Our investigation was to determine whether the system was useful as an "unattended" end-user terminal. It clearly is both extremely useful to novice end-users and highly appreciated by them. The modest improvements which we assume will be forthcoming from Cambridge are only the "icing on the cake". In our opinion, a user-friendly, end-user accessible MEDLINE subset system should be VERY high on the priority list for any medical library.

Appendix A-1

```
                    BiblioMed SURVEY TALLY
                       July 22, 1988


1.  YOUR PRIMARY AFFILIATION IS:            #
                                        RESPONSES      %

    a. Medicine                            25        54.3%
    b. Dentistry                            0          .0%
    c. Nursing                              4         8.7%
    d. Allied health                        2         4.3%
    e. Pharmacy                             1         2.2%
    e. Other                               14        30.4%
    n=                                     46


2.  YOUR PROFESSION IS:

    a. Physician                           13        25.0%
    b. Nurse                                3         5.8%
    c. Dentist                              0          .0%
    D. Other health pro                     4         7.7%
    e. educator                             1         1.9%
    f. Scientist/researcher                14        26.9%
    g. Student                             11        21.2%
    h. Librarian                            1         1.9%
    i. Other                                5         9.6%
    n=                                     52


3.  YOU WERE LOOKING FOR ARTICLES:

    a. By an author                        10        17.2%
    b. By title                             0          .0%
    c. On a subject                        44        75.9%
    d. in a journal code                    3         5.2%
    n=                                      1         1.7%
                                           58


4.  YOU NEEDED THE INFORMATION FOR:

    a. Patient care                         9        16.1%
    b. A paper or report                    9        16.1%
    c. A research project                  21        37.5%
    d. Keeping current                      6        10.7%
    e. To check a reference                 0          .0%
    f. Teaching/planning a course           5         8.9%
    g. Just curious                         3         5.4%
    h. Other                                3         5.4%
    n=                                     56


5.  THE INFORMATION YOU FOUND WAS:

    a. What you were looking for           16        32.0%
    b. More than you needed                 5        10.0%
    c. Some of what you needed             20        40.0%
    d. Not useful                           1         2.0%
    e. You could not find what you need     8        16.0%
    f. Other                                0          .0%
    n=                                     50
```

(QUESTIONS SIX AND SEVEN FROM NLM QUESTIONNAIRE NOT INCLUDED)

8. HAVE YOU USED ANY OF THE PRINTED PUBLICATIONS PRODUCED
FROM THE MEDLINE SYSTEM?

a. Yes	40	88.9%
b. No	5	11.1%
c. Don't know	0	.0%
n=	45	

9. IF YES, HOW DO THEY COMPARE WITH BiblioMed?

a. Printed are easier to use	4	12.1%
b. Printed are harder to use	19	57.6%
c. About the same	7	21.2%
d. Other	3	9.1%
n=	33	

10. HAVE YOU EVER USED ONLINE VERSION OF MEDLINE?

a. Yes, self	16	34.0%
b. Yes, librarian	24	51.1%
c. no	6	12.8%
d. don't know	1	2.1%
n=	47	

11. WHICH SYSTEM DO YOU PREFER?

a. MEDLINE etc.	9	25.0%
b. BiblioMed	16	44.4%
c. Done by library	2	5.6%
e. Don't know	9	25.0%
n=	36	

12. IF CD-ROM WERE NOT AVAILABLE, WHAT WOULD YOU DO?

a. Printed version	26	50.0%
b. Online version	7	13.5%
c. Ask library staff	8	15.4%
d. Ask friend/colleague	1	1.9%
e. Browsed stacks	4	7.7%
f. Nothing	4	7.7%
g. Other	2	3.8%
n=	52	

13. NEXT TIME YOU NEED INFORMATION, WHAT WOULD YOU DO?

a. Try BiblioMed again	34	66.7%
b. Printed version	4	7.8%
c. Online version	10	19.6%
d. Another source	3	5.9%
n=	51	

14. FREE OF CHARGE - HOW IMPORTANT?

a. Very	27	67.5%
b. Somewhat	8	20.0%
C. Relatively unimportant	4	10.0%
d. Would not have used	1	2.5%
n=	40	

Appendix A-3

15. HOW OFTEN DID YOU USE BiblioMed?

     a. First time   18   43.9%
     b. Once before   11   26.8%
     c. 3-5 times   8   19.5%
     d. 6 or more   4   9.8%
     n=   41

16. BiblioMed INSTRUCTION SCREENS WERE SUFFICIENT

     a. Strongly agree   12   27.9%
     b. Agree   19   44.2%
     c. Neutral   5   11.6%
     d. Disagree   5   11.6%
     e. Strongly disagree   2   4.7%
     n=   43

17. SPEED OF RESPONSE WAS SATISFACTORY

     a. Strongly agree   5   11.1%
     b. Agree   23   51.1%
     c. Neutral   7   15.6%
     d. Disagree   7   15.6%
     e. Strongly disagree   3   6.7%
     n=   45

18. THE MANUAL WAS USEFUL

     a. Strongly agree   1   2.6%
     b. Agree   15   38.5%
     c. Neutral   14   35.9%
     d. Disagree   8   20.5%
     e. Strongly disagree   1   2.6%
     n=   39

19. THE TIME SPAN (3 YEARS) WAS SUFFICIENT?

     a. Strongly agree   3   6.7%
     b. Agree   14   31.1%
     c. Neutral   5   11.1%
     d. Disagree   19   42.2%
     e. Strongly disagree   4   8.9%
     n=   45

20. COVERAGE OF THE DATABASE (500 JOURNALS) WAS SUFFICIENT

     a. Strongly agree   7   15.6%
     b. Agree   16   35.6%
     c. Neutral   5   11.1%
     d. Disagree   14   31.1%
     e. Strongly disagree   3   6.7%
     n=   45

21. BiblioMed WAS EASY TO USE?

     a. Strongly agree   11   24.4%
     b. Agree   22   48.9%
     c. Neutral   6   13.3%
     d. Disagree   4   8.9%
     e. Strongly disagree   3   6.7%
     n=   45

Log of Use From Menu Program

The versions of Bibliomed that we received for demonstration
purposes (2.00-2.02) consisted of separate programs for searching
the database and for doing the accompanying tutorial. In order
to provide patrons with easy access to both the search program
and the tutorial we developed a MENU PROGRAM that would present
those choices and then activate the selected program. In
addition, the menu program provided us with the opportunity to
obtain some USAGE INFORMATION on the programs. Finally, on pre-
selected dates, the menu program allowed us to require the user
to ENTER A PASSWORD in order to gain access to the search
program.

MENU PROGRAM

The menu program was written in BASIC and used the SHELL command
to load a secondary command processor and execute the user's
program choice. Using a menu program written in BASIC allowed us
a greater amount of control, security, and flexibility than would
have been available using a simple batch file. In addition, our
initial hardware configuration included a color monitor: BASIC
provided us with the means to construct a color scheme that
matched that provided by Bibliomed in its menus. The menu
program was included in a batch file that was called from the
computer's AUTOEXEC.BAT file. Following an exit from the menu
program,the batch file executed itself, creating a loop.

The initial menu displayed two options: the tutorial program and
the search program. A user could select the desired option by
entering the number corresponding to that option on the list.
Two hidden options were also available at this menu, one
providing for orderly shutdown of the system, the other providing
a maintenance exit. The former option was used by the night
staff prior to turning off the system. The program would close
its files and then park the heads on the hard disk drive. The
latter option was used for maintenance tasks such as data file
back-ups, listing the data file to hard copy, and exit to the
BASIC program editor for program changes.

USAGE INFORMATION

Selecting either the tutorial or the search program option would
present the user with two items prior to execution of the
selected program. Explanatory text would appear, followed by a
list of user categories (see end of table B-3). For the search
program, the user was required to enter a letter from the user
category list; the tutorial option allowed entry of only a
carriage return if the user wished to escape back to the initial
menu. The indicated user category, along with information on the
current date, time, and program selected, were then written to a
data file. Once the user information had been saved, the selected
program was executed.

ENTER A PASSWORD

A set of dates was chosen on which users would be asked to complete a questionnaire. A paper questionnaire was selected as the way to solicit feedback rather than an online questionnaire. In order to bring user and questionnaire together, we required the user to enter a password on those dates to gain access to the search program. The password prompt indicated to the user that the password could be obtained, along with the questionnaire, at the nearby Circulation desk. The password was written at the top of the questionnaire and was different for each of the selected dates. The list of dates and passwords was kept in a data file that was checked by the menu program during start-up. Entry of an incorrect password, or attempts to bypass the prompt with either a carriage return or control-C/control-break simply returned the user to the initial menu. Password checking was not case-sensitive.

Once in the search or tutorial programs, users would proceed as normal for those activities. The tutorial program would automatically terminate upon completion, allowing control to pass back to the library's menu program. The search program, however, did not automatically terminate. In practice, we had to rely upon users to recall the instructions at the program's entrance or to read the sign on the computer reminding them to use the quit option when done with searching. This was not a very reliable approach, made less so by the inclusion of an extra option menu in later versions of Bibliomed.

INFORMATION EXTRACTED

We wrote a second brief program, also in BASIC, that read the user characteristics data file and produced some summary descriptions. These summaries included: a day-by-day listing of the total number of users of each of the tutorial and search programs, including both a sub-total for each month and a final total for the entire demonstration period[1]; totals for each program used by class of user; totals for each program used by class of user by day of the week; and a figure that attempts to determine the number of times a user took the tutorial and then executed the search program.

In order to develop a figure that would describe the approximate number of occasions on which an individual used the tutorial and then used the search program, we assumed that a sequence of "tutorial use followed by search use" when both were done by an

---

[1] Tables follow and appear mostly as produced by the processing program except for the table numbering. The sensitivity values table (B-4) was constructed here from values produced by separate runs of the program. The day-by-day summary listing was not included.

individual of the same user category and within a given amount of time ("sensitivity value") represented an instance of an individual using both programs.[2] The magnitude of the "sensitivity value" can be set before the program processes the user characteristics file. In outline form, this filter appears as follows:

```
IF the tutorial program was used
    THEN IF the next program used was the search program
    AND  the next user was from the same class of user
         as the user of the tutorial program
    AND  that search program use occurred within a speci-
         fied number of minutes of the tutorial program
         use
         THEN count the pair of events as an instance of
              the same user taking the tutorial then going
              directly to the search program.
```

Results for different magnitudes of the sensitivity factor appear in table B-4.

It is well to keep in mind when looking at the tables that we did not have a highly-effective means available to ensure that each and every use of the BiblioMed programs was logged. Patron compliance with instructions together with informal staff monitoring lead to a higher proportion of users being logged between approximately 8:00 a.m. and 5:00 p.m. on weekdays than at other times.

---

[2] We did not attempt to assess instances of a user trying the search program and then taking the tutorial. Not only does the likelihood of this seem to be low, it also seems reasonable to predict that most of such cases would be caught by the "tutorial-search" sequence when the user again tried the search program. It is, however, another assumption.

Table B-1
Usage of Tutorial and Search Programs
Monthly summaries

Data gathered through June 21, 1988

```
February   T
           SSSSSSS

March      TTTTTTTT
           SSSSSSSSSSSSSSSSSSSSSSSSSSSSSSSSSSSSSSSS

April      TTTTTTTTTT
           SSSSSSSSSSSSSSSSSSSSSSSSSSSSSSSSSSSSSSSSSSSSSSSSSS

May        TTTTTTT
           SSSSSSSSSSSSSSSSSSSSSSSSSSSSSSSSSSSSS

June       TTTT
           SSSSSSSSSSSS
```

Each S or T equals 10 uses of the Search or Tutorial program.

Table B-2.
Program Used by Class of User

User Class	Tutorial	Search	Tutorial	Search
Faculty	58	225	20. 49%	79. 50%
Researcher	46	223	17. 10%	82. 89%
Classified	18	113	13. 74%	86. 25%
Hospital Student	31	122	20. 26%	79. 73%
Dent Student	3	4	42. 85%	57. 14%
Nurs Student	28	171	14. 7%	85. 92%
Med Student	19	188	9. 17%	90. 82%
AHlt Student	19	77	19. 79%	80. 20%
Licensed	35	105	25. 0%	75. 0%
Other	44	235	15. 77%	84. 22%
Totals	301	1463	17. 6%	82. 93%

Table B-3
Program Used by Class of User by Day of Week
Through June 21, 1988

		f	r	c	h	d	n	m	a	l	o		<Totals>
Sun	T	3	2	0	4	0	0	1	3	4	3	=>	20
	S	6	13	2	12	0	6	29	5	15	19	=>	107
													127
Mon	T	13	7	5	4	1	3	2	3	9	3	=>	50
	S	56	42	18	15	0	34	28	10	21	32	=>	256
													306
Tue	T	8	15	3	6	0	7	1	3	7	10	=>	60
	S	38	54	11	29	1	35	24	13	13	50	=>	268
													328
Wed	T	7	5	1	1	0	6	4	4	1	9	=>	38
	S	42	28	20	12	0	19	39	16	17	49	=>	242
													280
Thu	T	11	9	5	11	2	3	5	1	7	7	=>	61
	S	40	37	28	28	2	25	31	13	9	36	=>	249
													310
Fri	T	10	5	4	4	0	3	4	4	3	7	=>	44
	S	29	31	20	16	1	27	24	14	15	34	=>	211
													255
Sat	T	6	3	0	1	0	6	2	1	4	5	=>	28
	S	14	18	14	10	0	25	13	6	15	15	=>	130
													158
		f	r	c	h	d	n	m	a	l	o		<Totals>

User Category Legend
```
    f===>Faculty          d===>Dent Student      l===>Licensed
    r===>Researcher       n===>Nurs Student      o===>Other
    c===>Classified       m===>Med Student
    h===>Hospital St.     a===>AHlt Student
```

Table B-4
User Count by Sensitivity Value

Estimate of the number of users who took the tutorial
and then executed the search program based on the following time "sensitivity values".

Time value (minutes)	User Count
8	121
10	174
12	194
15	216

EVALUATION OF

BIBLIOMED

AT UNIVERSITY OF NEVADA

By *Joan S. Zenan*
  Mary Ellen Lemon
  Savitt Medical Library

  Lisa Leiden
  Office of Evaluation and
  Curriculum Services

  University of Nevada School of
  Medicine
  Reno, Nevada 89557-0046

EVALUATION OF
BIBLIOMED
AT UNIVERSITY OF NEVADA

Introduction

The University of Nevada School of Medicine participated in the National Library of Medicine's MEDLINE CD-ROM evaluation study as one of the three test sites for BiblioMed. This program is produced by Digital Diagnostics, Inc., in Sacramento, California. Their CD-ROM product is a subset of MEDLINE which contains approximately three years of journal article records from more than 500 English language journals, with an emphasis on clinical medicine. Abstracts are included for approximately 60% of the records and the database is updated quarterly.

BiblioMed is a user-friendly menu-driven system that easily retrieves records by searching on specific subjects, authors or journal titles. No prior knowledge of MEDLINE is assumed or felt needed by the vendor. Subjects, authors, or journal titles can be searched by selecting SEARCH or NEW SEARCH from the top of the screen. NEW SEARCH simply deletes any previous search results and begins a new search. Subjects are searched by typing a single word and pressing the enter key. BiblioMed defaults to an alphabetical listing of MeSH (Medical Subject Headings), and makes available the more than 15,000 MeSH headings that are used to index articles in MEDLINE. The user selects the most appropriate subject heading, further refining the search. If the word typed is not found in MeSH, BiblioMed automatically searches article titles for the word. For author or journal title searches, the user types in a last name or a unique title word and the program goes to the nearest match. Users can page up or down to find and mark the exact entry which fits their needs. Combinational (Boolean) operators AND or OR can also be used to refine the search results. Thus, subjects can be combined with other subjects (e.g., Students, Medical AND Stress, Psychological) and with author or journal title searches. Search results can be displayed by selecting DISPLAY CITATIONS at the top of the screen. Displays include author, title and journal source. Abstracts and MeSH headings can also be displayed by pressing the "A" key or the "M" key. Search results can be printed in full or abbreviated forms or downloaded to a formatted floppy disk by selecting PRINT at the top of the screen and choosing one of the four print/download formats.

Sites

The University of Nevada School of Medicine is community-based so most of the training sites for clinical work are in hospitals located some distance from the administrative and basic sciences parts of school. The Savitt Medical Library (Savitt) is located on the University of Nevada-Reno (UNR) campus and serves primarily year one and two medical students, all basic science faculty, and those affiliated with the Department of Family Medicine. Clerks, residents and clinical faculty located in Reno hospitals also make use of the collection and services of this library.

The Veterans Administration Hospital (VA) is located in downtown Reno. It is a 134 bed hospital with outpatient clinics. It is a training site for clerks and residents in internal medicine and surgery, and clerks in psychiatry. The medical library is located on the hospital grounds, in a trailer, and was not felt to be close enough to the wards by the Department of Internal Medicine for this test. Instead, BiblioMed was installed on a computer in their chief resident's office located near the hospital wards on the third floor.

The University Medical Center Library (UMCL) is located adjacent to the University Medical Center, a 399 bed hospital with outpatient clinics, in Las Vegas. It is a training site for clerks and residents in surgery, internal medicine and pediatrics. The library was selected as the test site because the Department of Pediatrics, the prime supporter of this test in Las Vegas, had its offices in the same building and expected its clerks and residents to use the CD-ROM in the library setting.

The Department of Family Medicine is located in a clinic building on the UNR campus across the street from the Savitt Medical Library. It is the training site for clerks and residents in family medicine and pediatrics.

Data Collection

Data was collected in three ways. A formal questionnaire (Appendix A), designed in conjunction with the School of Medicine's Office of Evaluation and Curriculum Services, was used at the Savitt Medical Library and the University Medical Center Library only. A log sheet, requesting date of search, searcher's status, search subject and purpose, and length of time to complete search, was used at Savitt, the VA and at University Medical Center. Focus interviews were conducted at the Department of Family Medicine and the VA.

The formal questionnaire was expected to elicit feedback on the mechanics of using the BiblioMed system as well as the suitability of its content for each user's needs. The log sheet was designed to tell who was using the system, what subject(s) they were searching, the purpose of their search, and how much time they spent searching. The focus interview was used to elicit feedback from practitioners in clinical settings about their use and application of the information they obtained from using the CD-ROM.

There were 63 questionnaires returned to the Savitt Medical Library and 12 to the University Medical Center Library. The log sheets had 293 entries from Savitt, 60 from University Medical Center, and 106 from the VA. Seven people participated in the focus interviews at the VA and the Department of Family Medicine.

Questionnaires

Formal evaluation forms were distributed to CD-ROM users at two test sites: one at Savitt Medical Library, located at the University of Nevada School of Medicine in Reno, where the evaluation period began on March 4th and ended June 15th, and one at the University Medical Center Library located adjacent to the University Medical Center in Las Vegas, Nevada, where the test period was May 16th through June 30th. The majority of formal questionnaires (63 of 75) were completed at Savitt Medical Library. The questionnaire addressed both first and multiple time users. Most of the following information is based on first time users' responses. Comments regarding multiple time user responses will be mentioned only when appropriate. A copy of the "CD-ROM Evaluation Report: Data and Comments," compiled by the School of Medicine's Office of Evaluation and Curriculum Services from the completed evaluation forms, is included in Appendixes B and C.

Savitt Medical Library, Reno

Overall, BiblioMed was very well received at the Savitt Medical Library. It was heavily used by a variety of users during the test period. One user, a medical student, even wanted to purchase the system for personal use. Seventy-three percent of the users indicated that they were familiar with some form of online database, either through their own searching or a mediated online search by a librarian. Some of the most interesting comments focused on the "speed" of response time of the database. While the majority of users (88%) rated the response time as satisfactory, there were numerous comments that said the response time was a "bit slow," especially when displaying citations. These comments are not surprising, but rather curious and amusing considering that five months ago many of these users had to resort to a manual search through *Index Medicus* or wait a day or two for a mediated online search by the librarian. Indeed, 67% now prefer using BiblioMed over a mediated online search (15.5%) or online searching on their own (14%). This preference may have been influenced by cost which was a very important factor for 54% of users and somewhat important to 35% of users in deciding which system to use.

On the question regarding the instructions on the BiblioMed screens, 90% of first time users found the screens clear and understandable. Several users, however, commented on confusion when using the "end" key, mistaking "end" for "quitting" the system entirely. This confusion has been a recurring complaint regularly communicated to the library staff.

Regarding the BiblioMed user manual, 63% of the first time users did not use it or did not find it helpful. Most comments indicated that the manual was not consulted. The manual was always available next to the CD-ROM station, as well as a brief instruction sheet adapted from the manual; however, most of the users asked the staff for help if they were having problems. On the question of the time span covered by BiblioMed (current three years), 63% felt this was sufficient. However, there were several comments that indicated some need for previous years, especially by those doing research.

Of all first time users, 67% were affiliated with the School of Medicine. This included medical students, graduate students, faculty and staff. Medical students and library staff also comprised a large portion (60%) of second time users. This was especially true in March and April when second year medical students were writing a paper for their pathology class.

Of the many reasons why first time users tried BiblioMed, 41% of the use was related to research, 22% for writing a paper or report, 13% to check a reference, and 11% for patient care decision making. These findings changed some for multiple time users, with research being 50% of use, a paper or report 38%, and patient care decision making 12%. No one did checking of references. Approximately 63% of both first and multiple time users searched by specific subject of broad topic. The listing of subjects on question #15 gave a good indication of the type of research being done. It also gave some clues to why BiblioMed was sometimes criticized for its lack of comprehensiveness and the reason for the request for other journals to be added to the database (especially *Journal of Physiology*). Aside from this concern, 30% of first time users found what they needed, 63% found some of what they needed, and 20% of multiple time users found what they needed and 80% found some of what they needed. From this response, we can infer that the system was more familiar and easier to use the second time around resulting in a better retrieval.

University Medical Center Library, Las Vegas

There were very few questionnaires (12) returned from the University Medical Center Library site due to the brief time the system was available for formal evaluation (7 weeks—May 16 through June 30). (Appendix C) However, there was very little overall difference in the response to questions. Of the users queried, 83% now prefer BiblioMed over printed indexes or online searching. Cost was still an important factor for 58% of the users. BiblioMed was rated as easy to use by 100% of the users.

In Las Vegas, 23% of the users that responded were residents, 23% were community physicians, 15% were teaching faculty, and another 23% were nurses. They too found many uses for BiblioMed including: 29% information related to patient care decision making, 24% planning or teaching a course, and 19% research. The subjects searched reflected these types of information needs, with 88% of the searches being done by specific subject or broad topic. In this clinical setting, there were no suggestions for other journals to be added to this database, and more than 92% of the users found either what they needed or some of what they needed.

User Logs

As mentioned above, formal evaluation forms were completed at two BiblioMed sites, and, in addition, log sheets were provided at both and at an additional clinical site in the VA Hospital. The log sheets allowed for the collection of some minimum data when users of BiblioMed were unwilling or unable to fill out the formal evaluation form. They were the only written source of data from the VA. At the Savitt Medical Library, the primary evaluation site, 293 users filled in the log sheet during the three and one half month test period. At University Medical Center, 60 users filled in the log sheet during a seven week trial period, and at the VA 106 responded over a three and one half month period.

All log sheet data were input into PC File, a database management program, and were reproduced in columnar reports with the following headings: date, status, subject, purpose and minutes. Pie charts were constructed in Lotus 1,2,3, using two of the variables from the logs, status of the user and the purpose of their search. Copies of the charts are included as Tables 1-6, and comments on each sites' data are included in the descriptions below.

Savitt Medical Library, Reno

The University of Nevada School of Medicine is a statewide, community-based medical school. The first two years of the medical curriculum are taught on the University of Nevada-Reno campus, and the last two years and the resident years take place primarily in Las Vegas and Reno hospitals, with all fourth-year students taking a four-week rotation in a rural community.

The Savitt Medical Library is located in the medical school complex and serves the schools' students, faculty and staff no matter where they are located. The library staff and its resources are available also to any Nevada citizen, though first priority is always the School of Medicine's needs. The Reno complex also houses all basic science departments, some clinical research laboratories, the Psychiatry Department, and a Family Medicine Center with clerks and residents across the street.

The library's primary on-site clientele are year one and two medical students, graduate students in basic science departments, and basic science faculty. Clerks who are rotating locally, residents who graduated from this school, and internal medicine faculty who want to keep up in the basic sciences use the library in the evening and on weekends. Family Medicine students and faculty come over when their in-house mini-library does not fill their needs. They do see out-patients and do have need for patient care management information. Several of their clerks remarked to library staff that BiblioMed had made their information gathering tasks much easier, and they were going to make sure their colleagues knew about it. They really liked the idea of having a MEDLINE CD-ROM system near where they would be doing patient care.

The log sheet statistics for status of users reflected very similar percentages to those found in the formal evaluation compilation. Those signing the log sheet were: medical students 37%, faculty 25%, graduate students 7%, library staff 13%, UNR undergraduates 13%, and other 5% (Table 1). Search purpose statistics were not as similar. Users listed patient care as their purpose about 12% of the time in the formal evaluation and only 4.5% on the log. Teaching or planning a course was listed 5% of the time in the evaluation and not at all on the log. The biggest discrepancy was in the area of research. The questionnaire showed 41% doing research while the log showed 71% (Table 2).

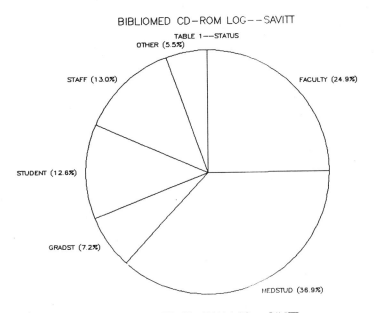

BIBLIOMED CD-ROM LOG--SAVITT
TABLE 1--STATUS

OTHER (5.5%)
STAFF (13.0%)
FACULTY (24.9%)
STUDENT (12.6%)
GRADST (7.2%)
MEDSTUD (36.9%)

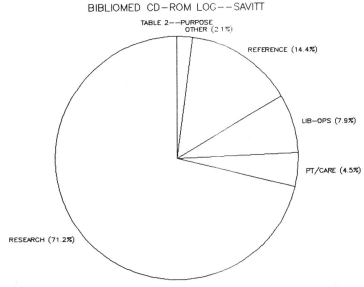

BIBLIOMED CD-ROM LOG--SAVITT
TABLE 2--PURPOSE
OTHER (2.1%)
REFERENCE (14.4%)
LIB-OPS (7.9%)
PT/CARE (4.5%)
RESEARCH (71.2%)

University Medical Center Library, Las Vegas

This library supports a number of the School of Medicine's clerkships and residency programs in Las Vegas, and provides library services to many of the smaller hospitals in the Southern Nevada area. It has a very good clinical journal collection which supports the patient care services in the hospital.

Comparing the log sheets to the formal evaluation data shows quite a difference in user status, however, because the numbers are so small—12 evaluation forms, 60 entries on the log sheets—it is difficult to come to many conclusions (Table 3). The library staff did not fill out the formal evaluation forms and so are not listed as one of the users, however they are 58% of the users on the log sheets. BiblioMed was not heavily advertised throughout the hospital, and access was limited to library hours. At least at first, it was most accessible to and most easily used by the library staff.

The purpose for doing a search was more in parallel for patient care which was about 28% on both the log and on the questionnaire. Teaching and course planning was listed 23.8% of the time on the questionnaire but not at all on the

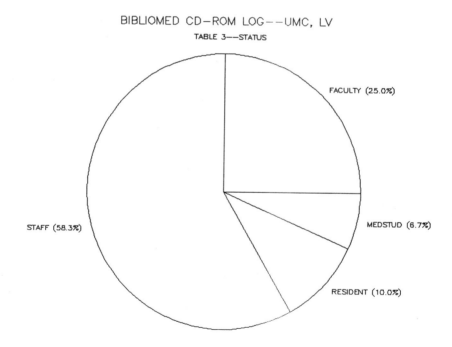

BIBLIOMED CD-ROM LOG--UMC, LV

TABLE 3--STATUS

FACULTY (25.0%)

MEDSTUD (6.7%)

RESIDENT (10.0%)

STAFF (58.3%)

log. Research accounted for 36.7% on the log and only 19% on the questionnaire. Reference on the log and keeping current on the questionnaire accounted for 23.3% and 19% respectively. Library operations were 8.3% of the purposes for searching (Table 4).

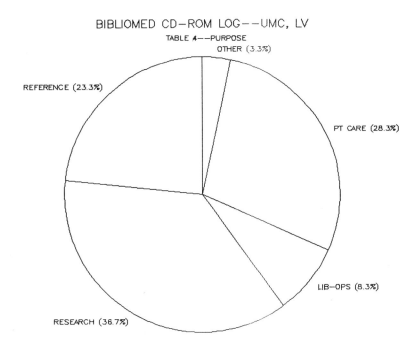

BIBLIOMED CD—ROM LOG——UMC, LV
TABLE 4——PURPOSE
OTHER (3.3%)
PT CARE (28.3%)
LIB—OPS (8.3%)
RESEARCH (36.7%)
REFERENCE (23.3%)

Veterans Administration Hospital, Reno

The VA Hospital is one of the School of Medicine's primary teaching sites. The Departments of Surgery and Internal Medicine have clerkships and residency programs located there. The library is physically located outside the main hospital in a modular building. Because of its physical distance from the patient care area the placement of BiblioMed on the 3rd floor of the hospital was the site of the choice. The 106 entries over three and one half months on their log sheets indicated that 51% of the users were residents, 40% were clerks, and 9% were clinical faculty (Table 5). The logs also showed that patient care was the purpose of more than 70% of the searches, while research accounted for 23% (Table 6).

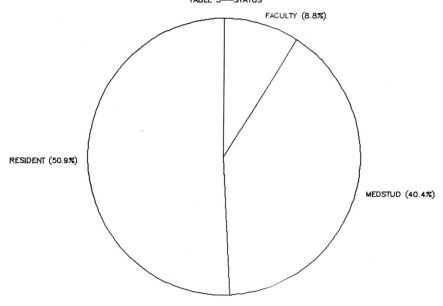

BIBLIOMED CD-ROM LOG--VA MED CTR

TABLE 5--STATUS

FACULTY (8.8%)

RESIDENT (50.9%)

MEDSTUD (40.4%)

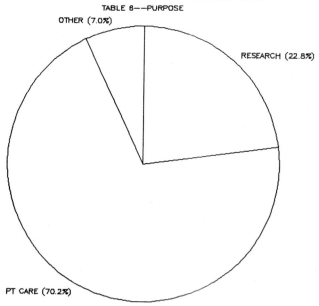

BIBLIOMED CD-ROM LOG--VA MED CTR

TABLE 6--PURPOSE

OTHER (7.0%)

RESEARCH (22.8%)

PT CARE (70.2%)

Focus Interviews

In September interviews were held at two clinical sites, the VA hospital and the Department of Family Medicine in Reno. The following paragraphs reflect the comments from seven individuals—two residency coordinators, a chief resident, two residents, a third year medical student (clerk), and two practicing physician/faculty members.

1. All but one resident felt that BiblioMed was good for a clinical setting, whether it was hospital or clinic-based. The resident who did not think it belonged in the hospital setting also did not like computers and preferred to "shoot" them! One physician also thought it would be useful in a rural clinic setting, as long as there was a library outreach service available to provide needed articles.

2. The residency coordinators felt BiblioMed or any of the other CD-ROM products would be most useful and helpful in clinical settings which were also teaching settings. They both felt the need of mediated searches by a librarian as a complement when comprehensiveness was an issue.

3. All interviewees used BiblioMed for patient care, especially diagnosis and treatment, whether it was for morning report, ward care or teaching of medical students in mini-rounds. One faculty member used it to learn so that he could be a better teacher on a particular topic.

4. The residents and clerk liked the system because it made finding relevant information for their presentations very easy and fast.

5. All felt abstracts were very important, especially in the non-library setting. Knowing the general content of an article helped them decide if they needed to make a trip or a phone call to the library.

6. The chief resident felt that for research purposes it would be helpful to have more journal titles and more years on the disk. One of the residency coordinators felt that more journals should be included which cover the "cutting edge" of clinical medicine.

Findings

The following statements reflect a synthesis of all the data collection instruments, analyses and personal interviews conducted by the authors.

1. BiblioMed was well received and most users felt it was easy to use.

2. A majority of users rated the response time as satisfactory or better.

3. Two-thirds of the users preferred BiblioMed over a mediated search or doing their own online searching. This may have been influenced by the fact that BiblioMed was free. Cost was an important (35%) or very important (54%) factor to the respondents.

4. The status of users varied by site. Savitt had its heaviest use by medical students (37%) and faculty (25%). The VA was mostly used by residents (61%) and clerks (33%), and the University Medical Center by faculty (25%) and library staff (58%).

319

5. The purpose of searches varied by site. At Savitt, patient care accounted for 4.5% and research 71% of use. At the VA 70% was for patient care and 22% was for research. At UMCL, 28.3% was for patient care and 36.7% was for research.

6. BiblioMed's on-screen instructions were clear and understandable to 90% of first time users. Confusion arose between "end" and "quit."

7. The user manual was not used or not found to be helpful by 63% of first time users.

8. The BiblioMed time span, three years, was sufficient for 63% of users.

9. Researchers requested more basic science journals and more back files.

Conclusion

The three test sites found BiblioMed useful for their settings. They each expect to continue using BiblioMed and look forward to updates which will include various planned enhancements. For now, BiblioMed is the CD-ROM MEDᴌINE program of choice for these Nevada sites.

Appendix A-1

<u>Instructions</u>: The MEDLINE CD-ROM system that you have just finished using is being tested on a trial basis at this library. Please complete this questionnaire in order to help us learn in greater detail how this system meets your needs. If you are a <u>first-time</u> <u>user</u> please <u>complete</u> the <u>entire</u> <u>questionnaire</u>; if you are a <u>second-time</u> <u>user</u>, please <u>skip</u> to item <u>12</u>. All responses will be kept confidential, only group data will be recorded in the summary report for the National Library of Medicine.

1. Have you previously used any of the following printed publications: INDEX MEDICUS; INTERNATIONAL NURSING INDEX; INDEX TO DENTAL LITERATURE; HOSPITAL LITERATURE INDEX? (Please check <u>one</u> response)

_____ YES (If "yes", go to Item 2) _____ NO (If "no", go to Item 3)

2. If you answered YES to Item 1, how do these printed indexes compare to the BIBLIOMED CD-ROM system that you just finished using? (Please check <u>one</u> response)

_____ EASIER TO USE _____ ABOUT THE SAME TO USE _____ HARDER TO USE

<u>COMMENTS</u>:

3. The BIBLIOMED CD-ROM system that you have just finished using is <u>not</u> an on-line system. Have you previously used an on-line version of MEDLINE (either by yourself or by having a librarian do a search for you)? (Check <u>one</u> response)

_____ YES, BY LIBRARIAN   _____ NO

_____ YES, BY MYSELF   _____ DON'T KNOW

     Please List: (_____)

4. Which of the following 4 sources of MEDLINE do you now prefer to use (Check <u>one</u> response)

_____ PRINTED MATERIAL (e.g. Index Medicus) _____ON-LINE MEDLINE
                                             By Librarian
_____ BIBLIOMED CD-ROM   _____ ON-LINE MEDLINE
                                             By Myself

5. The next time that you need to use MEDLINE information, which of the following same sources will you use? (Check <u>one</u> response)

_____ PRINTED MATERIALS   _____ ON-LINE MEDLINE
    (e.g. Index Medicus)   By Myself

_____ON-LINE MEDLINE   _____BIBLIOMED CD-ROM
    By Librarian

6. The BIBLIOMED CD-ROM system that you have just finished using has been provided free of charge to you.

How important was this to you in deciding to use this system, rather than an on-line version of MEDLINE? (Check <u>one</u> response)

_____ VERY IMPORTANT _____ SOMEWHAT IMPORTANT _____ NOT IMPORTANT

7. Were the instructions on the BIBLIOMED CD-ROM screens clear and understandable? (Check <u>one</u> response)

_____ YES   _____ NO

<u>COMMENTS</u>:

8. Was the rate at which the computer responded satisfactory? (Check <u>one</u> response)

_____ YES   _____ NO

<u>COMMENTS</u>:

9. Did the BIBLIOMED CD-ROM manual help you to use this system? (Please check <u>one</u> response)

_____ YES   _____ NO

<u>COMMENTS</u>:

10. Was the time-span of the references included in the BIBLIOMED CD-ROM sufficient for your needs? (Please check <u>one</u> response)

_____ YES   _____ NO

11. Overall, was the BIBLIOMED CD-ROM system easy to use? (Please check <u>one</u> response)

_____YES   _____ NO

<u>**COMMENTS**</u>:

12. My primary affiliation is with: (Please check <u>one</u> response)
<u>School of Medicine</u>:   <u>UNR:</u>

_____ Basic Science Faculty   _____ Faculty
_____ Clinical Science Faculty   _____ Staff
_____ Staff   _____ Graduate Student
_____ Student   _____ Undergraduate Student
_____ Graduate Student
_____ Resident

<u>Non-University</u>:

_____ MD   _____ RN   _____Other (Please List)

13. How often have you used the CD-ROM MEDLINE system? (Please check <u>one</u> response)

_____ FIRST TIME
     (If you are a first-time user, please complete the entire form)

_____ SECOND TIME   _____ 3-5 TIMES   _____ MORE THAN 5 TIMES

14. I used the BIBLIOMED CD-ROM system to find information on: (Please check <u>all</u> responses that apply)

_____ PATIENT CARE _____ RESEARCH PROJECT _____ PAPER OR REPORT

_____ CHECKING A REFERENCE   _____ KEEPING CURRENT

_____TEACHING/PLANNING A COURSE_____DID NOT NEED ANY INFORMATION,
                                                JUST CURIOUS
OTHER_____
                    (PLEASE STATE)

15. What was the subject or subjects of your search?

16. Were the journals included in BIBLIOMED CD-ROM sufficient for your needs? (Please check <u>one</u> response)

_____ YES   _____ NO (If no, please list the
                                      titles you would like to have included)

17. I was looking for articles by: (Please check <u>all</u> responses that apply)

_____ AUTHOR _____ TITLE _____ SUBJECT _____ JOURNAL _____ TOPIC

18. The information that I found on Bibliomed CD-ROM was: (Please check <u>one</u> response)

_____WHAT I NEEDED_____ SOME OF WHAT I NEEDED_____ NOT WHAT I NEEDED

<u>Please return your completed questionnaire to the reference desk.</u>

                        Thank you.

CD-ROM EVALUATION REPORT: Savitt Medical Library (Reno)

DATA AND COMMENTS

Ques. 1. Have you previously used any of the following printed publications: INDEX MEDICUS; INTERNATIONAL NURSING INDEX; INDEX TO DENTAL LITERATURE; HOSPITAL LITERATURE INDEX?

> **FIRST TIME USERS**
>
> YES = 51 (81%)
> NO = 12 (19%)

Ques. 2. If you answered YES to Item 1, how do these printed indexes compare to the Bibliomed CD-ROM system that you just finished using?

> **FIRST TIME USERS**
>
> 16 (30.8%) = Easier to Use
> 12 (23.1%) = About the same to Use
> 24 (46.2%) = Harder to Use

Comments: CD-ROM is fast, efficient and more effective by being able to cross reference topics. Except it is not very comprehensive. With the availability of computer search, hand text searching is too slow. CD-ROM is much faster & easier once learned. Much easier - 1 hour on MEDLINE CD-ROM equals 4 hours with index medicus. Computer is easier to use than it looks. The computer is easier to use and less time consuming. Index much harder. Very convenient & easy to use. Excellent system. If response time was 50% faster, it would be outstanding. May become easier once CD-ROM is utilized more. CD-ROM was much less laborious. Much harder to use index. Much slower & no abstract. Bibliomed CD-ROM surprisingly easy to use.

Ques. 3. The bibliomed CD-ROM system that you have just finished using is <u>not</u> an on-line system. Have you previously used an on-line version of MEDLINE (either by yourself or by having a librarian do a search for you)?

> **FIRST TIME USERS**
>
> 27 (45.0%) = YES, by Librarian
> 17 (28.3%) = YES, by Myself (grateful med = 4, home
>   computer, Northwest Univ. - U. of Chicago,
>   WolfPAC, GM, HLN)
> 16 (26.7%) = NO
> 0 (0.0%) = DON'T KNOW

Ques. 4. Which of the following 4 sources of MEDLINE do you now prefer to use?

FIRST TIME USERS

2 (3.4%) = Printed Materials (e.g. Index Medicus)
33 (56.9%) = Bibliomed CD-ROM
11 (19.0% = On-Line MEDLINE by Librarian
12 (20.7%) = On-Line MEDLINE by Myself

Ques. 5. The next time that you need to use medline information, which of the following same sources will you use?

FIRST TIME USERS

2 (3.4%) = Printed Materials (e.g. Index Medicus)
9 (15.5%) = On-line MEDLINE by Librarian
8 (13.8%) = On-line MEDLINE by Myself
39 (67.2%) = Bibliomed CD-ROM

Ques. 6. The BIBLIOMED CD-ROM system that you have just finished using has been provided free of charge to you.

How important was this to you in deciding to use this system, rather than an on-line version of MEDLINE?

FIRST TIME USERS

31 (54.4%) = Very Important
20 (35.1%) = Somewhat Important
6 (10.5%) = Not Important

Ques. 7. Were the instruction on the BIBLIOMED CD-ROM Screens clear and understandable?

FIRST TIME USERS

52 (89.7%) = YES
6 (10.3%) = NO

Comments: Somewhat confusing. Limiting topics required used of the documentation. Expectations didn't always do as told. I needed a little help getting started e.g. Mesh. Once I found out about the "End" command. I had much assistance from librarian. "F1" help keys could describe "where one can go" in addition to the specific response (e.g. flagging <u>another</u> mantron "END"). But it took a while to get used to the operating system. More user prompts would be helpful. No instructions to explain use of " End" key - difficult to locate and confusing in its role to move to headings. To me they were clear but I've used computers before. Excellent.

Ques. 8. Was the rate at which the computer responded satisfactory?

    FIRST TIME USERS

    50 (87.7%) = YES
     7 (12.3%) = NO

Comments: Bit slow - but perfectly acceptable. A little slow. Moving through long lists is very time consuming even with page down. The printing could have been faster for longer numbered citations. Perhaps the information could be downloaded to a disk and the disk taken home and reviewed. When searching for the author, it generally pulls up the author just after the one you want and you have to arrow up one or more to get the correct one. Abstract retrieval time should be sped up. Should be faster. Display citations moves too slow from one to next. S-L-O-W between abstracts. Mostly. It was a little slow in moving from reference to reference.

Ques. 9. Did the BIBLIOMED CD-ROM manual help you to use this system?

    FIRST TIME USERS

    19 (37.3%) = YES
    32 (62.7%) = NO

Comments: Didn't see it. It was present. Thx. Wasn't needed. Didn't look for it. What manual? Should have <u>read</u>. Didn't read it- just read the screen. Didn't read it. Very good manual. Did not use manual. Instructions were clear on screen. The librarian did. Didn't use. I didn't read it. I did not need the manual the screen commands were adequate. Used classmate for instruction. Not needed. Don't understand question.

Ques. 10. Was the time-span of the references included in the BIBLIOMED CD-ROM sufficient for your needs?

    FIRST TIME USERS

    34 (63.0%) = YES
    20 (37.0%) = NO

Comments: I wish that it could be more comprehensive of past articles older than 3 years. To 1966. Can't say - didn't finish search. Need other Journals i.e.: Journal of Physiology. Two years back is enough. Generally yes, however it would be beneficial to have been able to check back a number of years further for case reports. Needs to be back further. Previous years should be available. It would be helpful to have previous years available. Needs to back to mid 70's. Two years. Would be wise for backup disk to include previous years.

Ques. 11. Overall, was the BIBLIOMED CD-ROM system easy to use?

    FIRST TIME USERS

      56 (96.6%) = YES
       2 (3.4%) = NO

Comments: Once price is down for system, I look forward to personal purchase. Very easy. Printer problems.

Ques. 12. My primary affiliation is with:

FIRST TIME USERS		SECOND TIME USERS
8 (13.3%)	Basic Science Faculty	0 (0.0%)
6 (10.0%)	Clinical Science Faculty	0 (0.0%)
10 (16.7%)	Staff	0 (0.0%)
1 (1.7%)	Resident	0 (0.0%)
13 (21.7%)	Student	1 (20.0%)
2 (3.3%)	Graduate Student	0 (0.0%)
4 (6.7%)	Faculty	0 (0.0%)
1 (1.7%)	Staff	2 (40.0%)
4 (6.7%)	Graduate Student	1 (20.0%)
8 (13.3%)	Undergraduate Student	1 (20.0%)
0 (0.0%)	MD	0 (0.0%)
1 (1.7%)	RN	0 (0.0%)
2 (3.3%)	Other	0 (0.0%)

Comments: (Other) High School Research Students

Ques. 13. How often have you used the CD-ROM MEDLINE system?

FIRST TIME USERS		SECOND TIME USERS
26 (43.3%)	First Time	0 (0.0%)
9 (15.0%)	Second Time	0 (0.0%)
15 (25.0%)	3 - 5 Times	3 (60.0%)
10 (16.7%)	More than 5 Times	2 (40.0%)

Ques. 14. I used the BIBLIOMED system to find information on:

FIRST TIME USERS		SECOND TIME USERS
11 (11.0%)	Patient Care	1 (12.0%)
12 (13.0%)	Checking a Reference	0 (0.0%)
5 (5.0%)	Teaching/Planning a Course	0 (0.0%)
39 (41.0%)	Research Project (NIH grant work)	4 (50.0%)
6 (6.0%)	Keeping Current	0 (0.0%)
1 (1.0%)	Did not need any information, just curious	0 (0.0%)
21 (22.0%)	Paper or Report	3 (38.0%)
1 (1.0%)	Other	0 (0.0%)

Ques. 15. What was the subject or subjects of your search?

Comments: Potassium channels, calcium activated channels, sodium - calcium exchange, adolescent lactation, endothelial cells (cultured), pharmacological responses of these cells to drugs, bulimia, nutrition labeling, nutrient analysis via food frequency, epstein-barr virus, ferritin - iontophoresis horse raddish peroxidase, percutaneous suction diskectomy, child abuse, KIT (?), KP Campbell, G. Meissnell, DM Bers, Esophagus, Effect of reserpine on spontaneous activity of guinea pig portal veins, Ferritin: - iontophoretic injection and localization with EM, physician/patient relationship, self-mutilation, colposcopic examination, DX, & treatment. of anal warts, organ procurement and transplantation, cardiac electrophysiology, smooth muscle electro-physiology, mosquito venom, black fly venom, rypxococcus, t-cells of the immune system, bladder - physiology, opthalmoplegia & lesions to the medical longitudinal fasciculus in a patient with history of TIA, hypnosis, bunya, & adenoviruses, intercellular communication, tyrosine, colposcory/venereal warts MRI - parkinson's, holistic medicine, acupuncture and pain, assess. of nutritional status, Luge # - enzymes to organisms, Cooper, BW, infections in surgery, channels, substance P, smooth muscle, mathematical models, diagnosis, hypoglycemia: diagnosis, The ethical issues concerning workplace testing, Cost shifting medicine, ONR's anencephalic organ harvesting, author publications, myosin P in smooth muscle, burns - electrical, several, mechanical vertileta, pemphiqus, anorexia and multiple sclerosis, chloroquine effects on secretion, bladder-henrogenic control, mental retardation, preceptorship training, heat stress and growth (heat & development, Heat & hormones), hyperprolactinemia treatment w/surgery, laser surgery, long-term care of elderly, radiology, opthalmoplegia, glomerulonephritis, author search, hypoglycemia, pedunculeportre, Tiemos, Graybiel (author), lasers in surgery, monosodium glutamate, Authors - Kuriyama, H. and Bolton, T., smooth muscle currents, B cell lymphomas. (Verbatim Comments)

Ques. 16. Were the journals included in BIBLIOMED CD-ROM sufficient for your needs?

FIRST TIME USERS		SECOND TIME USERS
41 (73.2%)	YES	4 (80.0%)
15 (26.8%)	NO	1 (20,0%)

Comments: J. of Pediatrics, Sociology & Psychology, BBRC, J. Physiol.

Ques. 17. I was looking for articles by:

FIRST TIME USERS		SECOND TIME USERS
16 (19.1%)	Author	1 (12.5%)
7 (8.3%)	Title	1 (12.5%)
44 (52.4%)	Subject	5 (62.5%)
6 (7.1%)	Journal	1 (12.5%)
11 (13.1%)	Topic	0 (0.0%)

Ques. 18. The information that I found on Bibliomed CD-ROM was:

FIRST TIME USERS		SECOND TIME USERS
17 (29.8%)	What I Needed	1 (20.0%)
36 (63.2%)	Some of What I Needed	4 (80.0%)
4 (7.0%)	Not What I Needed	0 (0.0%)

Comments: Req'd earlier documents as well. For this search, the data bank is too limited.

Appendix C

Ques.5. The next time that you need to use MEDLINE informations which of the following same sources will you use.

    FIRST TIME USERS

       0 (0.0%) = Printed Materials (e.g. Index Medicus)
       1 (8.3%) = On-Line MEDLINE by Librarian
       1 (8.3%) = On-Line MEDLINE by Myself
      10 (83.3%)= Bibliomed CD-ROM

Ques.6. The BIBLIOMED CD-ROM system that you have just finished using has been provided free of charge to you.

How important was this to you in deciding to use this system, rather than an on-line version of MEDLINE?

    FIRST TIME USERS

       7 (58.3%) = Very Important
       3 (25.0%) = Somewhat Important
       2 (16.7%) = Not Important

Ques.7. Were the instructions on the BIBLIOMED CD-ROM screens clear and understandable?

    FIRST TIME USERS

      11 (91.7%) = YES
       1 (8.3%) = NO

Comments: Printing instructions not clear, due to previous computer experience, not sufficient prompting.

Ques. 8. Was the rate at which the computer responded satisfactory?

    FIRST TIME USERS

      12 (100.0%) = YES
       0 (0.0%) = NO

Comments: None

Ques. 9. Did the BIBLIOMED CD-ROM manual help you to use this system?

    FIRST TIME USERS

      8 (80.0%)
      2 (20.0%)

Comments: Librarian help was excellent, librarian helped, I didn't read it.

Ques.10. Was the time-span of the references included in the BIBLIOMED CD-ROM sufficient for your needs?

       FIRST TIME USERS

       11 (91.7%) = YES
        1 (8.3%) = NO

Comments: For this study but otherwise I usually require dates further back.

Ques.11. Overall, was the BIBLIOMED CD-ROM system ease to use?

       FIRST TIME USERS

       12 (100.0%) = YES
        0 (0.0%)   = NO

Comments: None

Ques. 12. My primary affiliation is with:

       FIRST TIME USERS

       0 (0.0%)   Basic Science Faculty
       2 (15.4%) Clinical Science Faculty
       0 (0.0%)   Staff
       3 (23.1%) Resident
       0 (0.0%)   Student
       0 (0.0%)   Graduate Student
       0 (0.0%)   Faculty
       1 (7.7%)   Staff
       0 (0.0%)   Graduate Student
       0 (0.0%)   Undergraduate Student
       3 (23.1%) MD
       3 (23.1%) RN
       1 (7.7%)   Other

Comments: (Other) physician assistant

Ques. 13. How often have you used the CD-ROM MEDLINE system?

       FIRST TIME USERS

       11 (84.6%) = First Time
        1 (7.7%) = Second Time
        1 (7.7%) = 3-5 Times
        0 (0.0%) = More than 5 Times

Ques. 14. I used the BIBLIOMED system to find information on:

FIRST TIME USERS

6 (28.6%)	Patient Care
0 (0.0%)	Checking a Reference
5 (23.8%)	Teaching/Planning a Course
4 (19.0%)	Research Project (NIH grant work)
2 (19.0%)	Keeping Current
1 (4.8%)	Did not need information, just curious
2 (9.5%)	Paper or Report
1 (4.8%)	Other

Comments: (Other) presentations to Dr. Little

Ques. 15. What was the subject or subjects of your search?

Comments: Medicaid, physician assistants, psoriatic arthritis (unable to find any citations), automatic implantable difibrillator, ultrufiltentim, meningitis, poncreolites & complications, cocaine, avascular necrosis RX & DX, cervical spine injury, placental pathology, pathology of cyclosporin toxicity. (Verbatim Comments)

Ques. 16. Were the journals included in BIBLIOMED CD-ROM sufficient for your needs?

FIRST TIME USERS

13 (100/0%) = YES
 0 (0.0%) = NO

Comments: None

Ques. 17. I was looking for articles by:

FIRST TIME USERS

0 (0.0%)	Author
1 (6.0%)	Title
13 (82.0%)	Subject
1 (6.0%)	Journal
1 (6.0%)	Topic

Ques. 18. The information that I found in BIBLIOMED CD-ROM was:

FIRST TIME USERS

6 (46.2%)	What I Needed
6 (46.2%)	Some of What I Needed
1 (7.7%)	Not What I Needed

Comments: None

333

EVALUATION OF

BIBLIOMED

AT CARLSON HEALTH SCIENCES LIBRARY, UNIVERSITY OF CALIFORNIA, DAVIS

By *Rebecca Davis*
    Carolyn Kopper
    Carlson Health Sciences Library
    University of California
    Davis, CA 95616

Evaluation Of BIBLIOMED
At Carlson Health Sciences Library,
University Of California, Davis

Introduction

This is a report of the evaluation of BIBLIOMED, a MEDLINE CD-ROM product tested at the Carlson Health Sciences Library during the period March 9 - May 31, 1988 and at the University of California Davis Medical Center Library during the period June 1 - July 22, 1988. The raw figures and percentages for responses to the evaluation form are included in Appendix A. Appendix B contains a checklist of system capabilities.

The Carlson Health Sciences Library was one of three libraries chosen to participate in the testing of BIBLIOMED as part of the nationwide testing of MEDLINE on CD-ROM products sponsored by the National Library of Medicine. The other two libraries testing BIBLIOMED were the University of Nevada (Reno) and the University of Oregon (Portland). Because the producer of BIBLIOMED maintains that it is uniquely suited to clinicians our test site was extended to include the Medical Center Library.

Serving both a veterinary and medical school, the Carlson Health Sciences Library (HSL) has over 200,000 volumes and 3,500 current subscriptions. Its staff of 35 includes six professional librarians. Approximately 700 database searches are performed yearly, 80% in the MEDLINE database. Other databases accessed include the Commonwealth Agricultural Bureaux (CABI), BIOSIS, and Psychological Abstracts. The Medical Center Library (MCL), located in the UC Davis Medical Center, serves a staff of clinicians and other hospital personnel with a collection of 23,000 volumes and over 800 periodical subscriptions. Two professional librarians head its staff of six. Approximately 1,000 database searches are performed yearly, almost all in the MEDLINE database.

In November 1987 the University of California system mounted the most current MEDLINE file for use by all of the UC health sciences libraries. The file can be accessed free of charge through the MELVYL online catalog and uses a command language patterned after that used for MELVYL.

BIBLIOMED is produced by Digital Diagnostics, Inc. of Sacramento, California. BIBLIOMED is a subset of the MEDLINE database which contains citations and abstracts to articles published in 525 clinically-related, English-language journal titles. The journal titles were selected from such standard sources as the Brandon-Hill List, the Library for Internists list published by the *Annals of*

Internal Medicine, and the list of journals indexed in the *Abridged Index Medicus.* A yearly subscription costs $975 and consists of one disk, updated quarterly and covering a 3-4 year period. An online tutorial is included. Towards the end of the testing period, the producers added an additional database to the disk. Called the AIDS database, it includes all citations related to the acquired immunodeficiency syndrome that have appeared in the MEDLINE database since 1980, regardless of journal title or language. This enhancement to BIBLIO-MED was not available soon enough to be included in the testing.

Testing Methodology

Throughout the remainder of this report, distinctions will be made between the testing process at the Carlson Health Sciences Library (HSL) and that at the Medical Center Library (MCL).

Hardware

The producer furnished the Phillips CM-100 CD-ROM player and an update to 640K for the library-owned Zenith 158 microcomputer with a 20MB hard disk and Hewlett-Packard Thinkjet printer. The entire configuration was secured to a portable table and placed in the vicinity of the Reference Desk, adjacent to the MELVYL/MEDLINE terminals and the card catalog. At MCL, the same hardware configuration was placed next to the MELVYL/MEDLINE terminals and the *Index Medicus.*

Publicity

Notices were placed in the campus newspaper and flyers announcing the test were included with the mailing of the HSL Newsletter. A large sign advertising the test was placed over the microcomputer. The sign was also used at MCL but the physical proximity of BIBLIOMED to the entrance of the library and word-of-mouth proved more than adequate to publicize its availability.

Availability

Because it was felt that the Reference Staff should be available to help users with BIBLIOMED, it was available only during the following hours at HSL when the Reference Desk was staffed:

Monday - Friday 9:00 a.m. - 5:00 p.m.

Monday - Thursday 7:00 p.m. - 9:00 p.m.

Saturday 1:00 p.m. - 5:00 p.m.

At MCL the system was available during the regular hours of the library. All of the users of both libraries were encouraged to try the system. No distinctions were made regarding categories of users. Users were initially asked to sign up to use the system in 30-minute slots; however, this was dispensed with very early in the test. The availability of MELVYL/MEDLINE terminals at both test sites lessened the competition for the BIBLIOMED station.

User Assistance

Each user of the system was encouraged to work through the short online tutorial provided by the producer. The tutorial was very useful in that it reduced the amount of time spent by reference staff explaining the system. During the testing period at HSL statistics were kept for the number of questions answered regarding BIBLIOMED. Over 130 such questions were logged regarding use of the system and hardware. The user documentation was tabbed, mounted on stiff cardboard and placed next to the terminal. Most users were not interested in the documentation and many even bypassed the online tutorial in favor of learning the system on their own. Additional online context-sensitive help was provided as part of the database.

Staff Training

Those persons who staffed the Reference Desk were given background information on the product and encouraged to experiment with it prior to the beginning of the formal testing. An additional copy of the user documentation was kept at the Reference Desk.

Problem Log

A problem log was also kept at the Reference Desk and used to record system glitches, comments and suggestions made by users. Staff were encouraged to record problems in detail to facilitate their correction by the producer.

Evaluation

The sample survey questions provided by the National Library of Medicine were used as the basis for the BIBLIOMED evaluation form. One of the other BIBLIOMED test sites was also consulted regarding their survey questions.

As originally envisioned, the evaluation form, which consisted of 16 questions, was to be mounted as part of the searching software. As a user logged onto the system, the first six questions would be asked online. When the user finished using BIBLIOMED and pressed QUIT the remaining 10 questions would appear. The responses to the evaluation questions were to be written to a separate online file that could be copied to a floppy or printed at the end of each day. The resulting online file could then be manipulated statistically at the end of the testing period.

The execution of the online evaluation form was problematic. Firstly, the online file that was set up to receive the responses to the form was so affected by system glitches that each time the program aborted and BIBLIOMED had to be rebooted, the contents of the online evaluation field were erased. During the first month or so of the testing period, system glitches were not uncommon. Secondly, most users responded to the first six questions when they began searching; however, instead of pressing QUIT when finished searching, many would simply walk away. Those who did press QUIT were more interested in seeking out the citations received during their search than in answering an additional ten questions. Also, because the librarian had not personally handed the user an evaluation form with a request that it be returned, there was little incentive to respond to the online form. For all of these reasons, the online evaluation form was eliminated and librarians distributed paper forms personally to users, with far better results.

Evaluation Results

A total of 73 forms were collected at HSL, with 28 collected at MCL. Approximately one form was collected for every two users of the system at HSL and one for every three users at MCL. Because of the smaller number of responses received from MCL, comparisons between the two test sites are made cautiously except in cases where there is a substantial difference in the response to a given question. The responses were manipulated using the Reflex database management software. See Appendix A for a copy of the evaluation form with raw figures and percentages.

As expected, the user population at HSL was far more diverse, with both the medical and veterinary departments well represented in addition to users from economics, law, zoology and psychology. The MCL users represented departments of the Medical Center including nursing and dietary services. User status was far more varied at HSL with a high percentage of graduate students. At MCL the highest percentage was for faculty.

Over half of the respondents at both sites indicated that they had performed their own database searches. We suspect that many of those responding are considering MELVYL/MEDLINE as an online source, so it should not be assumed that all who responded yes to this question have passwords and are accessing databases through outside vendors.

Most of those surveyed had never used BIBLIOMED before, with a higher percentage of first-time users at MCL. This difference between the sites in the number of people who had used the system was probably due to the fact BIBLIOMED was at HSL for close to three months, providing more opportunity to use the system.

The vast majority of users were looking for articles on a particular subject. As it is common for a user to request "titles" on a particular topic, one might assume that many of those indicating that they were looking for information by title were also searching by subject.

HSL users indicated most often that they needed information for a research project or report while those at MCL were most often planning to use the information to teach a class or for patient care. Given that the largest percentage of HSL respondents were graduate students, the focus on research and writing was expected. Likewise, the majority of the respondents from MCL were faculty members, thus the emphasis on teaching. The focus of the Medical Center accounts for the concern with patient care.

The question regarding the success of a search performed for various purposes must be considered in light of the user population at each site. Those at HSL have more need for information drawn from a broader set of journals than those covered by BIBLIOMED while those at MCL are more likely to be satisfied with the clinical orientation of the BIBLIOMED subset. Therefore, it was more likely that HSL users would have more instances of dissatisfaction with a search. Despite this consideration, however, over half of those responding indicated that their search was successful or very successful. Author searches seemed most problematic for HSL users. One-fourth of the author searches attempted were unsuccessful or less successful. However, all of the author searches attempted by MCL users were judged very successful. Title searches were similarly represented at both sites. Subject searches were largely successful at HSL, but even more so at MCL. The clinical nature of the journals in BIBLIO-MED probably accounts for this difference. Very little journal searching was attempted at HSL; however, those searches were largely unsuccessful. There were no journal searches performed at MCL.

BIBLIOMED was rated fairly high for ease of use at both sites with three-fourths of the MCL users giving it a rating of easy or very easy. This would seem to indicate that the producer's claim that it is an intuitive, "point and shoot" system is well founded.

The question regarding the usage of MELVYL/MEDLINE and its comparison to BIBLIOMED was unique to this university setting. Although the two systems are intended to be used in different ways, and despite the fact that funding for the development of a system such as MELVYL/MEDLINE would dwarf that available to a private producer, it was felt that there would be some value in asking users their opinion regarding how easy it was to learn the two systems. Regarding prior use of MELVYL/MEDLINE, twice as many HSL users had used the system than MCL users. There are a few factors that might account for this difference. At HSL there are five MELVYL/MEDLINE terminals that have been available to library users, whereas at MCL there are only two MELVYL terminals. So the HSL users have had more opportunity to have used MELVYL/MEDLINE. The amount of time available to an individual user to come into the library might also be less at MCL given the clinical and teaching duties of most of its staff.

In keeping with the above concern with the availability of MELVYL/-MEDLINE at HSL, it is not surprising that a higher percentage of HSL users found it easier to learn than BIBLIOMED. In contrast, more than a third of the MCL users found BIBLIOMED easier to learn. Regarding which system they would rather use, a third of the users at each site chose BIBLIOMED, citing the convenient display of subject headings and journal lists among the reasons for their choice. About one-fourth of the HSL users and one-fifth of the MCL users chose MELVYL/MEDLINE because of the ability to look for several words at one time, among other reasons. A substantial portion (over 40%) of the users at each site did not answer yes or no to this question. Many of the non-respondents indicated that they had no preference for one system over the other.

The instructions on the BIBLIOMED screen were considered to be clear and understandable by over 60% of the respondents at both sites. The time span covered by the database met the needs of over half of the respondents at both sites. A somewhat higher percentage of dissatisfaction with the time span at HSL explained why many HSL users expressed concern that older material was not available. Although about half of the respondents at each site were pleased with the response time of the system, there were substantial numbers at each site that indicated that the display of citations was too slow. Much higher satisfaction was expressed by MCL users regarding the ease of use of BIBLIOMED; however, MCL staff have indicated that a fair number of users were "walked through" a search. This is in keeping with their previous answers regarding its ease of learning. The response to the BIBLIOMED manual was quite interesting. About one-third indicated that it was useful. However, many users noted on the evaluation form that they did not use the manual. One could interpret this to mean either that the system is so user-friendly that a manual is superfluous, or that many users just wanted to learn the system as they searched. Reference staff observed that many of those who did not want to use the documentation asked more questions.

The two user groups provided contrasting answers to the question regarding satisfaction with the journal titles covered by BIBLIOMED. This dissimilarity in response reflected the different needs of the two groups—not surprising considering the difference in the two user groups. Over 80% of the MCL users were satisfied with the subset. However, only a little over 50% of the HSL users were satisfied with the subset. HSL users suggested the addition of several research-oriented journal titles. Several of the users who did not answer this question mentioned that they would need a list of the journal titles in order to ascertain its adequacy.

Comments by both sets of users focused primarily on system glitches responsible for several searches being aborted while displaying citations and the slowness of the display of retrieved citations. There was also some confusion regarding the use of Boolean searching and concern with the displaying of the least current citations first. The use of the END key to start a search was confusing to many users, as was the use of reverse highlighting in menu choices. However, some users felt that BIBLIOMED was better for first time users and the online display of possible subject headings was helpful.

Additional Comments

These comments represent a compilation of conversations with users, staff evaluation of the system and staff observations of users. Most of the problems encountered and mentioned here have been discussed with the producer.

The Test

The arrangements to secure the designation of HSL as a test site were in process some months before staff knew of the plans to mount MEDLINE at the University of California campuses. The producer of BIBLIOMED was justifiably concerned that BIBLIOMED would not compare favorably with a full-blown version of MEDLINE backed by funding from the National Library of Medicine and the university. We addressed this concern in two ways. The testing of the product was extended to the Medical Center Library—a setting more in keeping with the target market for BIBLIOMED; and at HSL every effort was made to ensure that the BIBLIOMED station had a functioning printer. As only two of the five MELVYL/MEDLINE terminals had printers, we knew that users were quite keen on being able to print citations and it was thought that this would make the BIBLIOMED station competitive with MELVYL/MEDLINE. This actually proved to be beneficial as shown by the estimated number of BIBLIOMED users (approximately 150 persons) at HSL.

The issue of librarian bias and its impact on the test is worth commenting on as we think it must certainly be experienced whenever a user-friendly version of an online source is produced. Librarians often feel that they know what is best for the user; and in the case of database access we think that one of the librarians' last frontiers of unquestioned expertise is affronted by database producers who claim that they also know what users want. In the case of MEDLINE there is a great temptation on the part of librarians to compare any user-friendly version of it with MEDLINE as accessed in full command mode by experienced searchers. An independently produced product such as BIBLIO-MED cannot possibly compete with the large online systems mounted on computing configurations with the latest capabilities and backed by research and development monies. The person who is interested in a user-friendly system usually has neither the time nor the inclination to learn full command access and really only wants a fair representation of the articles on a topic—not a comprehensive search. The impact of librarian bias on the testing of a product such as BIBLIOMED is first felt when staff do not feel compelled to really learn the capabilities of the product, assuming that their previous experience as an online searcher of MEDLINE will certainly enable them to learn the rudiments of something that purports to be simple enough for use by non-searchers. It is felt again in the way that users are informed that the system is available, whether staff present the system in a positive way. Many users rely on the advice of staff regarding the usefulness of library resources and they are influenced by staff attitudes towards a source of information. To be fair, it should also be acknowledged that the test site staff, realizing the possibility of bias, tried to emphasize the positive aspects of BIBLIOMED to users and encouraged them to use the system. As the direction of the online industry would indicate that user-friendly products are on the rise, we think it behooves librarians to adopt a more positive attitude towards their capabilities and usefulness for end-users.

Database Content

For its target population, BIBLIOMED appears to contain a reasonable subset of the clinically-related journals that will be most useful in a hospital setting. Most academic health sciences libraries have too great a need for research-oriented material to be able to justify an expenditure for such a subset.

Record Content

All of the essential components of a record are available on BIBLIOMED. It might be useful to include an update indicator so that a user could limit a search to those citations entered at the last quarterly update. Perhaps alternatively it would be useful to be able to limit searching by year.

MeSH Descriptors

Users responded well to being given a choice of MeSH headings. Staff also were very positive about the emphasis on the importance of the headings as they are often bypassed by end-users, usually to the user's detriment. Having the headings in a listing that only requires that the user determine the appropriate heading by choosing a term frees the user from having to know about such things as stopwords and bound headings. The automatic heading/subheading listing was also very useful in that it did not require the user to know the proper heading/subheading combination. The ability to explode terms was an excellent feature, especially being able to selectively explode part of a tree. The explosion capability is one of the hardest concepts to teach end-users, but BIBLIOMED makes the process much clearer.

Search Functions

All subject terms input are automatically searched as MeSH headings, and if no heading is found, titles are searched. This default is a good one for end-users in that it increases their chances for retrieval. It would not be useful to expand a search to abstracts, as experience has shown that the precision of the retrieved citations is greatly reduced. One of the aspects of the system that was consistently confusing to users was the use of the END key to start the system searching after a term had been input. Most users wanted to press ENTER or RETURN for this process. The producer's contention that pressing the END key is intuitive might need to be reconsidered. Boolean searching is not clearly presented and many users thought that they were confined to single topic searches. The process of combining terms is the backbone of database searching and should be more clearly indicated on the screen display. While some users managed to read the documentation or otherwise find out how to AND terms, it did not appear that the system was capable of ORing together two MeSH terms that were alphabetically separate. However, it was possible to OR terms that appeared in close proximity to each other on a MeSH listing. The

343

automatic truncation of input terms by the system is a helpful addition to end-users. This capability frees the end-user from having to consider the various permutations of a word. The system also allows user-truncated terms.

Output Capabilities (Display)

The display of citations was set to author, title and source, with options to display MeSH headings and the abstract. Many users expressed the desire to be able to display the titles of citations as an additional option to facilitate looking at more than one citation per screen. Several comments were also made concerning the slowness of the on-screen display. Many users became so impatient that they pressed the down arrow continuously, which had the effect of speeding up the display to the point that the information could not be read. One of the users suggested that when citations are retrieved the sector locations should also be retrieved and 50 citations should be loaded into memory. This would slow down the appearance of the initial set of 50 citations but would allow them to be displayed more quickly. Then the system could inform the user that it was retrieving the next 50 citations. The ability to scroll through the retrieved citations and mark certain records for printing was commented on favorably by many users.

Output Capabilities (Print)

A variety of formats were available for printing, including the bibliographic citation, the citation plus abstract, and the citation plus abstract and MeSH headings. The default for printing should be changed to the bibliographic citation. The current default to the citation plus abstract and MeSH headings was often not realized by most users and they felt especially burdened by the MeSH headings. Also, the concept of "report" was unfamiliar to many users. The system does not reliably print citations in the last-one-in, first-one-out order that most users have come to expect. In some instances the printing was only roughly in this order, in other instances citations were printed in chronological order. It would also be helpful if the printed output could be numbered to facilitate referral to a particular citation by the user.

Downloading

The downloading capability was faster than the on-screen display, but burdened the user with the full record, complete with MeSH headings. Alternative formats should be available.

User-Friendliness

BIBLIOMED is designed as a totally menu-driven system for the novice searcher. There is no command mode alternative. The menu choices are clearly presented and the lack of clutter on the screen display enables the user to focus more on the contents of the screen. One concern is the use of highlighting. Conventionally, the item chosen is highlighted, whereas in BIBLIOMED the item chosen is the only choice *not* highlighted. This made for some confusion as to what was really being chosen. The system always informs the user when it is searching for a term and when it is loading a set of citations. Function keys are not heavily used. Those keys used are clearly referred to on the screen. The online tutorial is well-done and greatly reduced the need for staff to teach users the rudiments of the system. It is provided as a menu choice on the welcome screen. The documentation for BIBLIOMED needs to be tabbed and indexed. Cross-references to all information concerning a certain capability should be added. At present, one would not be aware that while a simple explanation to journal searching is available, a more detailed one is also available. A clearer description of how to use the Boolean "AND" and "OR" would also be useful. A toll-free hotline has been established by the producer and is staffed by knowledgeable and helpful staff. The system can be used with no training, although the online tutorial is invaluable for introducing users to the system.

Appendix A-1

July 1988

BIBLIOMED EVALUATION

Carlson Health Sciences Library
University of California, Davis

Final Tally
HSL/n=73; MCL/n=28

PRE-SEARCH QUESTIONS

1) Department: HSL/ Medicine 33 (45%); Vet. Medicine 26 (36%)
      Psychology 3

2) Status:

	FAC	STF	GS	UG	SRA	PGR	RA	NON-UC
HSL/	8 (11%)	10 (14%)	29 (40%)	8 (11%)	1 (1%)	8 (11%)	3 (4%)	6 (8%)
MCL/	11 (39%)	6 (21%)	4 (14%)	2 (7%)	1 (4%)	1 (4%)	0 (0)	3 (11%)

3) Have you ever used any other online version of MEDLINE (either
   by yourself or by having a librarian process a search for you?
   Circle all that apply.

   a. yes, by myself - HSL/40 (55%); MCL/19 (68%)
   b. yes, librarian search - HSL/20 (27%); MCL/11 (39%)
   c. no - HSL/19 (26%); MCL/5 (18%)
   d. don't know - HSL/1 (1%); MCL/0

4) Have you ever used BIBLIOMED before ?

   No - HSL/60 (82%); MCL/26 (93%)
   Yes - HSL/13 (18%); MCL/2 (7%)
   If yes, how many times ? - responses invalid

5) How will you be looking for articles ?

   a. By an author - HSL/26 (36%); MCL/11 (39%)
   b. By title - HSL/8 (11%); MCL/9 (32%)
   c. On a subject - 66 (90%); MCL/26 (93%)
   d. In a journal - HSL/8 (11%); MCL/4 (14%)
   e. Other - HSL/1 (1%); MCL/1 (4%)

6) Why do you need the information ? Circle all that apply.

   a. Paper or report - HSL/32 (44%); MCL/11 (39%)
   b. Research project - HSL/48 (66%); MCL/19 (68%)
   c. Teaching/Planning a course - HSL/10 (14%); MCL/15 (54%)
   d. Keeping current - HSL/19 (26%); MCL/9 (32%)
   e. To check a reference - HSL/9 (12%); MCL/6 (21%)
   f. Patient care - HSL/5 (7%); MCL/11 (39%)
   g. Not needed, just curious - HSL/3 (4%); MCL/0
   h. Other - HSL/3 (4%); MCL/2 (7%)

POST-SEARCH QUESTIONS

1) How would you rate the success of your search ? (Please circle any letters that apply and indicate how successful you were in finding what you were looking for by circling the appropriate number ranging from 1 = Very Successful to 5 = Unsuccessful).

		1	2	3	4	5
a. By an author -						
n=24	HSL/	8(33%)	6(25%)	4(17%)	3(12%)	3(12%)
n=6	MCL/	6(100%)				

		1	2	3	4	5
b. By Title -						
n=13	HSL/	1(7%)	7(54%)	2(15%)	1(7%)	2(15%)
n=2	MCL/	2(100%)				

		1	2	3	4	5
c. On a Subject -						
n=59	HSL/	12(20%)	23(39%)	11(19%)	8(13%)	5(8%)
n=13	MCL/	1(8%)	8(61%)	2(15%)	1(8%)	1(8%)

		1	2	3	4	5
d. In a Journal -						
n=8	HSL/	0	1(12%)	5(63%)	0	2(25%)
n=0	MCL/					

		1	2	3	4	5
e. Other -						
n=2	HSL/	0	0	1(50%)	0	1(50%)
n=0	MCL					

2) How would you rate the ease of use of BIBLIOMED ? (Circle one)

Very Easy	1	2	3	4	5 Difficult
HSL/	19(26%)	29(40%)	12(16%)	8(11%)	5(7%)
MCL/	7(25%)	14(50%)	2(7%)	5(18%)	0

3) The library also has MEDLINE available through the MELVYL terminals. Have you ever used MELVYL/MEDLINE beofre ?

YES - HSL/46(63%)   NO - HSL/23(32%)   NO ANSWER - HSL/4(5%)
      MCL/ 9(32%)   MCL/19(68%)   MCL/0

If yes, how would you compare MELVYL/MEDLINE to BIBLIOMED regarding how easy they are to learn to use ? (Circle one)

a. MELVYL/MEDLINE is easier to learn - HSL/16(22%)
                                         MCL/ 5(18%)

b. BIBLIOMED is easier to learn   - HSL/15(21%)
                                         MCL/10(36%)

c. The two systems are about equal   - HSL/17(23%)
                                         MCL/ 4(14%)

4) Would you prefer to use BIBLIOMED or MELVYL/MEDLINE ? Please tell us the reason for your choice.

BIBLIOMED - HSL/23(32%)   MELVYL/MEDLINE - HSL/20(27%)
              MCL/ 9(32%)   MCL/ 6(20%)

                    NO ANSWER - HSL/30(41%)
                                MCL/13(46%)

PLEASE CIRCLE ONE RESPONSE FOR EACH OF THE FOLLOWING QUESTIONS:

5) The instructions on the BIBLIOMED screen were clear and understandable.

   a.Strongly Agree b.Agree c.Neutral d.Disagree e.Strongly Disagree

   HSL/   7(10%)   41(56%)   16(22%)   7(10%)   1(1%)
   MCL/   5(18%)   13(46%)   2(21%)   1(4%)   1(4%)

6) The time span (December 1984 - February 1988) covered by BIBLIOMED was sufficient for my needs.

   a.Strongly Agree b.Agree c.Neutral d. Disagree e. Strongly Disagree

   HSL/   8(11%)   33(45%)   14(19%)   14(19%)   1(1%)
   MCL/   6(21%)   13(46%)   5(18%)   2(7%)   1(4%)

7) The rate at which BIBLIOMED responded was satisfactory.

   a.Strongly Agree b.Agree c.Neutral d. Disagree e. Strongly Disagree

   HSL/   9(12%)   30(41%)   14(19%)   13(18%)   5(7%)
   MCL/   5(18%)   11(39%)   2(7%)   6(21%)   2(7%)

8) Overall, I found BIBLIOMED easy to use.

   a.Strongly Agree b.Agree c.Neutral d.Disagree e. Strongly Disagree

   HSL/   8(11%)   41(56%)   12(16%)   7(10%)   3(4%)
   MCL/   7(25%)   16(57%)   2(7%)   2(7%)   0

9) The BIBLIOMED Manual helped me to use the system.

   a.Strongly Agree b.Agree c.Neutral d.Disagree e. Strongly Disagree

   HSL/   6(8%)   19(26%)   31(42%)   8(11%)   1(1%)
   MCL/   5(18%)   5(18%)   9(32%)   3(11%)   0

10) The journals included in BIBLIOMED were sufficient for my needs. (BIBLIOMED covers a subset of over 500 English-language journals of the 3810 journals covered in MEDLINE).

YES - HSL/40(55%)   NO - HSL/20(27%)   NO ANSWER - HSL/13(18%)
      MCL/23(82%)   MCL/ 2(7%)   MCL/ 3(11%)

If you answer no, please indicate below the journals you would like included;

HSL: Bioessays; Evolution; IEEE Transactions in Biomedical Engineering; Journal of Lipid Research; Journal of Virological Methods; Molecular Immunology; Nucleic Acids Research; Biochemica Biophysica Acta; Biochemical and Biophysical Research Communications; IEEE Medicine and Biology; subject areas of veterinary medicine, ecology, toxicology and foreign titles.

Comments

HSL: BIBLIOMED is less frustrating for the first time user.
Couldn't understand how to combine searches in BIBLIOMED
Didn't like only being able to use one word at a time.
Citation display too slow (mentioned 7 times)
Search aborted while displaying (mentioned 6 times)
Likes MELVYL/MEDLINE because it has more journals.
Would like to display more than one citation per screen.
BIBLIOMED needs more journals.
BIBLIOMED prints least current citations first.
Likes BIBLIOMED's subject headings and journal listing.

MCL: Display of citations too slow (mentioned 2 times)
Wanted to be able to use more than one word to search.
Would like to have BIBLIOMED journal list by terminal.
MELVYL/MEDLINE is more flexible.

July 1988

EVALUATION OF CD-ROM VERSION OF MEDLINE DATABASE

The following evaluation checklist was developed by Nancy S. Hewison, Life Sciences Library, Purdue University, West Lafayette, Indiana, 47907, 317-494-2917 and is used with her permission.

Test Site: Carlson Health Sciences Library, University of California, Davis, CA 95616.

Producer: Digital Diagnostics, Inc.   Software Version : 2.01
          601 University Ave. Suite 255
          Sacramento, CA 95825
          800-826-5595

Database: BIBLIOMED   Date Evaluated   : June 1988

Price : $975 - BIBLIOMED
         $1150- BIBLIOMED + AIDS   How Often Updated: Quarterly
         $395 - AIDS

Description: BIBLIOMED is a subset of the MEDLINE database and contains over 500 English-language journal titles in clinical medicine. The database is designed to be used by clinicians needing current information and is designed so that the user can "point and shoot", that is, choose items from a menu. The user inputs a single word and is lead through a permuted display of MeSH terms. If no MeSH term is found the system defaults to title searching. Retrieved citations can be displayed on screen and printed as a set or the user can mark individual records for printing. Various formats are available for printing. The full record format is available for downloading. An AIDS database is also available on the same disk and differs from BIBLIOMED only in that it covers information back to the early 1980's and from the full list of MEDLINE journal titles. It is searched in the same way as BIBLIOMED. An online tutorial and system documentation is provided.

DATABASE CONTENT

1. Time Range: Stated _3/85 - 4/88_   Actual _11/84 - 1/88_

RECORD CONTENT

2. NLM Record Elements   (Searchable/Printable)

X/X	Author	0/0	Accession Number
X/X	Title	0/0	Update Code
0/X	Abstract	0/0	Author Address
X/X	Descriptor	0/0	English Abstract
0/0	Language (All English)	0/0	Registry Number
0/0	Year of Publication	0/0	Name of Substance
X/X	Source Journal	0/0	ISSN
0/0	Special List Indicator	0/0	Country of Publication

3. Record Elements Added by CD-ROM Producer - None Added

MeSH DESCRIPTORS

4. _x_ Displayable _x_ Printable _x_ Downloadable

5. MeSH Words Searched as Part of Unqualified Search _x_ Yes __ No

6. Single-Word Descriptors Protected _x_ Yes __ No

7. Multi-Word Descriptors:
   N/A Bound for Precison
   N/A Protected if Contain Stopwords or Commands
   N/A Commas
   N/A Hyphens
   N/A Apostrophes

   Note: The elements in this category are not applicable to BIBLIOMED because the user chooses a term from a list and so does not need to be concerned with format or stopwords.

8. Major/Minor Emphasis is _x_ Indicated in Records _x_ Searchable
   YES Can Search Both at Once
   YES Can Restrict to Major
   NO Can Restrict to Minor (Can't "not" out major descriptor)
   YES Major Descriptors are Posted to Minor Descriptors

9. Subheading Searching
   NO Main Heading with No Subheadings
   YES Main Heading with One Specific Subheading
   YES Main Heading with Several, Specified Subheadings
   YES Main Heading with All Possible Subheadings
   NO Main Heading with All Possible Subheadings Plus with none
   NO "Naked" Subheading

   Note: Once a MeSH term is chosen, that term is displayed with its subheadings and postings.

10. Consistency in Searching
    YES Major/Minor Emphasis Searched Identically for Single-Word and Multi-Word MeSH Headings
    YES Main Heading/Subheading Combination Searched Identically for Single-Word and Multi-Word MeSH Headings
    YES Major and Minor Headings Searched Identically (Except for Emphasis
    YES Major Heading/Subheading and Minor Heading/Subheading Searched Identically (Except for Emphasis)

11. Explosion YES Possible Using Term YES Works Correctly
    NO Possible Using Tree Number ___ Works Correctly

    Note: In addition to a standard explosion of a term, it is also possible to access the tree structure and selectively choose indented terms if all are not desired.

12. Check Tags Given Special Treatment ___ Yes _X_ No

   Note: Check tags are searchable as subject terms.

13. Review Articles Searchable _X_ Yes ___ No

   Note: The MeSH headings for reviews are searchable as subject
      terms.

SEARCH FUNCTIONS

14. Unqualified Search Term is Searched in All Fields ___ Yes _X_ No

   Note: All subject terms input by the user are automatically
   matched to a MeSH term. If no MeSH term is found the system
   defaults to title words.

15. Field Searching
   _X_ Qualification to Specific Field Possible

   Note: Can search titles directly by inputting term and pressing
   F10.

   YES Qualification to More Than One Field at a Time
   NO_ Post Qualification

16. Boolean Logic: _X_ AND _X_ OR ___ NOT/ANDNOT ___ OR NOT

   Note: To "AND" two concepts, the user must conduct two successive
   searches. Terms can be ORed together if they appear in proximity
   in the MeSH term display.

17. Order of Precedence for Evaluating Operators
   N/A AND before OR   N/A OR before AND   N/A Left to Right
   NO_ User Can Control by Nesting

18. Proximity Searching
   NO Same Field, Any Order
   NO Same Sentence, Any Order
   NO Same Sentence, Any Order, Immedicately Adjacent
   NO Same Sentence, Any Order, Within n Words
   NO Same Sentence, Same Order, Immmediately Adjacent
   NO Same Sentence, Same Order, Within n Words

19. Truncation/Wild Card: YES Right _NO_ Left _NO_ Within Word
   Symbol Used - :

   Note: The system allows the user to truncate any term entered and
   will automatically truncate most words.

20. Stopwords: _NO_ Stopwords Operational _NO_ List Provided

   Note: The user is not required to know about stopwords. However
   an internal stopword list is operational.

21. Search Helps and Timesavers
    YES Displaying Database Index (NBR, ROOT, EXPAND)

    Note: Each term input by the user generates a permuted display of
    MeSH terms that fall alphabetically close to the input term. The
    tree structure for a term can be viewed by pressing F2. All
    authors and all journals in the database have their respective
    lists from which users can choose.

    YES Displaying Particular Index
    YES Displaying Search History
    YES User Can Erase Prior Search Statement

    Note: If a term added to a search will produce zero results, the
    system gives the user the option of backing up to a previous
    search term. The system automatically displays the search history.

    NO Back-Referencing Sets
    YES Limiting Possible

    Note: Can limit by author, journal or by check tag, but not by
    date. A language limit is not necessary as the entire database is
    in English.

22. Ability to Combine Search Capabilities
    NO Truncation and Phrase/Adjacency Searching
    YES Truncation and Field Qualification
    NO Truncation and Nested Logic
    NO Nested Logic and Field Qualification
    NO Phrase Adjacency Searching and Field Qualification

OUTPUT CAPABILITIES

23. Display Capabilities/Flexibility
    YES Various Formats Available (Yes or No/User Can Specify)
        NO / NO Titles Only
        YES / YES Bibliographic Citation
        YES / YES Bibliographic Citation and Abstract
        YES / YES Full Record
        NO / NO Title and Descriptors
        ___ / ___ Other
    NO User Can Specify Which Set to Display
    YES User Can Specify Which Record to Display
    NO User Can Specify How Field Labels Are Displayed
    NO Order in Which Records are Displayed
        ___ Last-in-First-Out/Reverse Chronological Order ___ Other

        Note: The system displays in roughly reverse chronological
        order but also sometimes displays in chronological order.
        The full record consists of the bibliographic citation,
        abstract and MeSH headings.

        NO User Can Specify Sort

24. Print Capabilities/Flexibility
    YES Various Formats Avaliable (Yes or No/User Can Specify)
        NO /NO   Titles Only
        YES/YES Bibliographic Citation
        YES/YES Biblographic Citation and Abstract
        YES/YES Full Record
        NO /NO   Title and Descriptors
        ___/___ Others
    NO User Can Specify Which Set to Print
    YES User Can Specify Which Records to Print
    NO User Can Specify How Field Labels are Printed
        __ Abbreviated   __ Written Out   ___ Omitted

    NO Order in Which Records are Displayed
        __ Last-In-First-Out/Reverse Chronological Order   ___ Other
        __ User Can Specify Sort

Note: The system doesn't reliably print in reverse chronological order.

25. Downloading
    NO Various Formats Available (Yes or No/User Can Specify)
        NO/NO Titles Only
        NO/NO   Bibliographic Citation
        NO/NO   Bibliographic Citation and Abstract
        YES/NO Full Record
        NC/NO   Title and Descriptors
        ___/___ Other
    NO User Can Specify Which Set to Display
    YES User Can Specify Which Records to Display
    NO User Can Specify How Field Labels are Displayed
        __ Abbreviated   __ Written Out   ___ Omitted
    NO Order in Which Records are Displayed
        __ Last-In-First-Out/Reverse Chronological Order   __ Other
        __ User Can Specify Sort
    __ Speed of Downloading

Note: Downloading is faster than displaying but not as fast as downloading online. Only the full record format can be downloaded.

26. Downloaded Output Compatible With Word Processing Software YES

    Note: The downloaded citations are an ASCII file and can be imported into most word processing programs.

USER-FRIENDLINESS

27. Number of Modes Available: Novice: X Menu   ___ Command
                                Experienced: ___ Menu ___ Command

28. Menus
    YES Contain Appropriate Choices
    YES Expressed Meaningfully
    YES Ways to Undo/Escape From/Reverse Menu Choices
    YES "Quit" Always Available
    N/A Forgiveness re: Command Format
    N/A Abbreviated Forms of Commands

    Note: Has reverse highlighting, i.e. the desired command is <u>not</u>
    highlighted.

29. Commands
    N/A Easy to Remember
    N/A Ways to Undo/Escape From/Reverse Commands
    N/A "Quit" Always Available
    N/A Forgiveness re: Command Entry Format
    N/A Abbreviated Forms of Commands

    Note: The system is totally menu-driven.

30. Processing
    YES Message Displays on Screen to Show Processing in Operation
    YES User can Interrupt Processing

31. Time and Keystroke Saving Features
    NO Abbreviated Commands Possible
    YES Function Keys Utilized
    NO Search Strategy Can be Saved for Use with Multi-Disc Database

    Note: BIBLIOMED is complete on one disk. Function keys used are
    F10=title search, F1=help, F2=to view the tree structure.

32. Online Help
    YES Instruction/Tutorial Screen

    Note: The system has an online tutorial that guides the users
    through a subject and an author search in 5-7 minutes.

    YES Contextual/Point of Need Screens   YES Helpful
    N/A If More Than 3 Screens per Topic, Table of Contentts and Jump
    YES Error Messages Understandable and Enabling

    Note: Can press F1 at any time for contextual help.

33. Documentation
    YES Clearly Written and Understandable
    YES Logically Arranged
    NO Well-Indexed
    YES All Important Features of Software Explained
    YES Basic Instruction to Special Features of Database

    Note: There is no index. Information on how to "OR" is unclear.

34. Telephone User Support
YES Toll-Free Hotline
YES Staff Knowledgeable
YES Staff Follows up if Answer Not Immediately Known

Note: 800-826-5595

35. Use-Related Issues
YES Can be Used With Little or No Training
YES Can be Used Without Reading Manual
YES Can be Left for End-Users With Minimal Library Staff Input
YES Defaults Appropriate for End-Users
NO Non-Standard Entry Formats Yield Surprises

36. Special Features
NO Highlighting of Terms Searched   NO On Screen   NO On Printout
NO Material From Latest Update to Disk Identified in Record
NO Searchable

Note: Display of menu choices is very clear. General screen
display uncluttered. System automatically truncates terms input
by user. Has the option of limiting search to titles only.

EVALUATION OF

CORE MEDLINE/ EBSCO CD-ROM, SILVERPLATTER, AND KNOWLEDGE FINDER

AT

UNIVERSITY OF UTAH SPENCER S. ECCLES HEALTH SCIENCES LIBRARY

By *Nina E. Dougherty*
Mary E. Youngkin
Maureen O. Carleton
Catherine G. Cheves
Spencer S. Eccles Health
Sciences Library

Kathleen M. McCloskey
Hope Fox Eccles Clinical Library
University of Utah
Salt Lake City, UT 84112

Evaluation Of Core Medline/ EBSCO CD-ROM, SilverPlatter, And Knowledge Finder At University Of Utah, Spencer S. Eccles Health Sciences Library

Introduction

User satisfaction with CORE MEDLINE/EBSCO CD-ROM was evaluated both in a library setting and in a clinical situation at the University of Utah Health Sciences Center during the spring and early summer of 1988. The workstation was placed in the reference area of Eccles Health Sciences Library for four weeks and then in the office of the head nurse of the neurology unit at University Hospital for the next four weeks. The EBSCO MEDLINE core subset at the time seemed more appropriate for nurses and dentists than others since it extensively covered the nursing and dental literature and only minimally the general medical literature. In September, 1988, the workstation with a revised CORE MEDLINE/EBSCO CD-ROM product was returned to the neurology unit and placed in the open nursing station area for additional evaluation in a clinical setting. The new subset included 575 major health sciences journals, with minimal coverage of the nursing literature.

During the evaluation period users continued to have access to Silver-Platter MEDLINE CD-ROM which has been available since late 1987 in both Eccles Library and the Clinical Library in the hospital. Knowledge Finder was also available for a week during the EBSCO test period. Although it was located in the reference office for evaluation primarily by librarians, Macintosh users were encouraged to try it.

An atmosphere of active promotion of end-user searching of MEDLINE exists at the University of Utah. End-users have been encouraged to get their own passwords or to use (at cost) the library's passwords. In either case the library's equipment may be used at no charge. More recently users have been encouraged to use the CD-ROM systems. Information, demonstrations, training and assistance have been provided by vendors and librarians to groups and individuals as well as at the INFOFAIR held annually since 1983. The health sciences COLLEAGUE group account has 27 active passwords, mostly used on a departmental basis. Individuals and departments also have passwords to NLM, DIALOG, COMPUSERV and other systems. While end-user utilization of the library's passwords and equipment for online searching has dwindled since the introduction of free MEDLINE on CD-ROM, end-user online searching from offices has continued to grow.

Traditional online search service is provided for a charge by searchers at Eccles Library and the Clinical Library. The Clinical Library also provides free searches on topics related to management of a patient in the hospital. Since July, 1988, patient care team members have been able to transmit a request for a MEDLINE search to the Clinical Library after viewing a patient's record on the HELP patient information system. A MEDLINE printout and several selected articles are brought to the nursing station within an hour.

Computer literacy and use of computers appears to be reasonably prevalent among University of Utah health sciences faculty, researchers, administrators and students. Access to patient data in the hospital is via computer.

Methodology: Library Setting

The EBSCO CD-ROM workstation was located on a table immediately behind the reference desk. Participants in the study were recruited in two ways. Some users heard of the evaluation through publicity and specifically asked to use the system. Others were enlisted as they requested information or an online search at the reference desk. The librarian at the desk, after determining that the topic and other search parameters (such as years and journal coverage) were appropriate for the CORE MEDLINE/EBSCO CD-ROM product, encouraged the user to try the EBSCO CD-ROM. Some users wanted to try it and some still preferred to have a librarian do the search. Requesters at the desk were directed to the SilverPlatter or Knowledge Finder CD-ROM if more appropriate. It was assumed that pharmacy students would need the broader coverage of SilverPlatter, but some wanted to use EBSCO instead of waiting their turn for SilverPlatter.

Users of any of the three CD-ROM products during the four week period were asked to fill out an evaluation form, although repeat users during that time were not always given an evaluation form after the first time. The forms, which were altered slightly for each system, included the questions suggested by NLM as well as additional ones desired by local librarians.

Interviews were conducted with library staff members to ascertain what kind of help was needed by users and how much time it took. Instructions were to provide as much help as the user requested or appeared to need. The evaluation was not viewed as a test of end-users' ability to search a system with minimal help. A set of MeSH and the EBSCO MEDLINE CD-ROM manual were made available to the users.

The searches which requestors wanted librarians to do, or which librarians thought they should do, during the time period were tabulated and analyzed for characteristics distinguishing them from those users did themselves on CD-ROM.

Methodology: Clinical Setting

During the initial four weeks in the hospital neurology unit, the workstation was on the small desk of the small office of the head nurse. The equipment was located there for security reasons but made general use of the CD-ROM inconvenient. Only the head nurse and assistant head nurse used the CD-ROM. The same four-page evaluation form used in the library for EBSCO was given to them. Information about their usage, satisfaction and recommendations was primarily gained from an interview with each nurse. Some information was also acquired from four forms filled out by one of the nurses.

A reference librarian provided initial training to the head nurse who then took responsibility for training anyone else who might use the CD-ROM. A set of the printed MeSH tools was left with her. She was encouraged to call the Clinical Library any time she needed assistance. The Clinical Library also provided document delivery.

The workstation was removed from the head nurse's office after the four-week period and was not returned to the area until September, 1988, when space was provided for it on the counter of the nursing station in the open central area of the neurology unit. A decision was made to place the equipment in the open area even though no special security measures were available. Abridged one page evaluation forms, the manual, and a set of MeSH volumes were left next to the machine. An interview was conducted with the head nurse at the end of the first week. She again took responsibility for managing the CD-ROM system and providing training to those she felt would use it. She assumed that other nurses and clerks at the station, rather than medical students, residents and attending physicians, would want to use the CD-ROM.

Additional information about the usefulness in a clinical setting of immediate end-user access to MEDLINE, whether online or on CD-ROM, was gained through an interview with a cardiologist and the Head of the Clinical Library. The cardiologist searches COLLEAGUE online from his desk and also uses the Clinical Library SilverPlatter CD-ROM when visiting his patients in the cardiology unit adjacent to the library. Statistics and impressions on increasing end-user searching of the CD-ROM in the Clinical Library were obtained from the librarian.

Results: Library Setting

Thirty-six evaluation forms were turned in by EBSCO users, 24 by Silver-Platter users and five by Knowledge Finder users. Appendix A tallies the answers on the evaluation forms for all three systems. The report, however, will primarily discuss results of evaluation of the EBSCO CD-ROM. Appendix B shows some characteristics of requestors and search parameters for online searches performed by librarians during the four-week time period. There were 51 requests which resulted in librarians performing online searches at Eccles Library during the four weeks and a total of 65 searches undertaken by end-users on the three different CD-ROM products.

Twenty-two (61%) of the 36 evaluators of EBSCO in the library were students, with 13 being pharmacy students. Eight of the 36 users were affiliated with nursing in some capacity. Nurses seemed to have more multiple roles, such as simultaneously being a practicing nurse, Ph.D. student and teacher, than others. There were three students, two faculty members and a researcher from the School of Medicine. Five (four students, one faculty member) were from the College of Health and the rest of the 36 were from other areas of campus or off-campus. Thirty-six percent of the searches were for papers or reports, 20% for patient care, 20% for research projects and the remainder for keeping current and other purposes.

In contrast to users of CD-ROM during the evaluation period, 53% of those requesting mediated searches during the same time were faculty or researchers in the School of Medicine, who have the ability to pay for searches, who are accustomed to having searches done for them and who have limited time. Additional differences were that 81% of the requestors of mediated searches wanted citations from before 1986, and some wanted other databases searched.

A discussion of the implications of who is using CD-ROM, what their search success is, what is desired or needed in a MEDLINE subset and how users liked EBSCO CORE MEDLINE (spring, 1988, version) follows a description of the use of MEDLINE CD-ROM in the hospital neurology unit and by the cardiologist.

Results: Clinical Setting

The two nurses in the hospital neurology patient unit came to rely on being able to search MEDLINE on CD-ROM for a variety of purposes. The head nurse tended to search MEDLINE for nursing administration literature and the assistant head nurse to seek articles about diseases and care problems of patients in the unit. The latter articles were usually intended for the nurses in the unit but also might be given to the patients or their families, if appropriate. Both nurses found it convenient and useful to be able to immediately search MEDLINE to find answers for issues raised in the course of a conversation or to support their concerns as a member of a patient's care team. The EBSCO MEDLINE journal subset available in the spring was excellent for nursing administration literature but not adequate for the assistant head nurse when searching for clinical neurology literature. In September the revised journal subset with its minimal nursing literature coverage was no longer adequate for nursing administration and general nursing information literature needs. The new subset, however, seemed to be sufficient for clinical neurology topics. When using the earlier subset which emphasized the nursing literature, the two nurses rarely felt it was a waste of time because even if they weren't successful in finding what they were specifically looking for they usually found citations that were useful for other purposes.

Problems expressed by the nurses related to the EBSCO search interface and to the sheer bulk of a complete, dedicated CD-ROM workstation. The necessity to enclose phrases, including MESH headings, in quotation marks was difficult to remember. The inclination was simply to enter a phrase, which the EBSCO system interpreted as a series of words in an "or" rather than "adjacent" relationship. This was a particular problem if the phrase included the term "nursing." The need for quotation marks was dropped in the mid-September version of the EBSCO CD-ROM. Otherwise, the nurses felt the search interface was easy to use. The head nurse wanted to continue using the CD-ROM but was anxious to have it moved from her desk.

During the September, 1988, phase of testing the EBSCO CD-ROM in the neurology unit, more users had access to the workstation in the new location on the nursing station counter. In this second test phase the CD-ROM was used primarily by nurses in the unit. Nurses at stations on other floors also expressed interest. Four evaluation forms, mostly expressing delight with being able to use the system, were returned. One very computer-literate user had difficulty in locating his nebulous topic. The head nurse gave basic instruction to others on how to use the system and how to be reasonably specific in searching. She also tried to encourage use of the print Annotated MeSH which was placed next to the workstation. She said that some individuals encountering the workstation during hours she wasn't there told her that they read the manual to find out how to use the system. The head nurse had the impression that most new users were reading the tutorials on the CD-ROM. Users in the library, on the other hand, rarely used the manual or the tutorials, possibly because of the availability of a librarian to answer their questions.

The cardiologist who searches MEDLINE on COLLEAGUE from his desktop workstation, and who also uses the SilverPlatter CD-ROM in the Clinical Library had interesting observations. Although he searches MEDLINE frequently, and attended a brief library-sponsored training session on COLLEAGUE several years ago, he does not remember all the features and never uses subheadings or explosions in searching. Yet, without using MEDLINE as effectively as he might, he found the literature he located on MEDLINE to be very useful in his practice and supervision of housestaff. He felt he used SilverPlatter in an even less sophisticated manner, because the help screens were not visible on the monochrome screen in the Clinical Library, and still retrieved useful literature. He never uses a manual for a computer application, instead relying on help screens associated with the program.

The cardiologist searches MEDLINE online on COLLEAGUE for comprehensive searches for papers and research projects. He is more likely to use the SilverPlatter CD-ROM when he is on the ward near the Clinical Library although he dislikes having to change discs in order to search more than one year of MEDLINE on the SilverPlatter system. At times he is able to obtain enough information from an abstract that immediate access to the full article is not necessary. He recommends that there be more informative abstracts. Residents in the Cardiology Department receive training from him on how to search MEDLINE and a nudge to use the free SilverPlatter CD-ROM in preference to searching online. They do have access, however, to COLLEAGUE through the department Novell network.

Discussion

1. WHO ARE THE CD-ROM USERS?

Are the people using CD-ROM new users or are they people who usually use online MEDLINE? One indicator is whether the number of mediated online MEDLINE requests dropped during the evaluation period. There was only a slight decrease in the number of mediated search requests at Eccles Library during the evaluation period. There has, in fact, been no notable decline in requests for mediated searches at Eccles Library during the year in which SilverPlatter CD-ROM has been available to users. There was a difference in who was using CD-ROM at no charge during the evaluation period and who was requesting a search for which there was a charge. The major category of CD-ROM users was students. The major category of requestors of online searches during the same period was School of Medicine faculty and researchers.

The fact that MEDLINE CD-ROM was provided free of charge was important to the majority of EBSCO users, with it being an especially important factor to the students. Twenty-six of the 36 EBSCO users stated their being able to use CD-ROM free of charge was an important consideration. Seventeen of the 22 students using EBSCO CD-ROM stated that "free" was an important factor. Additional differences between those using CD-ROM and those requesting a search related to the desire to have more years and/or other databases searched; wanting a more comprehensive search; having less time; and being more willing to delegate the searching of MEDLINE to an "expert" searcher. Some of the CD-ROM users had their own passwords to search MEDLINE online. Convenience is presumably a factor in whether these people choose to use CD-ROM or an online system. When they are in the library they may use CD-ROM and when they are in their office they may search MEDLINE online from their desktop workstation.

An interesting phenomenon is that while the Eccles Library online search load has not changed since the provision of free CD-ROM, requests for free patient related searches and for searches for which there is a charge have both declined at the Clinical Library. This decrease in requests appears to be directly proportional to the increase in end-user use of CD-ROM in that library. This is not a case of users opting to do their own search at no cost instead of paying an intermediary to search for them. This is a case of their wanting to do their own search rather than having someone else do it.

The answers on the evaluation questionnaire may also provide an indication of whether the CD-ROM users represent new users or former online users. In fact, almost 70% of the CD-ROM users (all three systems) during the evaluation period stated they had used MEDLINE online before. Twenty-five percent of those who said they had used online before still preferred online, while 60% preferred CD-ROM, and the rest "didn't know." The librarians at Eccles Library felt that some users may not have correctly answered the question on whether they had used online before even though "online" was defined in the questionnaire. It has been noted that many of the CD-ROM users at Eccles Library during the past year haven't understood the distinction between CD-ROM and "online."

2. HOW SUCCESSFUL ARE THE CD-ROM USERS?

The majority of the users of the EBSCO MEDLINE CD-ROM felt they were successful to some degree in finding what they wanted. Forty-six percent stated that they found "some of what was wanted", 37% found "what I was looking for," 11% found "more than I needed," a psychologist, for whose topic the subset was inappropriate, said that it wasn't useful and one person was unsure. Their future success rate might be different since they received all the help they requested. As first time searchers they were also more receptive to help. An additional factor to consider is the true meaning of the answer, "I found what I was looking for." That answer may be more often selected by users who are less familiar with the literature on the topic and with MEDLINE, than by other users.

Information on how well the users actually did in using the CD-ROM is derived more from observations by the librarians than from other means, unlike an end-user search behavior study in 1985 which was designed to determine how successul end-users really were. Users in the current evaluation stated their topic on the questionnaire and were asked to provide a copy of their search strategy and results. The latter was not done consistently, nor does it reflect the assistance that might have been given to the user. Users tended to not use MeSH headings unless prompted. They very rarely selected the option on the menu of looking at MeSH headings. The neurology head nurse did become very conscious of the usefulness of MeSH headings and urged those she was helping to search for their terms in the MeSH volumes.

Whether they were successful or not, the majority of users of all three CD-ROM systems stated that the next time they needed such information they would use that particular CD-ROM system. There was some ambivalence on the part of EBSCO users who stated they had used online before as to whether they would use online or EBSCO CD-ROM in the future (Question 9). The questionnaire erroneously allowed only one answer for Question 9, rather than the multiple possibilities allowed for the question as to what they would do next time they needed that type of information (Question 11.) Of the 20 who stated they had used online before and answered Question 9 on what they preferred, seven said they preferred EBSCO CD-ROM, nine preferred online (seven doing their own), and four "didn't know". On the other hand, 31 of the 36 using EBSCO (when allowed to give multiple answers in Question 11) said that they would use EBSCO CD-ROM the next time they needed the same information.

3. WHAT IS THE IDEAL MEDLINE SUBSET?

An analysis of how satisfied the different professional categories of users were with what they found and with the journal subset yielded some surprising answers. It had been assumed that nurses would be more likely to find what they wanted and would be happier with the original EBSCO MEDLINE CD-ROM journal subset than other users. The only general medical journals in the subset were from the limited AIM list. There was little difference, however, between nurses and the other users in whether they felt they were successful in finding what they wanted. Four of the eight nurses said they had only found "some of what was wanted", three of the six from the School of Medicine said they found "what I was looking for", one medical student and two pharmacy students found "more than what was needed." There was also little difference between the users when answering the direct question of how satisfied they were with the journal subset. The majority of most users "agreed" or "strongly agreed" that the journal subset was sufficient. Nurses were among those who found the journal subset insufficient. When the subset was changed, it was no longer adequate for nursing topics. The limited time span (from 1986 to the present) was also of concern to one third of the users.

The revised 575 clinical journal subset provided by EBSCO in September appeared to be sufficient for many medical topics. For general hospital use, it would have to be supplemented by a subset covering hospital administration and nursing journals or by CINAHL and HEALTH as separate CD-ROM databases.

4. HOW EASY WAS EBSCO CD-ROM?

The majority of the users stated that EBSCO MEDLINE CD-ROM was easy to use. They planned to turn to it the next time they needed to search MEDLINE. A feature they especially liked was the ability to limit citations to those in journals held by the library.

Librarians assisting the users noted that they did have difficulty with moving through the system which required constant switching from one screen to another. This appeared to be the most difficult technical problem, which the librarians tried to ameliorate by demonstrating the proper process to each new user. Screen change messages were simpler and clearer in the new version in September. Users also tended to easily get a "fatal error" message in the earlier version. The wording of the message, which was changed in the September release, made the user insecure. Users appeared to get the message usually because they failed to follow the instructions on the screen. The other notable problem was the need to enclose a phrase in quotation marks in order to search it as a phrase rather than separate words searched in an "or" relationship. This was also changed in the new version. A phrase that was entered was now searched as a phrase.

Conclusions

Health sciences users at the University of Utah want to search MEDLINE on their own, no matter how successful or unsuccessful they truly are or think they are. Students, especially, want to be able to search MEDLINE without charge. CD-ROM is a medium for free, local end-user searching of MEDLINE that can realistically be provided to users at the University of Utah. Being able to search a disc containing several years of a limited subset of MEDLINE is more convenient than having to individually search multiple discs for a more comprehensive MEDLINE subset. A limited subset, however, may not meet the needs of all of the patient care team in a clinical setting and certainly does not meet the needs of all of Eccles Library users.

Users who have their own passwords for online searching will probably use the most convenient means of searching MEDLINE at any one time or for a particular information problem. If they are in or near the Eccles Library or Clinical Library and if the CD-ROM workstation is available, they may use the CD-ROM for a particular problem. They will probably also continue to use an online system.

How easy or effective the software for one CD-ROM product is versus that for another may be a moot point in the near future. The companies producing the different MEDLINE products are actively responding to user problems and suggestions but making continual improvements.

We wish to acknowledge the invaluable assistance with the project that was provided by Mary Ann Lambert, RN, Head Nurse, Neurology Nursing Station, University Hospital.

CD-ROM EVALUATION, Eccles Health Sciences Library, University of Utah
April-June, 1988

ANSWERS ON COMPLETED EVALUATION FORMS for:

1. EBSCO at Eccles Library (36 completed forms)
2. EBSCO at nursing station (Head nurse and assistant head nurse used
     multiple times. One filled out forms, the other was interviewed.)
3. Silver Platter (24 completed forms)
4. Knowledge Finder (5 forms completed by users. Primarily being
     evaluated by librarians)

The EBSCO CORE MEDLINE CD-ROM product was assigned to Eccles Library
for evaluation. During the same time period, however, the Silver Platter
MEDLINE CD-ROM was available for the full time and Knowledge Finder for a
week. Since users were asked to fill out evaluation forms when using any of
the products, the answers on the forms for the additional products are
included in this report.

	EBSCO Library	EBSCO Hospital	Silver Platter	Knowledge Finder	TOTAL
Total Forms:	36	2 users	24	5	67
QUESTIONS:					
1. Primary affiliation:					
a. Medicine	6	-	6	3	15
b. Dentistry	-	-	-	-	-
c. Nursing	6	2	5	-	13
d. Pharmacy	13	-	5	-	18
e. College of Health	5	-	2	-	7
f. Other Univ Utah	2	-	3	2	7
g. Other (non-UU)	4	-	3	-	7
2. Profession					
a. Physician	3	-	1	3	7
b. Nurse	8	2	7	-	17
c. Dentist	-	-	-	-	-
d. Other health profess.	4	-	3	1	8
e. Educator	3	1	1	1	6
f. Scientist/researcher	4	-	6	2	12
g. Student	22	2	11	-	35
h. Other	5	-	1	1	7
3. Looking for articles:					
a. By author	-	-	3	2	5
b. Under a title	3	-	4	1	8
c. On a subject	36	[all]	21	5	62
d. In a journal	2	-	1	-	3
e. Other	-	-	-	1	1

	EBSCO Library	EBSCO Hospital	Silver Platter	Knowledge Finder	TOTAL
4. Needed for:					
a. Patient care	13	[yes]	1	1	15
b. Paper or report	24	-	14	4	42
(Student paper)	(20)	-	(7)	-	(27)
c. Research project	14	-	8	4	26
d. Keeping current	8	[yes]	3	2	13
e. To check a reference	2	-	2	1	5
f. Teaching/plan course	3	[yes]	1	1	5
g. Other	5	[yes]	3	1	9
5. Information found was:					
a. What was looking for	13	sometimes	12	3	28
b. More than needed	4	sometimes	2	-	6
c. Some of what needed	16	sometimes	7	1	24
d. Not useful	1	-	2	1	4
e. Other	1	-	-	-	1
6. Used any of print versions					
a. Yes	28	1	24	3	56
b. No	4	1	-	2	7
c. Don't know	3	-	-	-	3
7. If yes, used print, is PRINT:					
a. Easier to use	10	-	8	-	18
b. Harder to use	9	1	14	2	26
c. About same	6	-	2	-	8
d. Other	1	-	-	-	1
8. Have used online version					
a. Yes, by myself	10	-	10	2	22
b. Yes, librarian search	11	2	8	3	24
c. No	13	-	4	1	18
d. Don't know	1	-	1	-	2
9. If have used online, prefer					
a. Online, own	7	-	-	2	9
b. EBSCO	7	1			8
Silver platter			16		16
Knowledge Finder				2	2
c. Online, librarian	2	-	-	-	2
d. Don't know	4	1	2	-	7
10. If this CD-ROM not available today, would have					
a. Used printed version	20	1	17	1	39
b. Used online version	10	1	3	2	16
c. Asked library staff	12	1	5	2	20
d. Asked friend, colleague	4	-	-	-	4
e. Browsed in stacks	9	-	6	1	16
f. Nothing	1	1	1	-	3
g. Other (2 said "cried")	2	-	3	-	5

	EBSCO Library	EBSCO Hospital	Silver Platter	Knowledge Finder	TOTAL
11. Next time will:					
a. Try this CD-ROM	31	2	24	5	62
b. Try printed	10	-	4	1	15
c. Try online	10	-	4	3	17
d. Another source	1	-	1	1	3
12. How important is no charge for use of CD-ROM in deciding to use it as opposed to online.					
a. Very important	22	-	17	3	42
b. Somewhat important	4	-	6	2	12
c. Relatively unimportant	9	2	1	-	12
d. Wouldn't use online	1	-	-	-	1
13. How often have you used this CD-ROM product?					
a. First time	31	(used repeatedly	11	5	
b. Once before	2	during this	2	-	
c. 3-5 times	3	evaluation)	4	-	
d. 6 or more times	-		7	-	
14. How many discs did you use today? (Only applicable for Silver Platter)					
a. 1 disc			8		
b. 2 discs			3		
c. 3 discs			6		
d. 4 discs			6		
15. Instructions on screens sufficient for use:					
a. Strongly agree	8	2	5	1	
b. Agree	17	-	13	4	
c. Neutral	8	-	5	-	
d. Disagree	2	-	-	-	
e. Strongly disagree	-	-	1	-	
16. Response rate satisfactory					
a. Strongly agree	9	-	9	1	
b. Agree	16	-	14	2	
c. Neutral	8	-	5	2	
d. Disagree	2	1	-	-	
e. Strongly disagree	-	-	1	-	
17. Manual was helpful					
a. Strongly agree	2	-	1	-	
b. Agree	2	-	6	1	
c. Neutral	17	1	13	4	
d. Disagree	7	-	1	-	
e. Strongly disagree	1	-	-	-	
Wrote, "didn't use"	5	1	2	-	

	EBSCO Library	EBSCO Hospital	Silver Platter	Knowledge Finder	TOTAL
18. Changing discs is easy. (Didn't have this on our questionnaire because was designed for EBSCO)					
19. Time span sufficient:					
a. Strongly agree	5	-	6	-	11
b. Agree	19	1	11	1	32
c. Neutral	2	-	-	-	2
d. Disagree	8	-	6	2	16
e. Strongly disagree	1	1	1	2	5
20. Found product easy to use					
a. Strongly agree	10	-	8	-	
b. Agree	18	2	13	5	
c. Neutral	4	-	1	-	
d. Disagree	3	-	1	-	
e. Strongly disagree	-	-	-	-	
21. Additional question for EBSCO and Knowledge Finder: (Described journal subset) Was journal subset sufficient for your needs today?					
a. Strongly agree	7	-	-	1	
b. Agree	15	1	-	1	
c. Neutral	9	1	-	1	
d. Disagree	3	-	-	1	
e. Strongly disagree	1	-	-	1	

ONLINE SEARCH REQUESTS, Eccles Health Sciences Library, April 11-May 10, 1988

Characteristics of requestors and search parameters are listed for online searches that were performed by librarians during the month in which the EBSCO MEDLINE CD-ROM product was being evaluated at Eccles Library. Librarians suggested to users with appropriate search requests that they use a CD-ROM product first or instead of having an online search done. Some users with appropriate requests still elected to have their search done online. Only the online or CD-ROM searches done during the month the EBSCO product was tested at Eccles Library are in this tabulation.

CHARACTERISTIC:	ONLINE SEARCH by librarian * 51 searches	CD-ROM SEARCH by user 65 searches
1. Primary affiliation:		
a. Medicine, School of	27	15
b. Nursing, College of	1	9
c. Pharmacy, College of	2	18
d. Health, College of	3	7
e. Other University of Utah (UU)	3	7
f. Other: Non-UU, health professional	4	7
g. Other: Non-UU, non-health prof.	6	0
2. Profession/status		
a. Physician	24	7
b. Nurse	0	15
c. Other health professional	2	8
d. Educator	26	5
e. Scientist/researcher	29	12
f. Student	8	33
g. Other (lawyers, etc)	6	7
3. Databases requested		
a. MEDLINE	43	65
b. BIOSIS	1	
c. Chem Abs	4	
d. CINAHL	1	
e. HEALTH	1	
f. Psyc Abs	3	
g. SDILINE	1	
h. SPORT	1	
i. SSCI	1	
j. TOXLINE	4	
4. Years requested:		
a. 1986 -	8	
b. 1983 -	6	
c. 1980 -	7	
d. 1978 -	9	
e. 1975 -	2	
f. 1972 -	2	
g. 1970 -	2	
h. 1966 -	8	

371

EVALUATION OF THE

EBSCO CD-ROM CORE MEDLINE SYSTEM

AT THE UNIVERSITY OF ILLINOIS

AT CHICAGO

By   Peter Vigil
     Vislava Tylman
     Kimberly Laird

Library of the Health Sciences,
Information Services
University of Illinois at Chicago
Chicago, IL 60612

Evaluation Of The EBSCO CD-ROM Core Medline System At The University Of Illinois At Chicago

Introduction

The EBSCO CD-ROM CORE MEDLINE System contains a "core" of 600 journal titles emphasizing clinical medicine and nursing from the MEDLINE database. It covers the last 2-3 years and has approximately 250,000 citations, 50% with abstracts. The system configuration consists of a KAYPRO 286 microcomputer, a Magnavox RGB Display 80 color monitor, a Hitachi CD ROM player, and a STAR printer. The system runs under DOS 3.2.

The entire system is menu driven, has an extensive tutorial and provides the user with options throughout the dialogue to receive help messages.

EBSCO's CORE MEDLINE has three interface levels. All three are similar with increasing levels of complexity and power options. Level 1, or Patron, provides the user with several input lines. The relationship among lines is a Boolean AND operation. Terms input on a single line default to a Boolean OR operation. Phrase queries or adjacency are executed by using quotes, and brackets may be used to execute an inclusive AND operation within the same line. The number of characters that terms can be apart when brackets are used is controlled by a system administration option.

The second level, Patron2, offers the above but also provides another series of input lines for subject headings, journal titles, and authors. The third section, Advanced, contains the same input sections as Patron2, but in addition has an input section on the bottom for combining previous search queries in logical Boolean expressions. It is necessary, however, to consult a different screen to identify the previous search statements.

The system provides several index files for MESH headings, authors, & journal titles. The user has the option of entering input directly or selecting from a menu option by scrolling through the index.

The system has the ability to store searches by patron ID, run SDIs, target journals specific to the institution's local collection, and initiate ILLs. The local journal and ILL component were not used by UIC.

The system was placed 20 feet from the reference desk and within view of library personnel at the desk. It was made available during all the hours reference coverage was provided. A quick guide was developed to allow the patron to get started through the menus. The EBSCO user manual was kept at the work-station and a policy and brief instruction manual prepared by LHSIS was also placed at the workstation. This included a notice of a 15-minute limit when ano-ther patron was waiting, how to get from the DOS prompt to start the system, downloading options, the on site print limit (25 citations), the three interface levels and the availability of 2 weekly one-hour seminars on using the system. There was also a highly visible sign at the workstation and at the reference desk informing patrons of the seminars. Signs were posted throughout the library in-forming patrons of the system's availability. Various notices and announce-ments were also included in the LHS monthly newsletter NEWS NOTES.

Methodology

Two questionnaires were utilized to address the reaction of both new users and experienced users. The questionnaire for new users was intended to compile data on users' profiles and their satisfaction with the system. A second instru-ment was used to find out how the users were interacting with the system. It was not realistic to combine the two questionnaires, since a minimum level of experience would be required before the users could be expected to engage in any "advanced" information retrieval techniques, such as using MESH explos-ions, combining sets, etc.

The new user questionnaire was distributed from April through July, and the experienced user questionnaire from June through August.

Results

A copy of the questionnaires and the tabulated results are attached to this report as Appendixes A and B. One hundred and two questionnaires of the new user type were returned; and twenty-three of the experienced user. When the system was installed, it seemed there was some reluctance to use it. Although signs were placed about the library and at our INDEX MEDICUS locations, the unit more or less remained idle for the first week. However, as patrons began to use the system, its popularity accelerated and within a short time there were often patrons waiting in line.

Highlights of the results are as follows. Over three-fourths of the respon-dents were affiliated with UIC. Over a third were physicians. Ninety-two percent were interested in a subject. Eighty-eight percent found some information useful to their needs. Almost a third had searched MEDLINE as an end-user before, and two thirds had had a mediated MEDLINE search in the past. There was a two to one preference to search themselves, and 72%, given various options such as using print or another online searching system, would prefer to use EBSCO CORE MEDLINE. Ninety-four percent would have used the printed INDEX MEDICUS, if the CORE MEDLINE had not been available. Free access was an important consideration to the vast majority of the users.

Sixty-one percent were regular microcomputer users, 33% were regular user of the the library's online catalogs, and 20% used the UIC Academic Data network electronic-mail system.

On the system capabilities and documentation, the users were satisfied with system speed, the brief guide, EBSCO's manual, and the menu screens. Most felt reference assistance made it possible for them to use the system. Overall, 86% felt the system is easy to use, only 4% disagreed and 6% strongly disagreed. The least satisfactory aspect of the system concerned the time span; 32% disagreed or strongly disagreed that the years covered were sufficient.

This last indication was also confirmed with the experienced user questionnaire. Seventy-five percent of respondents indicated if a choice had to be made they would prefer more years of coverage rather than more journal titles.

Since only 23 users filled out the "experienced user" questionnaire it appeared that the users were rather reluctant to consider themselves experienced. Further, those that did indicated by their answers that they are rather naive with the system's capability.

One of the indicators of expertise and/or experience is the use of multiple sets in searching. Although eight respondents indicated that they used multiple sets and 12 indicated using at least 2 sets or more, there was apparently some confusion on their part, since only 2 reported using the Advanced level, which is necessary to do multiple set searching. No doubt they were referring to individual search query lines in the patron1 and patron2 levels.

Discussion

By all accounts from the reference staff, the level of use by the patrons of the system was quite naive. Although, the patrons overwhelmingly indicate that it is easy to use, their reluctance to identify themselves as "experienced" users attests to their awareness of their minimal level of expertise.

They would like to learn more but most are not willing to take the time to attend the one-hour seminars or go through the online tutorial. The staff observed very few using the tutorial session. Moreover, it would appear that the patrons will search broadly and select what they want rather than pursue options that will provide precision. As expected the users were quite confused by the whole notion of Boolean expressions and algorithmic problem solving.

Patron1 and Patron2 levels are easy to use but users did not understand or forgot the need to use quotes or brackets on the input lines. Often they executed a search with 4 terms that logically should be ANDed, but since the quotes or brackets were omitted and terms were input on two lines, the search executed was (A OR B) AND (C OR D) rather than the exact A AND B AND C AND D! Although the user had selected valid terms, they are combined incorrectly, yielding faulty results. Indeed this has been our frequent observation.

It is interesting, however, that this omission of the proper Boolean expression sometimes corrects another mistake; that of using too many terms or terms that are really extraneous. In other words a query with multiple subconcepts will be restrictive but since the users are incorrectly ORing these subconcepts, the effects counter each other.

There was very little use of the Advanced level interface. Proper use of this level implies a rather sound understanding of Boolean logic that both observation and documentation indicate the searchers did not have. Perhaps in time more users would eventually use the advanced level; but this seems unlikely without formal instruction.

In the comments the users mentioned their concern with having to execute several steps between menu screens and query profile screens. This was improved, however, with newer releases of the interface, which made greater use of function keys. Other comments were mainly for more resources, backfiles, more terminals, different databases, remote access, etc.

Conclusion

The users found the system easy to use, and although many required assistance to get started, help required was minimal. As long as the users kept the searches simple they were able to retrieve "something" on their topic. Search precision was virtually nonexistent. Rather, the searchers retrieved broad sets and then selected from these sets the items they wanted to print. It was apparent, however, that they recognized their naive use, both by comments and by their reluctance to identify themselves as experienced. Comments such as "I would like to learn more," "I'm not using the potential of the system," "I'm only using very minimal basics," "I wish the system could teach me more," etc., from the experienced user questionnaires, indicated their own awareness of their limitations.

Appendix A-1

6. Have you used an online version of MEDLINE (either yourself or by having a librarian process a search for you)?

   a. yes, by myself, which system or/and vendor   30

   b. yes, librarian search   64

   c. no   16   d. don't know   4

   (Circle all that apply)

7. If yes, you've used online MEDLINE, which system do you prefer?

   a. online, own search   27

   b. CD-ROM MEDLINE (EBSCO)   31

   c. online, librarian   15

   d. don't know   14

   (Circle one only)

8. Next time do you need this sort of information, what will you do?

   a. try EBSCO MEDLINE   73

   b. try a printed version   10

   c. try an online version   16

   d. try another source   6

9. What is your regular (several times a week) computer use?

   (Check all that apply)

UIC ADN Network	Y 20	N 30	Don't know 6
Library's LUIS/LCS	Y 33	N 28	Don't know 5
Microcomputer	Y 62	N 23	Don't know 3
Other	Y 11	N 18	Don't know

   Which system _____

10. If this MEDLINE CD-ROM system had not been available today, what would you have done?

(Enter all that apply)
a. used a printed version   96
b. used an online version   13
c. asked a library staff member   27
d. asked a friend or colleague   4
e. browsed through the stacks   24
f. nothing   5
g. other   6

PART II. SYSTEM EVALUATION - NOVICE

1. How often have you used EBSCO CD-ROM MEDLINE?
   a. 1st time   60   b. once before   17   c. 3-5 times   18

2. EBSCO MEDLINE is provided free of charge to library users. How important a consideration was this in your decision to use this system, instead of an online version of MEDLINE?
   a. very important   73
   b. somewhat important   11
   c. relatively unimportant   7
   d. would not have used an online version of MEDLINE   9

Enter one only (on the following 5 point scale) for questions 3-9.

SCALE: A   B   C   D   E
         Strongly   Strongly
         Agree   Agree   Neutral   Disagree   Disagree

3. The rate at which the computer responds is satisfactory.
   A 36   B 40   C 8   D 4   E 1

4. The brief user guide helped me to use the system.
   A 25   B 34   C 17   D 13   E 7

5. The EBSCO Medline manual helped me to use the system.
   A 17   B 28   C 13   D 11   E

6. Reference assistance made it possible for me to use the system.
   A 23   B 20   C 25   D 8   E 8

7. The time span covered by EBSCO MEDLINE was sufficient for my needs.
   A 22   B 33   C 11   D 17   E 16

8. Overall, I found EBSCO MEDLINE easy to use.
   A 40   B 35   C 13   D 4   E 6

9. Instructions on EBSCO MEDLINE screens were sufficient for my use.
   A 36   B 28   C 9   D 8   E 6

10. Have you taken the 1 hour instruction to the system?
    YES   13   NO   87

If the answer to 10 is NO, could you be interested in attending a session? (You may sign up at the reference desk.)
    YES   37   NO   36

OPTIONAL: We are planning a follow-up questionnaire for users who advance with the system. We therefore need your name to correlate this data with the next phase.

NAME: _____

DEPARTMENT: _____   TELEPHONE: _____

EXPERIENCED USER QUESTIONNAIRE
N=23

Please fill out this questionnaire if you have used Micro computer based MEDLINE at least three times.

1. Did you previously fill out the Novice User Questionnaire?

        Yes 15   No 8

If yes, may we have your name to correlate the two questionnaires?

        Name _____

If no, we would appreciate your completing the Novice User Questionnaire.

2. How many times have you used this system?

        3-5   13   5-10 5   10 +   1

3. Which level interface are you using:

        Patron 1   13
        Patron 2   7
        Advanced   2

4. Did you obtain a password?

        Yes 11   No 19

5. Identify your level of use with the following and circle the appropriate response.

    A. Single term searching

        frequently 1   occasionally 5   rarely 5   never 8   don't know

    B. Phrase searching e.g. "online retrieval"

        frequently 12 occasionally 4   rarely 1   never 3   don't know 3

    C. Use of the online author index

        frequently 1   occasionally 8   rarely 3   never 11   don't know

    D. Use of the online journal title index

        frequently 1   occasionally 2   rarely 2   never 1   don't know

    E. National Library of Medicine Subject Headings (printed version)

        frequently 9   occasionally 2   rarely 4   never 7   don't know 1

F. Use of the online index for identifying medical subject headings

frequently 3   occasionally 3   rarely 1   never 12   don't know 3

G. Exploding medical subject headings

frequently 2   occasionally 5   rarely 2   never 7   don't know 7

H. Use of multiple sets, i.e. making more than 1 set, then combining with a Boolean Logic expression e.g. 1 and 2, etc.

frequently 5   occasionally 2   rarely 1   never 10   don't know 3

I. How many sets per search have you averaged?

2-3   10   3-5   2   5-10   don't know   9

J. Did you use the set history display function i.e., entering a question mark?

frequently   occasionally   rarely   never 17   don't know 4

K. Did you use the store search capability?

frequently 1   occasionally 2   rarely 1   never 14   don't know 3

6. What feature of the system do you like best?

_____

7. What feature do you like least?

_____

8. What additional features would you like?

_____

_____

_____

9. This system is limited to covering 500 more journals and the last 2 years. If you have to make a choice would you rather see

increased journal coverage   4   choose
or   only
more years of coverage   18   one

10. Additional comments

_____

_____

_____

BILOXI, MISSISSIPPI VA MEDICAL CENTER'S EXPERIENCE WITH

MEDLINE ON EBSCO CD-ROM

By *Christiane J. Jones*
Gwen G. Vanderfin
Pamela B. Howell

Library Service
VA Medical Center
Biloxi, Mississippi 39531

BILOXI, MISSISSIPPI VA MEDICAL CENTER'S EXPERIENCE WITH MEDLINE ON EBSCO CD-ROM*

Introduction

The Veterans Administration Medical Center at Biloxi, Mississippi is unique to this study in that it is a government facility with hospital-based health care practitioners. The 1,140 bed medical center is comprised of two hospitals located nine miles apart, and outpatient clinics at Mobile, Alabama and Pensacola, Florida. Residents and allied health students enhance the care provided by more than 1,600 employees.

Library Service has a longstanding reputation as a vital support to patient care, education and research activities at Biloxi. The heart of the library program has been traditional information services provided through outreach to the user at the point of need. In recent years, Library Service has added various microcomputer hardware and software classes and a microcomputer learning center. However, this was the first experience with either end-user searching or CD-ROM.

Methodology

Biloxi chose to formally evaluate the EBSCO CD-ROM product. Library users who had previously expressed interest in end-user searching or new technologies were randomly assigned to either the experimental group or the control group of 15 persons each. The purpose was to determine if a formal educational intervention prior to using the system affected use of or satisfaction with the system, or overall library staff time assisting users.

Participants in the experimental group received a one-hour introduction to basic techniques of end-user searching and CD-ROM technology. A reference librarian gave the introductions in groups of three so that each participant had hands-on experience during the session. The same librarian individually showed participants in the control group how to turn on the system and/or get to the tutorial.

The CD-ROM system was placed in the microcomputer learning center and scheduled for use like other systems in the center. The librarian was avail-

*This reflects the author's personal views and in no way represents the official view of the Veterans Administration or the U.S. Government.

able to provide additional assistance to both groups as needed. Basic written instructions on how to get started and sample searches were also available to participants of either group.

All participants in both groups were involved in direct patient care activities. There were no researchers, educators, residents or students in either group, although the system was available to them on a walk-in basis. As would be expected, both groups in the formal evaluation needed information primarily for patient care and keeping current.

Participants completed evaluation forms after each use of the system. The forms were adapted from the prototype provided by the National Library of Medicine. After a participant's first use of the system, he/she completed a full questionnaire (see Appendix A). After each subsequent use, the participant completed a shortened questionnaire specific to the search just completed (see Appendix B). This time-saving change was made in consideration of the participants' patient care responsibilities, but provided useful data related to differences in use patterns.

Findings

Participants who received formal training prior to using the system were more comfortable with subject searching than participants who were not formally trained. They occasionally searched by author, title or journal but tended toward more complex subject searching. Participants who were not formally trained also searched more often by subject but were more likely to try author, title or journal. (Figure 1)

Participants who were formally trained also appear to be more satisfied with their search results. (Figure 2)

Participants from both groups were similar in their previous use of INDEX MEDICUS. However, there were significant differences in their comparisons of use between printed versions of INDEX MEDICUS and MEDLINE on CD-ROM. (Figure 3)

Figure 1

TYPES OF SEARCHES

	Formally Trained	Not Formally Trained
Author	5%	18%
Title	5%	12%
Subject	85%	56%
Journal	5%	14%
Other	—	—

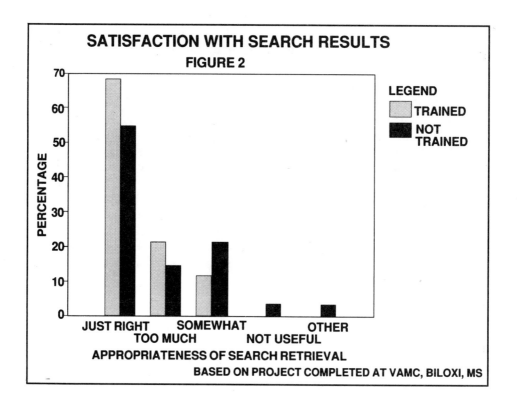

SATISFACTION WITH SEARCH RESULTS

FIGURE 2

All participants in both groups had used an online version of MEDLINE. Only 23% of the formally trained group had searched themselves while none in the group non-trained had searched himself/herself. System preference could have been influenced by previous use of online MEDLINE as well as the formal training. (Figure 4)

The majority of participants from both groups indicated they would have asked a library staff member for the information needed if the CD-ROM system had not been available, with other options being less important. Over 80% from

Figure 3

COMPARISON WITH PRINTED INDEX MEDICUS

	Formally Trained	Not Trained
Easier	—	70%
Harder	90%	30%
Same	10%	—
Other	—	—

Figure 4

SYSTEM PREFERENCE

	Formally Trained	Not Trained
Online, own search	20%	—
MEDLINE ON CD-ROM	50%	20%
Online, librarian search	20%	30%
Don't know	10%	50%

each group indicated that they would try CD-ROM the next time they needed similar information.

Participants indicated that cost of information was very important to them. In reality, it isn't a consideration at all since affiliated users are not charged for any services including online searching. This cost consideration most likely reflects an awareness of the high costs of medical care.

Statements related to EBSCO's MEDLINE were given a numerical rating based on A-5, B-4, C-3, D-2, E-1. Although overall ratings were good, several of the comments were related to these factors. (Figure 5)

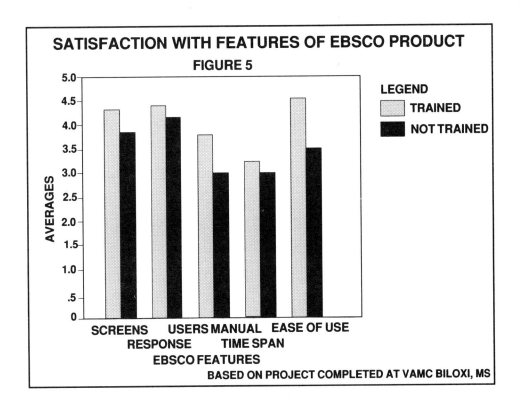

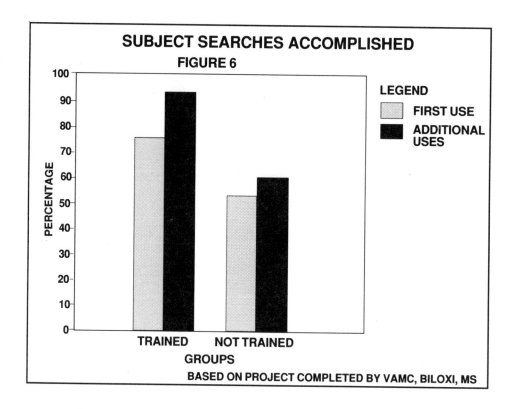

SUBJECT SEARCHES ACCOMPLISHED

FIGURE 6

LEGEND
FIRST USE
ADDITIONAL USES

GROUPS

BASED ON PROJECT COMPLETED BY VAMC, BILOXI, MS

Data comparing first-time users to additional users revealed interesting comparisons between the two groups. As would be expected, trained first-time users performed more subject searches than non-trained first-time users. The same held true for additional system uses. However, the percentage of subject searches performed during additional uses of the system increased at a greater rate among trained users than non-trained users. (Figure 6)

Trained first-time users appear to be as successful as additional users in finding the information they needed. Untrained users in our evaluation appear to be more satisfied with search results the first time they used the system than with additional uses. (Figure 7)

With additional uses of the system, trained participants became less likely to return to printed INDEX MEDICUS if CD-ROM were not available. There was no change with additional uses among non-trained participants. (Figure 8)

Although both groups required significant library staff assistance, the groups varied in their pattern of assistance. Staff time averaged 19 minutes per system use for trained participants, including prorated class time, compared to 29 minutes per use for non-trained participants. After-class assistance averaged 16 minutes per use for the 38% that required additional assistance.

Following the 8-week formal evaluation in the library, the CD-ROM system was moved to two patient care areas for two weeks each. The outpatient clinic and a medical inpatient ward were chosen because physicians in each area are internists, but they provide different types of care. Physicians in each area

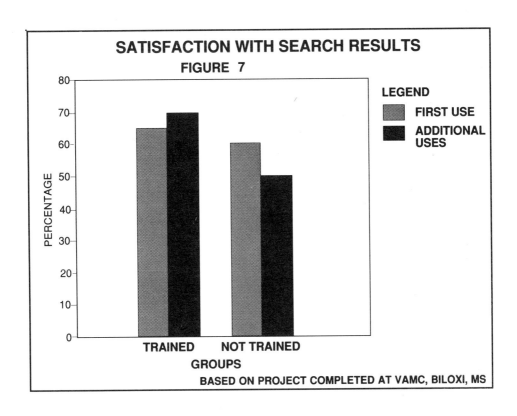

SATISFACTION WITH SEARCH RESULTS
FIGURE 7

LEGEND
FIRST USE
ADDITIONAL USES

BASED ON PROJECT COMPLETED AT VAMC, BILOXI, MS

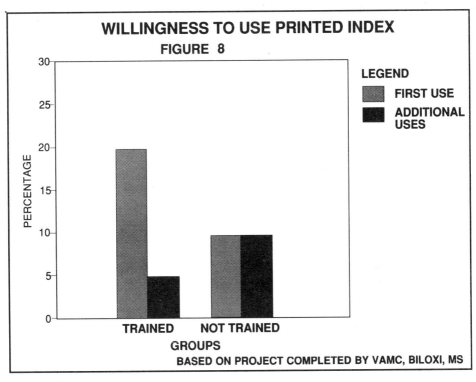

WILLINGNESS TO USE PRINTED INDEX
FIGURE 8

LEGEND
FIRST USE
ADDITIONAL USES

BASED ON PROJECT COMPLETED BY VAMC, BILOXI, MS

received the formal introduction to basic online searching and CD-ROM as a group at their staff meetings. A focus group was held with physicians in each area following the two-week evaluation periods.

Physicians in the outpatient clinic had previously requested a CD-ROM product for that site. Funds were not available at the time, but the request was kept under consideration, and the test system was subsequently placed there for evaluation. The system was used only once during the two-week period. Reasons given for not using the system fell into two categories: lack of time; no need for information. The one system user, who had initiated the original request for a CD-ROM product, was disappointed that the system was not full-text, but felt the abstracts were of some help.

All system uses on the medical ward were for patient-related problems. Seventy-five percent of the physicians used the system at least once. Twenty percent of them had participated in the formal evaluation in the library. The consensus was that there was no real advantage to having the system located on the ward, but there were several distinct disadvantages:

(1) The librarian was not available to provide assistance.

(2) Articles needed were in the library.

(3) The ward atmosphere was not always conducive to searching.

Conclusion

From our findings, it appears that user education is essential to successfully introducing CD-ROM technology. Users who are given formal training are more comfortable with complex searching and more satisfied with search results. This could be from either the real educational value of the introduction or the increased confidence in their own abilities and the system. User education also lessens library staff time spent assisting users, but more importantly provides a pattern of assistance which is easier to manage.

An additional conclusion is that MEDLINE on CD-ROM does not appear to have significant advantages for a medical center with strong, well-established library services and no major teaching responsibilities. Health care providers whose primary responsibilities are direct patient care still prefer the library and its services. Technology-oriented users would take advantage of the system but prefer it in the library setting along with other information services. This attitude might change if the CD-ROM system were interfaced with the hospital information system and online access to library resources.

The real potential we see for the current EBSCO MEDLINE is in small health care facilities where there is no library or librarian, or the "library" is a shelf of books and journals in someone's office. ABRIDGED INDEX MEDICUS is suitable for this type of institution. The CD-ROM system would provide access to the index as well as the searching capability. Barriers to this concept would be product cost, user education, and access to journal articles. User education and journal articles could be obtained through state health sciences information networks with a mission to improve access to information and/or through an established library.

EBSCO MEDLINE ON CD-ROM EVALUATION QUESTONNAIRE

NAME _____ DATE _____

<u>INSTRUCTIONS</u>

This EBSCO MEDLINE on CD-ROM systems is being tested by the Biloxi VA Medical Library. We would like you to fill out this questionnaire in order to help us find out who is using the system, and how useful it is to you. Thank you!

1. My primary affiliation is: (select one)

    a. Medicine   e. Rehabilitation Medicine
    b. Dentistry   f. Allied Health
    c. Nursing   g. Other (please specify _____)
    d. Surgery

2. My profession is: (select one)

    a. Physician   d. Psychologist
    b. Nurse   e. Researcher/Educator
    c. Dentist   f. Resident/Student
                                 g. Other (please specify_____)

3. I was looking for articles: (select all that apply)

    a. by an author
    b. under a title
    c. on a subject
    d. in a journal
    e. other

4. I needed the information for: (select all that apply)

    a. patient care   e. to check a reference
    b. a paper or report   f. teaching/planning a course
    c. a research project   g. not needed, just curious
    d. keeping current   h. other

5. The information I found was: (select one)

    a. what I was looking for
    b. more than I needed
    c. some of what I needed
    d. not useful
    e. other

6. Have you used any of the printed publications produced from the MEDLINE system (e.g. INDEX MEDICUS, HOSPITAL LITERATURE INDEX)?

   a. yes   b. no   c. don't know

7. If yes, you've used printed versions, how do they compare to EBSCO's MEDLINE on CD-ROM? (select one)

   a. easier to use
   b. harder to use
   c. about the same to use
   d. other

8. Have you used an online version of MEDLINE (either yourself or by having a librarian process a search for you)? (select all that apply)

   a. yes, by myself
   b. yes, librarian search
   c. no
   d. don't know

9. If yes, you've used online MEDLINE, which system do you prefer? (select one)

   a. online, own search
   b. EBSCO's MEDLINE on CD-ROM
   c. online, librarian search
   d. don't know

10. If this MEDLINE CD-ROM system had not been available today, what would you have done? How would you have found the needed information? (select all that apply)

   a. used a printed version
   b. used an online version
   c. asked a library staff member
   d. asked a friend or colleague
   e. browsed through the stacks
   f. nothing
   g. other _____

11. Next time you need this sort of information, will you: (select all that apply)

   a. try EBSCO MEDLINE on CD-ROM
   b. try a printed version
   c. try an online version
   d. try another source

12. EBSCO's MEDLINE on CD-ROM is provided free of charge to library users. How important a consideration is the cost of information retrieval to you? Would you be willing to pay for this service?

    a. very important
    b. somewhat important
    c. relatively important

13. How often have you used EBSCO's MEDLINE on CD-ROM?

    a. first time
    b. once before
    c. 3-5 times
    d. 6 or more times

Enter ONE only (on the following 5 point scale) for questions 15 through 19.

SCALE:	A	B	C	D	E
	Strongly Agree	Agree	Neutral	Disagree	Strongly Disagree

15. _____ Instructions on EBSCO's MEDLINE screens were sufficient for my use.

16. _____ The rate at which the computer responds is satisfactory.

17. _____ The EBSCO MEDLINE user's manual helped me to use the system.

18. _____ The time span covered by EBSCO's MEDLINE was sufficient for my needs.

19. _____ Overall, I found EBSCO's MEDLINE on CD-ROM easy to use.

Comments/Recommendations: (Enter here anything you would like to add about EBSCO's MEDLINE on CD-ROM.)

EBSCO MEDLINE ON CD-ROM SEARCH EVALUATION

NAME _____ DATE _____

I. I was looking for articles: (select all that apply)

    a. by an author   d. under a title
    b. on a subject   e. other
    c. in a journal

2. The information I found was: (select one)

    a. what I wanted   d. not useful
    b. more than I needed   e. other
    c. some of what I needed

3. If this MEDLINE CD-ROM system had not been available today, what would you have done? How would you have found the needed information? (select all that apply)

    a. used a printed version   e. browsed through the stacks
    b. used an online version   f. nothing
    d. asked a friend or   g. other _____
       colleague

4. Next time you need this sort of information will you: (select all that apply)

    a. try EBSCO MEDLINE on CD-ROM c. try an online version
    b. try a printed version   d. try another source

5. How often have you used EBSCO's MEDLINE on CD-ROM?

    a. once before
    b. 3-5 times
    c. 6 or more times

Comments/Recommendations

CAMBRIDGE AND SILVERPLATTER CD-ROM SYSTEMS

AT MEHARRY MEDICAL COLLEGE LIBRARY A SURVEY OF INITIAL AND REPEAT USER RESPONSE

By   *Martha Earl*
Cheryl Hamberg
Mary Nichols
Adalyn Watts

Meharry Medical College Library
1005 D. B Todd Blvd.
Nashville, TN 37208

CAMBRIDGE AND SILVERPLATTER CD-ROM SYSTEMS AT MEHARRY MEDICAL COLLEGE LIBRARY: A SURVEY OF INITIAL AND REPEAT USER RESPONSE

Introduction

Among the goals of librarianship, the provision of information to the library user, as quickly and thoroughly as possible, remains central. In addition, academic librarianship stresses educating users to accomplish their own research and satisfy their own information needs. Among physicians and health professionals, in particular, the need for quick information retrieval has been noted (14). The development of CD-ROM technology offers medical librarians the opportunity to transfer those ideals into a reality. Because successful achievement of those goals means different things to different users, success of CD-ROM searching must be evaluated both objectively and subjectively. Various studies have recorded impressions of user response (2, 6, 10) while others have formally surveyed users and user reaction (1, 7, 9). At Meharry we undertook to evaluate two CD-ROM systems (Cambridge and SilverPlatter) both formally, by using a survey, and informally, by recording the impressions of the librarians. This paper describes the methods, results, and conclusions of the formal study.

A survey of the literature not only revealed numerous observations on the use of CD-ROM in libraries but three especially pertinent studies involving Compact Cambridge MEDLINE. The UCLA Biomedical Library (7) used a formal survey as did Indiana University Medical Sciences and Optometry Libraries (1), although the latter included other end-user systems besides CD-ROM. Though not a formal study, the observations of the librarians at the State University of New York Health Science Center at Syracuse concerning Compact Cambridge were highly relevant (2). Also pertinent were the Houston Academy of Medicine-Texas Medical Center Library's survey of user response to Quick Search, a subset of MEDLINE, (9), and Carol Tenopir's summary of surveys of user response to Infotrac, a general interest database on laser disc (12).

These user surveys provided a precedent for the types of responses we might expect from Meharry end-users on similar questions although other questions would differ. We assumed that users would try the CD-ROM systems and that some would utilize the CD-ROM more than once. We assumed survey respondents would fill out the questionnaires as honestly as possible.

Methodology

For use as the survey instrument, Meharry modified the user questionnaire suggested by the National Library of Medicine and devised a similar follow-up questionnaire for repeat users. Copies of the questionnaire are appended (Cambridge forms differ only by the product name). Using the initial questionnaire, Meharry investigated the types of users, the perceived success of their searches, the ease of use of the CD-ROM system, the method (CD-ROM, online, or manual) preferred, and the preferred CD-ROM system. With the follow-up questionnaire, we assessed whether use became easier, searches became more successful, and the CD-ROM system availability changed users' approaches and attitudes toward searching.

Classes were held weekly and by appointment for anyone interested in learning to use the CD-ROM systems. In addition, librarians and one student assistant supervised searches when users needed assistance. Librarians distributed questionnaires randomly to trained users actually involved in the process of searching on one of the CD-ROM systems.

However, the collection of forms was influenced by matters of time and access. At Meharry we acquired the Cambridge system in November 1987 and began end user training. When the SilverPlatter system arrived in March 1988, many patrons were already trained in the use of Cambridge. In addition, until the last month of the survey, only the Cambridge system was available in the evenings after the reference office closed. We have since been able to relocate the SilverPlatter system to the public area where both systems reside in lockable security cabinets; the need for security for equipment is essential (11). In the meantime far more repeat users utilized Cambridge than SilverPlatter. Plus, we observed that some people trained on Cambridge opted to reuse that system despite later training on SilverPlatter. We compensated for this inequity by emphasizing training on SilverPlatter as soon as access to that system improved.

Another factor inhibiting the collection of forms was shortage of personnel to train CD-ROM users. Librarians, overwhelmed by patron demand for training, sometimes neglected to hand out the surveys. Even if the CD-ROM systems and surveys were available in the evenings, librarians were not. When students taught their fellow students how to use the CD-ROM systems, surveys were seldom completed. Nevertheless, we collected twenty-six Cambridge and twenty-seven SilverPlatter initial forms and nineteen Cambridge and seven SilverPlatter follow-up forms.

Results

To measure user types on the initial survey we asked that patrons relate primary affiliation, profession, search goal (author, subject, title, journal), search reason, search instructor, index familiarity, CD-ROM system use frequency, and computer literacy. The follow-up form only requested primary affiliation, profession, search goal, search reason, and CD-ROM use frequency. Responses could be multiple for profession, search goal, search reason, search instructor, and index familiarity but were single for primary affiliation and CD-ROM use frequency. Not all those surveyed answered all the questions. The results are presented in Tables I through VIII. The different groups of survey respondents are represented on the tables as Cambridge initial (CC-I), SilverPlatter initial (SP-I), Cambridge follow-up (CC-F), and SilverPlatter follow-up (SP-F). The abbreviation SG stands for survey groups. The survey question (q) relevant to the subject of the table is indicated in parentheses after the title of the table; question numbers unique to the follow-up form are indicated by an "f" after the question number.

Results enable us to describe the majority of surveyed users. They were affiliated with medicine, were students searching on a subject for the purpose of a report or research project, were trained by librarians, were familiar with *Index Medicus,* and felt comfortable with computers. Most respondents to the initial questionnaire were first time users while most respondents to the follow-up survey had used the system more than three times.

Next we measured search success. On the initial survey form we asked that patrons mark responses to describe the information found and whether English abstracts of foreign documents were useful. On the follow-up form we asked for a similar description of the search results plus how the number of articles through which a patron browsed to locate what s/he needed had changed with repeated use of the CD-ROM system. Results are noted on Tables IX through XI. We measured use of English abstracts of foreign documents under search success due to our observations that such abstracts were useful to some researchers but useless to others. The ability to eliminate such records was an indication of some degree of search sophistication. The measurement of number of documents browsed indicated how efficiently repeat users were finding what they needed. A change in articles browsed could indicate a change in search techniques and coupled with the response to whether or not they found what they needed could indicate needs for further training in refinement of search methods.

The results can be summarized as follows. Among initial survey respondents, over half found what they were seeking, but a significant number (33% of Cambridge and 16% of SilverPlatter users) found only some of what they sought. The percentage of Cambridge follow-up users finding only some of what they sought was consistent with initial survey results while the percentage increase for SilverPlatter follow-up users may be skewed by the small number of respondents. Concerning English abstracts of foreign documents, equal numbers of the majority of users either found them useful or were neutral on the subject. Only a few felt strongly that the English abstracts of foreign documents were not useful. Concerning change in the number of articles browsed, 58% of Cambridge repeat users were looking through fewer documents while 32% were looking through more and 10% had not changed. For SilverPlatter repeat users 50% had not changed while 33% had decreased, and 17% had increased. However, one must note from Table VII that SilverPlatter repeat users had less experience than Cambridge repeat users. Nonetheless, one can state that most repeat users continued to find what they needed but browsed fewer articles to do so.

Third, we tested ease of use. On the initial survey form patrons responded to experience with online MEDLINE, number of discs used, the rate of system response, utility of the manual, ease of changing discs, ease of use overall, and adequacy of staff assistance. On the follow-up survey repeat users answered questions on the change over time in the speed of finding information and the ease of use of the system. We determined that patron familiarity with searching MEDLINE online would be a factor in ease of use of searching the CD-ROM system. The speed of finding information could indicate success in learning system commands as well as in improving search technique. We also asked whether searching itself had become easier for repeat users. Results are presented in Tables XII through XX.

One can note the following concerning ease of use. Among initial survey respondents, half of all users had not used MEDLINE online. Of those with experience with MEDLINE online, 32% had accomplished their own online searches, while 68% had had searches performed by librarians. Concerning the number of discs used, the majority used three or four discs; most found changing discs easy. The majority also found the rate of system response satisfactory, staff assistance adequate, and the system easy to use overall. While the majority (51%) gave the manual a neutral rating in helpfulness, 37% found it useful and 12% not useful. For the repeat users all but two were finding what they needed quickly, and all but one found searching easier over time. Interestingly, one replied that the ease of the search depended on the topic.

Fourth, we measured the method preferred by users. The initial survey asked for patrons' comparison of CD-ROM to printed indexes and to online MEDLINE, what alternatives to CD-ROM would they use, what would they try next time, how important was price, and how adequate was the time span covered by the CD-ROM discs. Repeat users were asked which method (CD-ROM, printed index, online) they preferred. Results are displayed on Tables XXI through XXVII.

Results reveal use of both MeSH headings and textwords. Concerning the comparison of the printed indexes to the CD-ROM system, roughly 43% found the printed indexes easier to use than the CD-ROM while 47% found the CD-ROM easier to use; 6% found them to be about the same. However, roughly 70% would prefer the CD-ROM to online searching, and 78% would try the CD-ROM the next time they needed a literature search. An additional 7% would go to the printed indexes, and 9% would try online. The strong majority (90%) indicated that the availability of the CD-ROM without charge was important; two even indicated that they would not use an online search. As for the time span being sufficient, most agreed that it was. In the absence of the availability of the CD-ROM, 43% would use the printed indexes, 28% would ask staff for help, 19% would browse the stacks, and 8% would try online while 7% would ask a colleague, do nothing, or other. For the follow-up users, only one user showed no preference; 95% of Cambridge and 100% of SilverPlatter users preferred the CD-ROM system.

Next we compared the users' approach. On the initial questionnaire we asked whether text words or MeSH headings were used. On the follow-up survey we asked the same question plus whether the use of textwords versus MeSH headings had changed with time. Users were allowed multiple responses to the first but not to the second question. Tables XXVIII and XXIX display results.

Results can be summarized as follows. Initial survey respondents used MeSH headings more than textwords. However, though follow-up users reported that they were using MeSH headings more since when they had started using the system, their answers to what they were utilizing on the actual search in progress revealed they were using more textwords than MeSH headings.

Sixth, we measured the attitude of repeat users toward library searching. We asked survey respondents whether, since the availability of the CD-ROM system, they had used or had wanted to use the library more, and why or why not. Results are displayed in Tables XXX through XXXIII.

The majority wanted to and did use the library more due to the CD-ROM's availability. However, whereas 92% wanted to use the library more, only 81% did so. The majority (53%) said that the CD-ROM caused them to use the library more because they could find what they needed faster, 26% because they could browse, and 21% because using the CD-ROM is fun. Of those who said that they wanted to use the library more due to the CD-ROM but had not yet, 61% were busy with other concerns, 22% found library hours inconvenient, 5% found distance a problem, and 10% felt uncomfortable using the CD-ROM.

Finally, we compared the two CD-ROM systems. We examined all responses except primary affiliation, profession, search goal, search reason, index familiarity, alternate method, MeSH versus textword, instructor, usefulness of English abstracts, and computer literacy. We determined these responses to be irrelevant for the following reasons. Most people, regardless of profession or affiliation or computer literacy, were not involved in choosing the system on which they were trained. Users had search goals, strategies, and reasons unrelated to the system. English abstracts of foreign documents were the same on either system. However, all other responses can be useful to compare Cambridge and SilverPlatter systems. Results are arranged as before in order of user types, search success, ease of use, method preferred, approach, and attitude.

First, considering user types we will compare the CD-ROM systems in terms of use frequency. Among Cambridge initial survey respondents, 50% were using the system for the first time, 19% had used it once before, 31% had used it more than three times. In contrast, among SilverPlatter initial survey respondents, 74% were first-time users, 15% were second-time users, and only 11% had used it three or more times. Among Cambridge follow-up users 89% had used it more than three times with 58% of those using it more than six times. Among SilverPlatter follow-up users, few that they were, 57% had used it more than three times. These discrepancies have been explained previously by the limited access to SilverPlatter and the longer and more open access to Cambridge.

In terms of search success, we compared the percentage of users who found the information they sought, how this differed with repeated use of the systems, and amount of change in browsing. Certainly some search topics yield more records than others. However, an overall change in whether users found what they were seeking using a particular system could reflect how well they had learned to manipulate that system. Also, we could use change in the amount of browsing to compare systems due to the different formatting of screens. On Cambridge one viewed one record at time and proceeded to the next. On SilverPlatter parts of different records appeared on the same page. We observed this caused confusion to some patrons, especially SilverPlatter users already familiar with Cambridge. Concerning information found, 54% of initial Cambridge respondents and 61% of follow-up users found what they were seeking. 13% of Cambridge initial respondents and 6% of follow-up users found more than they needed while 33% of initial and follow-up users found only some of what they needed. Among SilverPlatter users, 68% of initial and 67% of repeat users found what they sought, 16% of initial users found too much, and 16% of initial and 33% of follow-up users found some of what they needed. Cambridge users appeared to have found what they sought better with repeated use, going from 54% to 61%. However, 67% of SilverPlatter users on both surveys said they found what they sought. Considering change in the number of articles through which repeat users browsed, 58% of Cambridge users browsed through less compared to 33% of SilverPlatter users. 32% of Cambridge and 17% of Silver-Platter users browsed through more while 10% of Cambridge and 50% of SilverPlatter users did not change the perceived amount through which they browsed.

To compare ease of use between the two systems we examined online experience, number of discs used, speed of system response, manual usefulness, ease of changing discs, overall ease, adequacy of staff assistance, speed of use, and ease of search. Experience with online searching was similar for users of each system with differences statistically insignificant. Sixty-nine percent of Cambridge survey participants used three or fewer discs compared to 67% of SilverPlatter users. These findings were also statistically insignificant. Comparing rate of response only one Cambridge user (4%) found rate of response unsatisfactory. However, the response rate was satisfactory to 96% of SilverPlatter users compared to 92% of Cambridge users. Regarding the usefulness of the manual 39% of Cambridge users and 35% of SilverPlatter users found the manual useful while 61% of Cambridge users and 42% of SilverPlatter users were neutral. However, 23% of SilverPlatter users disagreed with the statement that the manual was useful. As for ease of changing discs 87% of Cambridge users and 96% of SilverPlatter users found changing discs easy. Nine percent of Cambridge and 4% of SilverPlatter users were neutral on the subject while 4% of Cambridge users disagreed that changing discs was easy. As for overall ease of the system, 92% of Cambridge and 96% of SilverPlatter users found the systems easy to use; the remaining 8% and 4% respectively were neutral. Regarding staff assistance, 96% of both Cambridge and SilverPlatter respondents found assistance adequate, with the remaining 4% neutral. Among repeat users 89% of Cambridge and 100% of SilverPlatter users found they searched more quickly with repeated use. Similarly 95% of Cambridge and 100% of SilverPlatter users found searching easier with repeated use of the systems; 5% of repeat Cambridge users said search ease depended on search strategy.

To compare the CD-ROM systems by method users preferred, we examined preference for printed index or online versus CD-ROM system, system they would use next time, importance of fees, adequacy of time span, and system preferred by repeat users. Regarding printed index versus CD-ROM, results of the initial survey showed that 35% of Cambridge users found the printed indexes easier versus 50% of SilverPlatter users. Roughly equal numbers (47% of Cambridge users and 46% of SilverPlatter users) found the printed indexes harder to use than the CD-ROM while 9% of Cambridge users and 4% of SilverPlatter users said they were the same. Another 9% of Cambridge users marked the "other" category. Among initial survey respondents who were familiar with online searches, 55% of Cambridge and 83% of SilverPlatter users preferred the CD-ROM system to an online search. Thirt-six percent of Cambridge users preferred to do their own searches online. Eight percent of Silver-Platter users preferred the librarian do the online search. Nine percent of Cambridge and 8% of SilverPlatter users did not know whether they preferred an online or CD-ROM search. For the method they would use next time Cambridge users replied that 87% would use CD-ROM, 7% would use printed indexes, 7% would try online while SilverPlatter users replied that 73% would use CD-ROM, 8% would use printed indexes, 11% would try an online search, and 8% would try another method. As for the importance of fees in using a CD-ROM system 64% of Cambridge versus 81% of SilverPlatter users replied fees were very important. Twenty percent of Cambridge and 7% of SilverPlatter users said they would not use an online search. Twelve percent of Cambridge and 7% of SilverPlatter users replied that charge was relatively unimportant. Considering adequacy of time span covered by the discs, 87% of Cambridge users and 93% of SilverPlatter users agreed that the time span was adequate for their needs. One should note that Cambridge discs covered 1982 through 1988 while SilverPlatter discs covered 1983 through 1988. Four percent of Cambridge and SilverPlatter users disagreed that the time span was adequate while the remaining 9% and 4%, respectively, were neutral. Lastly, concerning the system preferred by repeat users, 95% of Cambridge and 100% of SilverPlatter users preferred the CD-ROM to online, printed indexes or other methods of research. The remaining 5% of Cambridge users had no preference.

Next we compared the CD-ROM in terms of user attitude by examining changes in library use and reasons the CD-ROM has or has not changed library use. Since beginning to use the CD-ROM, 79% of Cambridge and 86% of Silver-Platter users had used the library more and 21% of Cambridge and 14% of SilverPlatter users had utilized the library the same amount. No one had used the library less. But 95% of Cambridge and 83% of SilverPlatter users wanted to use the library more while 5% and 17% respectively wanted to use the library about the same amount as before they used the CD-ROM. Among Cambridge users who wanted to use the library more, 29% said they could find what they needed faster, 28% liked to browse the abstracts in their fields, and 23% thought searching was fun. Among like SilverPlatter users 75% could find what they needed faster, 13% liked to browse, and 13% thought searching was fun. Of those who wanted to use the library more due to the CD-ROM but had not yet, 8% of

Cambridge users and 20% of SilverPlatter users said they did not feel confident using the CD-ROM. The other reasons (distance, library hours and other concerns) were not reflective of the CD-ROM system and thus were not considered in the comparison of the two systems.

Conclusions

We can draw various conclusions from the results of the study concerning user types, perceived search success, ease of use of the CD-ROM system, method preferred, and preferred CD-ROM system. Conclusions can also be drawn concerning whether use became easier, searches more successful, and whether CD-ROM availability changed users' approaches and attitudes.

That most users were medical students searching on a subject for the purpose of a report or research project comes as no surprise since Meharry is an academic medical center. In addition, although Meharry is open to the community, use of the CD-ROM is restricted to Meharry faculty, students, and staff. Neither is it surprising in light of extensive user education that most users were familiar with *Index Medicus* and were trained by librarians. That most users felt comfortable with computers may reflect the greater computer literacy of students compared to older groups. Roughly 40% of respondents were faculty or staff and 60% were students. Perhaps those more computer literate opted to try the CD-ROM system while the less computer literate preferred manual or online (through an intermediary) methods and were, thus, not included in survey results. (Librarians are encouraging all users to try the CD-ROM for appropriate information requests.) Sixty-two percent of users were searching for research or report purposes, 10% for patient care, 9% for current awareness, and 19% for other reasons. Rambo also found among his Quick Search respondents that 60% were involved in research while 20% needed information for patient care (9). In contrast, MEDLARS is used only 27% of the time for research but 36% for patient care (13). In the medical school setting, CD-ROM can well serve health professionals for whom research is the primary search motivation.

Considering search success we could draw the following conclusions. Our results were similar to results at UCLA (7), SUNY (2), Houston (9), and with Infotrac (12) in that users were satisfied with their searches. As at UCLA and SUNY, at Meharry over half found what they were looking for while a third found some of what they were looking for. Users did perceive that their searches were more complete than they could have been (2), a fact which did concern librarians. Yet, as Carol Tenopir remarked, despite librarians' worries, for most users what they do get is enough (12). Search technique did change with continued use of the system for 80% of repeat users; 52% browsed fewer articles to find what they needed while 28% browsed more. Whatever this may indicate in terms of technique, repeat users were experimenting and changing their methods in searching. Perhaps classes in advanced search techniques could allay the concerns of librarians about user search thoroughness. However, that most users continue to find what they need while browsing fewer articles indicates that such concerns may be unwarranted for the majority of users. Perhaps users who browse more articles do need more user education. Rietdyk asserted that inadequate search techniques may require more time at the terminal (10) while Rambo found that 38% of Quick Search survey respondents wanted further training (9). Or perhaps some simply prefer to browse more records. The ability to browse at one's own pace is an advantage of CD-ROM over online (10). More research would be necessary to discern how browsing reflects on search technique.

One can also note that most users utilized three or four discs. Bonham and Nelson indicated that most of their respondents only wanted records dated from one to five years back (1). We concur with them that time span offered by the CD-ROM systems is sufficient for most users (1).

As for English abstracts of foreign documents, most users were either neutral or found them useful. One can conclude that English abstracts of foreign documents should continue to be included in CD-ROM products intended for use in research areas.

Concerning ease of use, we can conclude that users at Meharry found the CD-ROM systems easy to use. Garfinkel noted that speed is a critical issue for CD-ROM users (6). Survey respondents found changing discs easy and system response adequate. The overwhelming majority of users of both systems rated overall ease of use of the CD-ROM systems as high.

As for the manuals, we can conclude that of those who used them, more found them useful than not useful (37% versus 12%). However, 51% were neutral on the subject, indicating the probable percentage of users who never opened them. It may not be that the manuals were undesirable to most users but rather that they preferred one-on-one instruction.

Librarians agree that some amount of instruction is necessary to use MEDLINE on CD-ROM. Few librarians have found that they can rely on vendor-supplied aids, such as manuals, or on the user friendliness of software (4). Pearce at Columbia found that users typically required fifteen to twenty minutes of explanation from the librarian and almost invariably had more questions while searching (8). Bonham and Nelson indicated that half of their respondents preferred one-on-one instruction and needed brief written instructions (1). Librarians at SUNY did most of their training one-on-one and in small groups and emphasized that instruction is necessary (2). At Meharry we also trained users one-on-one and in small groups. Users not only needed instruction in use of MESH headings (2) and search techniques but also in computer terminology (7) and system capabilities (8). As Glitz stated, a major problem is that users try textwords instead of MeSH headings despite thorough user education (7). However, we found repeat users employing MeSH headings more often. Once users realize that retrieval is greater when they use MeSH headings, they apparently utilize them. Librarians can continue to encourage users to ask questions as they perform searches (2).

As for the method preferred by users, results demonstrate a strong preference for the CD-ROM. While 43% actually found the printed indexes easier to use versus 47% who found the CD-ROM easier, 78% of initial survey respondents and over 90% of repeat users would try the CD-ROM next time. That 43% found the printed indexes easier to use could indicate patrons quite comfortable with *Index Medicus* and/or computer shy. Nevertheless, as Glitz found in 85% of her respondents, most would try the CD-ROM again (7). Garfinkel indicated that patrons would choose CD-ROM over free online searching (6). One hardly needs to state that preference for CD-ROM was overwhelming. As patrons become familiar with CD-ROM in libraries, they may come to expect CD-ROM to be available for their use, creating a greater demand for CD-ROM products. And certainly one can conclude that if CD-ROM is available, patrons will use it.

A major factor in the positive response to CD-ROM was its availability without cost. Bonham and Nelson found that most of their survey participants would use an end-user system frequently if it were free and easily accessible (1). Indeed, Dodson also stated that CD-ROM is well-suited to end-user searching since there is not cost penalty (5). There may be queuing lines at some libraries (10) though we have only occasionally had that experience at Meharry. Cost is so important that if the CD-ROM were unavailable, only 8% would try online methods. If CD-ROM is to gain and maintain a strong foothold in libraries, searching must remain a free service for end-users.

Looking at users' approach to searching, that most used MeSH headings more often indicates their familiarity with MeSH prior to trying the CD-ROM system. This was the result of extensive user education and the common sense of those who retrieved better results when they used MeSH headings (2). We reiterate that training in search techniques and use of MeSH headings is essential.

Considering the attitude of repeat users, the majority wanted to and did use the library more due to the availability of the CD-ROM. This is significant for librarians. SUNY reported that the CD-ROM improved public relations (2). At Meharry only 10% of those who wanted to use the library more but had not, listed feeling uncomfortable using the CD-ROM as a reason. Certainly those 10% needed more instruction. However, the 81% who wanted to use the library more and had done so signified the powerful role of the CD-ROM in changing the attitude of library patrons toward searching and frequenting the library. Patrons liked browsing the records and enjoyed searching on the CD-ROM. The majority came to the library more often because they perceived that they could find what they needed more quickly. The evolving ability of CD-ROM to put very recent data in the hands of researchers when they need it is a step toward fulfilling one of the primary goals of librarianship—to get the information to the researchers as quickly and efficiently as possible. By drawing people to the library to learn how to find that information on the CD-ROM system, the system helps to fulfill a primary goal of academic librarianship—to help the users to find the information for themselves. Certainly whether or not they use anything else in the library, they will use the CD-ROM and find information. As Chen remarked, CD-ROM is real; it works incredibly well (3).

Comparing the CD-ROM systems, one can note various differences. Most of these differences were minor. Slightly more SilverPlatter than Cambridge users replied that they found what they were seeking. Similarly although over 90% of both groups find system response satisfactory and the system to be easy to use overall, more SilverPlatter than Cambridge users were pleased. Silver-Platter users found the discs easier to change than Cambridge users. Cost mattered more to SilverPlatter than Cambridge users; this correlates with a slightly larger percentage of students among the SilverPlatter user group. More Silver-Platter than Cambridge repeat users listed speed of finding information as a motivation for using the library more; yet the disparity in the sizes of the repeat user groups may make such a comparison inconclusive. However, Cambridge also came out ahead in some areas. Cambridge users found the manual marginally more useful than SilverPlatter users. Significantly, 35% of Cambridge users versus 50% of SilverPlatter users found the printed indexes easier to use than the CD-ROM system.

For the patron unfamiliar with computers or searching, the menus on Cambridge may make searching easier than searching on SilverPlatter. This assertion seems to be supported by the replies of survey respondents familiar with online searching. Of those, 83% preferred SilverPlatter to online compared to 55% of Cambridge users. Of Cambridge users 36% preferred to do their own searches online. In general, experienced searchers preferred SilverPlatter while inexperienced searchers preferred Cambridge. However, one wonders with Garfinkel if they were clear concerning the difference between online and CD-ROM searching (6). Yet, 87% of Cambridge and 73% of SilverPlatter initial users would try CD-ROM again with 7% of Cambridge and 11% of SilverPlatter users wanting to try an online search; that fewer SilverPlatter users were satisfied with their initial CD-ROM searching and more wanted to try online could suggest either greater or less computer literacy than Cambridge users. Obviously among repeat users, who liked the CD-ROM well enough to use it again, 95% of Cambridge and 100% of SilverPlatter users preferred the CD-ROM to online. Since libraries serve both inexperienced and experienced end-users, CD-ROM producers can consider more on-screen instructions for the noncomputer-literate end-user plus features more like online for experienced searchers. In general, end-users of both systems preferred CD-ROM to online or manual methods.

Nevertheless, the CD-ROM is not a replacement for online or manual methods. Rather it is a complement, but a complement which can replace online or manual methods for a significant number of users and do that with a high degree of user satisfaction.

The capacity of CD-ROM to draw researchers to the library and to the most current and useful information is nothing short of revolutionary. Such a revolutionary tool in the information age can be strongly embraced and guided by library and information specialists who can help researchers find the world on silver discs.

REFERENCES

1. Bonham, Miriam D., and Nelson, Laurie L. "An Evaluation of Four End-user Systems for Searching MEDLINE," *Bulletin of the Medical Library Association* 76(April 1988): 171-180.

2. Capodagli, James A.; Mardikian, Jackie; and Uva, Peter A. "Medline on Compact Disc: End-user Searching on Compact Cambridge," *Bulletin of the Medical Library Association* 76(April 1988): 181-183.

3. Chen, Ching-chih. "Libraries and CD-ROM," *Microcomputers for Information Management* 2(1985): 129-134.

4. Crane, Nancy, and Durfee, Tamara. "Entering Uncharted Territory: Putting CD-ROM in Place," *Wilson Library Bulletin* 62(December 1987): 28-30.

5. Dodson, Carolyn. "CD-ROMs for the Library," *Special Libraries* 78(Summer 1987): 191-194.

6. Garfinkel, Simson L. "Columbia's Contagious CD-ROM Fever," *CD-ROM Review* 3(July 1988): 27-29.

7. Glitz, Beryl. "Testing the New Technology: MEDLINE on CD-ROM in an Academic Health Sciences Library," *Special Libraries* 79(Winter 1988): 28-33.

8. Pearce, Karla J. "CD-ROM: Caveat Emptor," *Library Journal* 113(February 1, 1988): 37-38.

9. Rambo, Neil. "Quick Search Survey Results," *Library Lines* 1(January 1988): 3.

10. Rietdyk, Ron J. "Creation and Distribution of CD-ROM Databases for the Library Reference Desk," *Journal of the Amer-ican Society for Information Science* 39(January 1988): 58-62.

11. Roose, Tina. "The New Papyrus: CD-ROM in Your Library?" *Library Journal* 111(September 1, 1986): 166-167.

12. Tenopir, Carol. "Infotrac: a Laser Disc System," *Library Journal* 111(September 1, 1986): 168-169.

13. U.S. Department of Health and Human Services, Public Health Service, National Institutes of Health, National Library of Medicine. *Long Range Plan. Report of Panel 2: Locating and Gaining Access to Medical and Scientific Literature* Bethesda, MD: National Technical Information Service, 1986.

14. Wertz, R.K. "CD-ROM: a New Advance in Medical Information Retrieval," *Journal of the American Medical Association* 256(December 26, 1986): 3376-3380.

Appendix A-1

```
         SILVERPLATTER MEDLINE CD-ROM EVALUATION QUESTIONNAIRE

Instructions:

 This MEDLINE CD-ROM SilverPlatter system is being tested by
Meharry Medical Library.  We would like you to fill out this
questionnaire in order to help us find out who is using the
system, and how useful it is to you.  Please circle your answers
and return this form to the reference librarian.  Thank you!

1.  My primary affiliation is (enter one only):  a.  Medicine,
b.  Dentistry, c.  Basic sciences, d.  Graduate school,
e.  Allied health, f.  Administration, g.  Nursing, h.  Other

2.  My profession is (enter all that apply):  a.  physician,
b.  nurse, c.  dentist, d.  other health care professional,
e.  educator, f.  scientist/researcher, g.  student,
h.  librarian, i.  administrator, j.  other

3.  I was looking for articles (enter all that apply):
a.  by an author, b.  under a title, c.  on a subject, d.  in a
specific journal, e.  other

4.  I needed the information for (enter all that apply):
a.  patient care, b.  a paper or report, c.  a research project,
d.  keeping current, e.  to check a reference, f.  teaching or
planning a course, g.  a grant proposal, h.  not needed, just
curious, i.  other

5.  If I was looking up a subject, I used (enter all that apply):
a.  a text word, b.  more than one text word, c.  a MESH heading,
d.  more than one MESH heading

6.  The information I found was (enter one only):  a.  what I was
looking for, b.  more than I needed, c.  some of what I needed,
d.  not useful, e.  other

7.  I received training from (enter all that apply):
a.  a librarian, b.  a student, c.  a faculty member, d.  other,
e.  I did not receive training, f.  I did not find training
necessary

8.  Which of the following printed publications have you ever
used (enter all that apply)?  a.  Index Medicus,
b.  International Nursing Index, c.  Index to Dental Literature,
d.  Hospital Literature Index, e.  I have not used any of the
above, f.  I cannot remember
```

9. If you have used the printed indexes, how do they compare to SilverPlatter MEDLINE (enter one only)? a. easier to use, b. harder to use, c. about the same to use, d. other

10. Have you used an online version of MEDLINE (MEDLINE over the telephone), either yourself or by having a librarian process a search for you (enter all that apply)? a. yes, by myself, b. yes, librarian search, c. no, d. do not know

11. If you have used online MEDLINE, which system do you prefer (enter one only)? a. online, own search, b. SilverPlatter MEDLINE, c. online, librarian search, d. do not know

12. If this MEDLINE CD-ROM system had not been available today, what would you have done (enter all that apply)? a. used a printed index, b. used an online version, c. asked a library staff member, d. asked a friend or colleague, e. browsed through the stacks, f. nothing, g. other

13. Next time you need this sort of information, what will you do (enter all that apply)? a. try SilverPlatter MEDLINE, b. try a printed version, c. try an online version, d. try another source

14. SilverPlatter MEDLINE is provided free of charge to library users. How important a consideration was this in your decision to use this system, instead of an online version of MEDLINE (enter one only)? a. very important, b. somewhat important, c. relatively unimportant, d. would not have used an online version of MEDLINE

15. How often have you used SilverPlatter MEDLINE? a. first time, b. once before, c. 3-5 times, d. 6 or more times

16. SilverPlatter MEDLINE contains material on five discs covering five years from 1983 to 1987. How many discs did you use today? a. 1, b. 2, c. 3, d. 4, e. 5

Enter one only (on the following 5 point scale) for questions 18 through 25. Write the letter next to the question number.

SCALE: A   B   C   D   E
        Strongly   Strongly
         Agree   Agree   Neutral   Disagree   Disagree

18.   The rate at which the SilverPlatter system responds is satisfactory.

19.   The SilverPlatter MEDLINE manual helped me to use the system.

20.   Changing SilverPlatter MEDLINE discs is easy.

21.   The time span covered by SilverPlatter MEDLINE was sufficient for my needs.

22.   Overall, I found SilverPlatter MEDLINE easy to use.

23.   I feel like I am comfortable with computers.

24.   I think staff assistance was adequate.

25.   English abstracts of foreign documents were useful to me.

SILVERPLATTER MEDLINE CD-ROM FOLLOW-UP QUESTIONNAIRE

Instructions:

This MEDLINE CD-ROM system is being tested by Meharry Medical Library. We would like you to fill out this follow-up questionnaire in order to help us find out who the repeat users of the system are and how useful it is to you. Please circle your answers and return this form to the reference librarian. Thank you!

1. My primary affiliation is (enter one only): a. Medicine, b. Dentistry, c. Basic sciences, d. Graduate school, e. Allied health, f. Administration, g. Nursing, h. Other

2. My profession is (enter all that apply): a. physician, b. nurse, c. dentist, d. other health care professional, e. educator, f. scientist/researcher, g. student, h. librarian, i. administrator, j. other

3. I was looking for articles (enter all that apply): a. by an author, b. under a title, c. on a subject, d. in a specific journal, e. other

4. I needed the information for (enter all that apply): a. patient care, b. a paper or report, c. a research project, d. keeping current, e. to check a reference, f. teaching or planning a course, g. a grant proposal, h. not needed, just curious, i. other

5. If I was looking up a subject, I used (enter all that apply): a. a MESH heading, b. more than one MESH heading, c. a text word, d. more than one text word

6. Since I have started using the CD-ROM, for subject searching I generally (enter one only): a. use text words more often than MESH headings, b. use MESH headings more often than text words, c. use MESH headings and text words about the same amount of time, d. it depends on the search topic

7. The information I found was (enter one only): a. what I was looking for, b. more than I needed, c. some of what I needed, d. not useful, e. other

8. With repeated use of the CD-ROM system, I find what I need on the CD-ROM (enter one only): a. more quickly, b. more slowly, c. in about the same amount of time

9. Also, with repeated use of the CD-ROM system, I find that the number of articles through which I have to browse to find what I need has generally (enter one only): a. increased, b. not changed much, c. decreased

10. When I search for articles, I generally prefer to use (enter one only): a. the CD-ROM system, b. the printed indexes, c. an online (MEDLINE over the telephone) search by the librarian, d. I have no preference

11. Since the library has made the CD-ROM system available, I use the library (enter one only): a. more, b. less, c. about the same

12. Also, since the library has made the CD-ROM system available, I want to use the library (enter one only): a. more, b. less, c. about the same

13. How often have you used the CD-ROM system? a. once before, b. 3-5 times, c. 6 or more times

14. Since you have been using the CD-ROM more often, do you find that searching has become generally (enter one only): a. easier over time, b. more difficult over time, c. has not changed, d. do not know, e. depends on the search topic

15. If the CD-ROM system has changed how much I use the library, it is because (enter all that apply): a. I can find what I need faster, b. I can browse the abstracts in my field, c. the CD-ROM is fun to use, d. the CD-ROM has not changed how much I use the library

16. If I want to use the library more due to the CD-ROM system and have not yet, it is because (enter all that apply): a. the library is too far away, b. library hours are inconvenient, c. I am too busy with other things, d. I do not feel confident using the CD-ROM

TABLE I

PRIMARY AFFILIATION
(QUESTION No. 1)

SG*	MED SCHL	DENT SCHL	BASIC SCI.	GRAD SCHL	ALLIED HEALTH	ADMIN	NUR	OTHER	TOTAL
CC-I	20	1	0	3	0	0	0	2	26
SP-I	15	5	2	3	1	0	0	1	27
CC-F	12	0	1	5	0	0	0	1	19
SP-F	5	0	1	0	1	0	0	0	7
TOTAL	52	6	4	11	2	0	0	4	79

*NOTE: In this and subsequent tables, "SG" denotes the SURVEY GROUPS who answered questions about their experience on one of the two CD-ROM systems. "CC" stands for COMPACT CAMBRIDGE and "SP" stands for SILVERPLATTER. The "I" after them refers to the answers given by users after their initial use of a system. "F" refers to the survey answers as reported by users after they had used a system two or more times.

TABLE II

PROFESSION (QUESTION No. 2)

SG	MD	RN	DDA	OHCP	EDUC	SCI/RES	STU	LIB	ADM	ETAL	TOTL
CC-I	4	0	1	0	1	5	20	0	0	0	31
SP-I	6	0	2	0	2	7	16	0	0	0	33
CC-F	3	0	0	0	1	6	14	0	0	0	24
SP-F	1	0	0	0	0	2	4	0	0	0	7
TOTL	14	0	3	0	4	20	54	0	0	0	95

OHCP = Other health care professionals
LIB = Librarian
ETAL = Other

TABLE III

SEARCH GOAL (QUESTION No. 3)

SG	AUTHOR	TITLE	SUBJECT	SPECIAL JOURNAL	OTHER	TOTAL
CC-I	5	3	22	1	1	32
SP-I	2	4	24	2	0	32
CC-F	5	4	17	3	0	29
SP-F	1	0	7	0	0	8
TOTAL	13	11	70	6	1	101

TABLE IV

SEARCH REASON   (QUESTION No. 4)

SG	PT.	REPORT	RES.	CURR.	REF.	CLASS	GRANT	FUN	ETAL	TOTL
CC-I	5	12	14	5	5	1	2	1	1	46
SP-I	4	12	13	3	0	2	1	0	1	36
CC-F	5	13	11	4	1	0	2	4	1	41
SP-F	0	4	4	0	0	2	1	0	0	11
TOTL	14	41	42	12	6	5	6	5	3	134

PT = Patient care
REPORT = Report/Paper
RES. = Research
CURR. = (Keeping) Current
REF. = Checking a reference
CLASS = Required coursework
FUN = Searching for fun, curiosity
ETAL = other

TABLE V

SEARCH INSTRUCTOR   (QUESTION No. 7)

SG	LIBR.	STUDENT	FACULT.	OTHER	NO TRAIN	NO NEED	TOTL
CC-I	22	7	0	0	1	0	30
SP-I	27	0	0	0	0	0	27
TOTAL	49	7	0	0	1	0	57

TABLE VI

INDEX FAMILIARITY   (QUESTION No. 8)

SG	IM	INL	IDL	HLI	NONE	CAN'T RECALL	TOTAL
CC-I	21	0	1	0	2	1	25
SP-I	23	1	4	2	2	0	32
TOTAL	44	1	5	2	4	1	57

IM = <u>Index Medicus</u>
INL = <u>Index to Nursing Literature</u>
IDL = <u>Index to Dental Literature</u>
HDL = <u>Hospital Literature Index</u>

TABLE VII

CD-ROM SYSTEM USE FREQUENCY
(QUESTION No. 15)

SG	FIRST TIME	ONCE BEFORE	3-5 TIMES	>6 TIMES	TOTAL
CC-I	13	5	5	3	26
SP-I	20	4	2	1	27
CC-F	0	2	6	11	19
SP-F	0	3	2	2	7
TOTAL	33	14	15	17	79

TABLE VIII

COMPUTER LITERACY   (QUESTION No.23)

SG	STRONGLY AGREE	AGREE	NEUTRAL	DISAGREE	STRONGLY DISAGREE	TOTAL
CC-I	8	8	6	2	0	24
SP-I	12	9	4	2	0	27
TOTAL	20	17	10	4	0	51

TABLE IX

INFORMATION FOUND   (QUESTION No. 6)

SG	WHAT WAS SOUGHT	MORE FOUND	SOME FOUND	NOT USEFUL	OTHER	TOTAL
CC-I	13	3	8	0	0	24
SP-I	17	4	4	0	0	25
CC-F	11	1	6	0	0	18
SP-F	4	0	2	0	0	6
TOTAL	45	8	20	0	0	73

TABLE X

ENGLISH ABSTRACTS USEFUL
(QUESTION No. 25)

SG	STRONGLY AGREE	AGREE	NEUTRAL	DISAGREE	STRONGLY DISAGREE	TOTAL
CC-I	7	2	11	2	1	23
SP-I	9	3	10	2	1	25
TOTAL	16	5	21	4	2	48

TABLE XI

CHANGE IN ARTICLES BROWSED
(QUESTION No. 9F)

SG	INCREASED	NOT CHANGED	DECREASED	TOTAL
CC-F	6	2	11	19
SP-F	1	3	2	6
TOTAL	7	5	13	25

TABLE XII

ONLINE EXPERIENCE
(QUESTION No. 10i)

SG	BY MYSELF	LIBRARIAN	NONE	DO NOT KNOW	TOTAL
CC-I	4	8	15	0	27
SP-I	5	11	14	0	30
TOTAL	9	19	29	0	57

TABLE XIII

NUMBER OF DISCS (QUESTION No. 16)

SG	1	2	3	4	5	6+	TOTAL
CC-I	10	3	5	3	1	4	26
SP-I	4	8	6	0	9	0	27
TOTAL	14	11	11	3	10	4	53

TABLE XIV

RATE OF SYSTEM RESPONSE
(QUESTION No. 18)

SG	STRONGLY AGREE	AGREE	NEUTRAL	DISAGREE	STRONGLY DISAGREE	TOTAL
CC-I	14	8	1	1	0	24
SP-I	20	6	1	0	0	27
TOTAL	34	14	2	1	0	51

TABLE   XV

USEFULNESS OF MANUAL
(QUESTION No. 19)

SG	STRONGLY AGREE	AGREE	NEUTRAL	DISAGREE	STRONGLY DISAGREE	TOTAL
CD	8	1	14	0	0	23
SP-I	6	3	11	2	4	26
TOTAL	14	4	25	2	4	49

TABLE XVI

EASE OF CHANGING DISCS
(QUESTION No. 20)

SG	STRONGLY AGREE	AGREE	NEUTRAL	DISAGREE	STRONGLY DISAGREE	TOTAL
CC-I	11	9	2	1	0	23
SP-I	18	8	1	0	0	27
TOTAL	29	17	3	1	0	50

TABLE XVII

OVERALL EASE
(QUESTION No. 22)

SG	STRONGLY AGREE	AGREE	NEUTRAL	DISAGREE	STRONGLY DISAGREE	TOTAL
CC-I	14	8	2	0	0	24
SP-I	20	6	1	0	0	27
TOTAL	34	14	3	0	0	51

TABLE XVIII

ADEQUACY OF STAFF ASSISTANCE
(QUESTION No. 24)

SG	STRONGLY AGREE	AGREE	NEUTRAL	DISAGREE	STRONGLY DISAGREE	TOTAL
CC-I	18	4	1	0	0	23
SP-I	25	1	1	0	0	27
TOTAL	43	5	2	0	0	50

TABLE XIX

USE SPEED   (QUESTION No. 8)

SG	MORE QUICKLY	MORE SLOWLY	SAME	TOTAL
CC-F	17	0	2	19
SP-F	6	0	0	6
TOTAL	23	0	2	25

TABLE XX

SEARCH EASE (QUESTION No. 14)

SG	EASIER	MORE DIFFICULT	NO CHANGE	DO NOT KNOW	TOPIC	TOTAL
CC-F	18	0	0	0	1	19
SP-F	6	0	0	0	0	6
TOTAL	24	0	0	0	1	25

TABLE XXI

PRINTED INDEX VERSUS CD-ROM (QUESTION No. 9i)

SG	EASIER	HARDER	SAME	OTHER	TOTAL
CC-I	8	11	2	2	23
SP-I	12	11	1	0	24
TOTAL	20	22	3	2	47

TABLE XXII

ONLINE VS CD-ROM (QUESTION No. 11)

SG	ONLINE, SELF	CD	ONLINE, LIBRARIAN	DO NOT KNOW	TOTAL
CC-I	4	6	0	1	11
SP-I	0	10	1	1	12
TOTAL	4	16	1	2	23

TABLE XXIII

ALTERNATE METHOD
(QUESTION No. 12)

SG	PRINT	ONLINE	STAFF	PEER	STACKS	NOTHING	OTHER	TOTAL
CC-I	16	2	9	1	6	1	0	35
SP-I	16	4	12	1	4	0	2	39
TOTAL	32	6	21	2	10	1	2	74

TABLE XXIV

NEXT TIME   (QUESTION No. 13)

SG	CD USED	PRINT	ONLINE	ANOTHER	TOTAL
CC-I	26	2	2	0	30
SP-I	27	3	4	3	37
TOTAL	53	5	6	3	67

TABLE XXV

CHARGE   (QUESTION No. 14)

SG	VERY IMPORTANT	SOMEWHAT IMPORTANT	RELATIVELY UNIMPORTANT	WOULD NOT USE	TOTAL
CC-I	16	5	3	1	25
SP-I	22	2	2	1	27
TOTAL	38	7	5	2	52

TABLE XXVI

TIME SPAN (QUESTION No. 21)

SG	STRONGLY AGREE	AGREE	NEUTRAL	DISAGREE	STRONGLY DISAGREE	TOTAL
CC-I	12	8	2	1	0	23
SP-I	14	11	1	1	0	27
TOTAL	26	19	3	2	0	50

TABLE XXVII

SYSTEM PREFERRED (QUESTION No. 10F)

SG	CD BEST	PRINT	ONLINE/ LIBRARIAN	NO PREF.	TOTAL
CC-I	18	0	0	1	19
SP-I	7	0	0	0	7
TOTAL	25	0	0	1	26

TABLE XXVIII

MESH HEADINGS VERSUS TEXTWORDS (QUESTION No. 5)

SG	TEXT WORD	>TEXTWORD	MESH HEADING	<MESH	TOTAL
CC-I	6	10	19	11	46
SP-I	4	8	20	8	40
CC-F	13	13	4	5	35
SP-I	1	4	1	3	9
TOTAL	24	35	44	27	130

TABLE XXIX

MESH HEADING USE CHARGE OVER TIME
(QUESTION No. 6F)

SG	MORE TEXT	MORE MESH	SAME	SEARCH TIME	TOTAL
CC-F	3	10	2	3	18
SP-F	3	2	0	1	6
TOTAL	6	12	2	4	24

TABLE XXX

LIBRARY USE (QUESTION No. 11F)

SG	MORE	LESS	SAME	TOTAL
CC-F	15	0	4	19
SP-F	6	0	1	7
TOTAL	21	0	5	26

TABLE XXXI

DESIRE TO USE LIBRARY (QUESTION No. 12F)

SG	MORE	LESS	SAME	TOTAL
CC-F	18	0	1	19
SP-F	5	0	1	6
TOTAL	23	0	2	25

TABLE XXXII

CD-ROM LIBRARY USE CHANGE REASONS
(QUESTION No. 15F)

SG	FASTER	BROWSE	FUN	NOT CHANGED	TOTAL
CC-F	17	10	8	0	35
SP-F	6	1	1	0	8
TOTAL	23	11	9	0	43

TABLE XXXIII

LIBRARY NONUSE REASONS   (QUESTION No. 16F)

SG	ASSISTANCE	HOURS	OTHER CONCERNS	CD	TOTAL
CC-F	1	3	8	1	13
SP-F	0	1	3	1	5
TOTAL	1	4	11	2	18

EVALUATION OF

MEDLINE ON
SILVERPLATTER CD-ROM

EXPERIENCE OF THE
GEORGE WASHINGTON UNIVERSITY
HIMMELFARB HEALTH SCIENCES LIBRARY

By *Anne M. Linton*
Elaine R. Martin
Shelley Bader

Himmelfarb Library
George Washington University
Medical Center
2300 Eye St. NW
Washington, DC 20037

EVALUATION OF MEDLINE ON SILVERPLATTER CD-ROM: EXPERIENCE OF THE GEORGE WASHINGTON UNIVERSITY HIMMELFARB HEALTH SCIENCES LIBRARY

Introduction

The SilverPlatter CD-ROM workstation was set up in a public area midway between the Reference and Circulation desks on the main floor of the Himmelfarb Library. This location is clearly visible to patrons as they enter the Library and as they exit both the stairs and elevator from the 2nd and 3rd floor stacks. Both Reference and Circulation staff can easily provide assistance to this location. Circulation staff primarily assisted patrons with paper jams and similar mechanical problems, while Reference staff provided help with system use and search formulation. The system was set up as a self-service search station, available all hours that the Library is open. Six discs, covering MEDLINE from January 1983 through the second quarter of 1988, were put out for patron use during the evaluation period (mid-February - July 1988). The station itself was dedicated to the SilverPlatter MEDLINE CD program, which could only be exited by rebooting. Staff observed that, many days, the station was in use nearly all of the seventeen hours that the Library is open. Evaluation forms were placed at the station and a decorative box was provided for completed evaluation forms. Patrons are accustomed to seeing a CD workstation in that area since the Library had evaluated both the Cambridge and BRS/Colleague MEDLINE CD-ROM products and ISI's *Science Citation Index* compact disc version.

Comparison with miniMEDLINE

The Library also has the miniMEDLINE program available for all Medical Center patrons. This program, mounted on an on-campus minicomputer, provides users with menu-driven access to references in 417 journals owned by the Himmelfarb Library. Its major emphasis is current clinical and educational literature from 1986 to the present. The program is updated monthly. Four dedicated miniMEDLINE terminals are located in an area adjacent to the Reference desk. The miniMEDLINE program is also available via dial access and through the University's local area network.

Evaluation Instrument

The Library modified the evaluation form provided by the National Library of Medicine to condense the number of questions asked and to add comparative questions regarding miniMEDLINE and SilverPlatter (Appendix A).

Instruction in Use of CD-ROM

The Reference staff thoroughly acquainted themselves with the system and instructional manual provided and concluded that a simpler, briefer guide to searching SilverPlatter's CD MEDLINE was needed. A four-page set of instructions was developed (Appendix B). Copies of this guide were provided at the workstation along with the SilverPlatter manual and discs. Additional signs regarding disc changing procedures and printing were placed near the keyboard of the workstation. A decision was made to provide individual assistance to users rather than attempting to schedule specific training sessions. This decision was based on the staff's experience in training miniMEDLINE users. Busy clinicians and students can rarely set aside the time for additional training sessions in their schedules. Moreover, they usually prefer to learn new systems when they actually need to use them to meet a specific information need. Articles promoting the availability of the SilverPlatter MEDLINE system were placed in the Library newsletter and the Medical Center's weekly internal newsletter. In addition, signs and flyers directing users to the system were placed throughout the Library.

Observations and Results

Reference librarians observed that the system was regularly used during the evaluation period. They made a particular effort to encourage users to complete the evaluation form. As is frequently the case when evaluations are voluntary, only 52 completed forms were turned in. (See results in Appendix C.) Eighty-five percent of the respondents were Medical Center faculty, staff or students. The remaining 15% was evenly divided between other University users and non-University users. Of the Medical Center users, 22% were comprised of research faculty and 29% comprised of medical students. The particular interest by researchers in the CD version of MEDLINE is corroborated by the fact that 67% of the users indicated research as the purpose of their searches.

Reference librarians informally observed that most clinicians headed directly for the miniMEDLINE terminals and seemed satisfied with the program's content. In contrast, many research staff expressed frustration at the limited scope and coverage of the miniMEDLINE program. They were quite pleased to learn that they could search the complete MEDLINE file back to 1983 on the SilverPlatter CD-ROM. Comments on evaluation forms regarding the comprehensiveness and breadth of the SilverPlatter CD MEDLINE further corroborate this observation. The fact that the Library does not own all of the journals included on the compact discs did not bother most researchers since they are generally more willing to wait for interlibrary loans than clinicians.

All respondents said they were able to find relevant references using the SilverPlatter system. Forty-three percent of the searches were completed by using Medical Subject Headings, 36% by words in titles, 16% by author, 2% by journal, and 3% by some other method. Almost all users had checked another source before beginning a search on SilverPlatter. Seventy percent of respondents indicated that the program was easy to search and 49% stated that the prompts were clear. Most users were clearly pleased with both the search process and their search results. This fact surprised the Library's reference staff at first since they had evaluated both the Cambridge and BRS/Colleague compact disc versions of MEDLINE previously. These other programs had seemed easier to use to staff already trained in the art of online searching. However, the staff's previous experience in teaching patrons to use miniMEDLINE had taught them that trained searchers approach a user-friendly search system with very different expectations from end-users!

Conclusions

Several factors contributed to the users' overall favorable experience with the SilverPlatter CD MEDLINE. First, the program provides excellent online help screens. They are clearly-written, full of examples, and accessible at any time during the search process. Users were often seen to leave their search in process to check a fine point of searching and then return to the point where they had left off. Second, many users approached the SilverPlatter program with a very positive attitude. They were nearly all familiar with online searching. Forty-eight percent had had the Library run MEDLINE searches for them previously; 74.5% had used miniMEDLINE. Moreover, they were generally the type of individuals who are unafraid of computers and willing to seek out and learn new technologies. The fact that SilverPlatter's "FIND" prompt puts them directly and immediately in search mode was very inviting. These users enjoyed the opportunity to explore both the MEDLINE database and a new search program at their leisure. They often only wanted help from Library staff when they hit a major obstacle to their search. Third, the SilverPlatter CD MEDLINE provided users with a chance to browse through large numbers of references and a variety of topics without having to worry about online costs or print charges. While a sign was posted telling users to limit their search time to 15 minutes if others were waiting, this rule rarely had to be enforced. The SilverPlatter users seemed to be a very civilized group and worked out any scheduling conflicts among themselves amicably.

Library Reference staff was surprised to note the high percentage of searches completed using Medical Subject Headings. They observed that many users began their searches with free-text terms and only turned to Medical Subject Headings if frustrated with their free-text results or if convinced by Reference staff that their use would result in more relevant retrieval. Two features of the SilverPlatter CD MEDLINE probably combat this reliance on free-text searching at the expense of Medical Subject Headings. First, the index to the MEDLINE database is always available online. Users reviewing the index may highlight any highly-posted term for the system to search automatically. Second, users may also highlight any term in a relevant record for automatic searching. Thus, it is easy to identify significant Medical Subject Headings on SilverPlatter CD MEDLINE and even easier to search them since no rekeying is involved. Free-text searching can thus serve as a gateway to Medical Subject Headings on SilverPlatter. Reference staff found this highlight-and-search feature to be a very positive aspect of the program. With the proliferation of user-friendly search systems online and within the Library itself (One respondent stated that he uses miniMEDLINE, BRS/Colleague, and SilverPlatter!), users are tempted to rely solely on free-text methods of searching rather than learn each system's unique way of entering Medical Subject Headings. This reliance on free-text can be frustrating for researchers who need to see everything written on a topic as well as for clinicians and students who miss important articles by choosing to search the wrong synonym or not enough synonyms for a concept.

User familiarity with a search system seems to play a real role in successful use of the system. One respondent indicated a preference for miniMEDLINE because he/she was more familiar with it. Another respondent volunteered that the SilverPlatter program became easier to use with each use. These sorts of reactions are to be expected in any environment where users acquainted with one system are introduced to another. User adaptability to new search systems should prove to be an interesting area of study as libraries make various CD products from multiple publishers, all with different searching systems, available.

Eighty-one percent of the respondents felt that the CD-ROM covered a sufficient number of years. A suggestion to have the system go back to 1980 was made. The lack of retrospective coverage in miniMEDLINE is often a source of user frustration. Researchers preferred the comprehensiveness of SilverPlatter CD MEDLINE with regard to both journal coverage and time. No one commented on the fact that SilverPlatter was not as current as miniMEDLINE or MEDLINE, although users did repeatedly ask just how recent the material included on the CDs was.

All respondents indicated that they would like to see the system in the Library permanently. Sixty-two percent would be willing to pay for the service, while another 7% said that it would depend on the cost.

Problems Observed

The process of changing discs proved problematic for many users. Additional signs were placed near the workstation keyboard offering directions, and staff watched for problems so that they could offer users assistance. This problem was alleviated by daisy-chaining multiple disc players to the workstation. Three discs could then be accessed from a single menu. Since the MEDLINE database from 1983 to June 1988 consists of 6 discs, the process of changing discs could not be entirely eliminated. The cost of so many disc players would be prohibitive for this and many other libraries. Nonetheless, users do not want to be bothered with changing discs. No one accidentally walked off with a disc. However, one user accidentally placed the disc in the floppy drive. After the staff carefully extricated the disc from the drive, they taped the door shut. This solution was not entirely satisfactory since 3 or 4 regular users of the program utilized its downloading capability to load their search results into file management programs on computers in their offices.

While the SilverPlatter CD MEDLINE was well-received by both Library staff and users, it still has several draw-backs.

First, the screen display in search mode is confusing. If a user enters the phrase "myocardial infarction," the program lists separate postings for both "myocardial" and "infarction" in statements 1 and 2 respectively before giving postings for the these words adjacent to each other in search statement 3. First-time users often think that they have done something wrong since the program does not immediately respond to the phrase that they have typed.

Second, references display one immediately after the other. This results in references being split across screens, making abstracts and descriptors harder to read. Users of the program sometimes forget which title goes with which abstract or descriptors when they are faced with the last half of one record and the first half of another.

Third, several procedures require the use of the TAB key. Many users had difficulty locating and using this key. Consequently, they would display all of the records from a large set when they only wanted to review a few, or they had trouble selecting and searching words from records during the highlight-and-search process. Both procedures require the user to press the TAB key.

Fourth, while the SilverPlatter CD MEDLINE provides access to every field on the MEDLINE record and permits users to limit search retrieval by year, language, species, etc., it does not permit users to "explode." Several users of the program requested the Library to run MEDLINE searches for them so that they did not have to enter every drug in a specific therapeutic category or every disease affecting a body system. Many researchers are interested in doing broad searches in order to assess the amount and type of research going on in a particular field and would welcome the "explode" capability.

Fifth, users were often confused by the need to type a number sign (#) before set numbers that they were using to combine concepts. For instance, when "anding" search sets 1 and 2, they might simply type "1 and 2," thereby retrieving records with numbers 1 and 2 in them instead of their concepts.

Finally, the fact that the 3 discs for 1985 through 1987 do not each correspond to a single year but instead represent overlapping time periods provided an additional frustration to program users.

Summary

The staff and users of the Library retained a very positive impression of the SilverPlatter CD MEDLINE. It is viewed as an important adjunct to the Library's other information resources. The limits on the Library's miniMEDLINE database due to computer storage capacity severely restrict its coverage and, therefore, its utility as an extensive research tool. Yet miniMEDLINE provides widespread and immediate access to clinical references for multiple users across the Medical Center campus. On the other hand, the SilverPlatter CD MEDLINE provides single user access to the entire MEDLINE file back to 1983. It is a valid alternative for the core of researchers at the Medical Center.

Appendix A

MEDLINE ON CD-ROM

1. CIRCLE ONE OF THE FOLLOWING TO INDICATE YOUR STATUS:

GWU MED. CENTER		GWU Non-Medical	Non-GWU
Faculty, patient care	Staff of _____	Faculty	Faculty
Faculty, research or teaching		Student, graduate	Student
Faculty, allied health	Student, medical	Student, UG	Law firm
Intern/Resident/Fellow	Student, graduate		
Nursing staff	Student, allied health		Other_____

    PURPOSE OF SEARCH: _____

2. WHICH PRODUCT DID YOU USE? ___SILVER PLATTER ___CAMBRIDGE

3. WERE YOU ABLE TO FIND RELEVANT REFERENCES ON YOUR TOPIC? Y / N

4. DID YOU SEARCH FOR REFERENCES BY ___AUTHOR ___TITLE WORDS
   ___MEDICAL SUBJECT HEADING ___JOURNAL ___OTHER_____?

5. WHAT SOURCES DID YOU CHECK PRIOR TO SEARCHING THE CD-ROM
   ___INDEX MEDICUS ___miniMEDLINE ___OTHER_____?

6. WAS THE DATABASE EASY TO SEARCH?

   EASY   DIFFICULT
   1   2   3   4   5

7. DID YOU FIND THAT THE PROMPTS PROVIDED TO HELP YOU SEARCH
   WERE CLEAR AND EASY TO FOLLOW?

   CLEAR   NOT CLEAR
   1   2   3   4   5

8. DID THE CD-ROM COVER A SUFFICIENT NUMBER OF YEARS FOR
   YOUR SEARCH? Y / N

9. WOULD YOU LIKE TO SEE THIS PRODUCT IN THE LIBRARY
   PERMANENTLY?   Y / N

   IF YES, WOULD YOU PAY TO USE THIS SERVICE? Y / N

10. HAVE YOU EVER HAD THE LIBRARY RUN A MEDLINE SEARCH? Y / N

11. HAVE YOU EVER USED miniMEDLINE? Y / N

   IF YES, WHICH SYSTEM DO YOU PREFER ___miniMEDLINE OR
   ___SILVER PLATTER OR ___CAMBRIDGE? WHY? _____

   _____

12. HOW OFTEN HAVE YOU USED THE SILVER PLATTER CD-ROM?
   ___FIRST TIME ___1-2 TIMES ___3-5 TIMES ___6+ TIMES

COMMENTS:

Guide to Searching SilverPlatter MEDLINE

To Begin Your Search

Hit the F7 key to restart MEDLINE.

At the FIND: prompt, you may type the following:

1. A **term** consisting of any combination of characters or numbers, e.g. hepatitis or 5-ASA.
2. A **phrase**, e.g. hepatitis antibodies.
3. A **root**, indicated by the truncation symbol *, e.g. hepati* retrieves all words that begin with those 6 letters (hepatic, hepatitis, etc.).
4. A **Medical Subject Heading** which must be entered as follows:
    Ex. hepatitis-antibodies-* in mesh
    The phrase "in mesh" tells the system to search for this in the subject heading field. Truncate with * to retrieve a heading with all possible subheadings. If the heading is a single word, end with a hyphen:
    Ex. hepatitis- in mesh
5. An **author's name** entered last name first as follows: koop-ce* or koop-c* if the middle initial is not known. For fastest searching, include the phrase "in au", e.g. koop-ce* in au.
6. A **previous search request**, using a number sign (#) and the number assigned by the system, e.g. #8. This number can be used interchangeably with the search term. Reasons for reusing a request are: to combine it with other terms; to show or print previous results; or to repeat a search in another segment of the database after an XCHANGE of discs.

```
SilverPlatter v1.3.     MEDLINE (R) 1985-1987 DISC 3
IMMMMMMMMMMMMMMMMMMMMMMMMMMMMMMMMMMMMMMMMMMMMMMMMMMMMMMMMMMMMMMMMMMMMMMI
: No.  Request                                              Records  :
:                                                                    :
: #1:  HEPATITIS                                              2130   :
: #2:  5-ASA                                                    10   :
: #3:  HEPATITIS                                              2130   :
: #4:  ANTIBODIES                                            11761   :
: #5:  HEPATITIS ANTIBODIES                                    300   :
: #6:  HEPATI*                                                5506   :
: #7:  HEPATITIS-ANTIBODIES-*                                 >76    :
: #8:  HEPATITIS-ANTIBODIES-* in MESH                          84    :
: #9:  KOOP-C*                                                >8     :
: #10: KOOP-C* in AU                                            8     :
: #11: #8                                                      84    :
:                                                                    :
:                                                                    :
:                                                                    :
:                                                                    :
:                                                                    :
HMMMMMMMMMMMMMMMMMMMMMMMMMMMMMMMMMMMMMMMMMMMMMMMMMMMMMMMMMMMMMMMMMMMMMM:
FIND:

Type a search request, then press RETURN. To SHOW records found, press F4.
```

To Combine Terms

You may combine terms using:

   OR   retrieves all records that contain either or both terms
anywhere in the record.

            Ex. drug or abuse

This strategy retrieves any records that mention either drug or
abuse. Both terms may or may not be present in the same record.

   AND   retrieves all records that contain those terms anywhere in
the record.

            Ex. drug and abuse

This will retrieve records that contain these two words, but also
locates records that contain drug and sexual abuse where the 2
terms may be unrelated.

   WITH   retrieves all records in which those terms appear in the
same field.

            Ex. drug with abuse

This will retrieve records that contain both words in a single
field such as in the abstract field.

   NEAR   restricts retrieval to terms located in the same
sentence. By adding a number to near, you can specify exactly
how close the terms should be to one another.

            Ex. drug near abuse
                    or
                 right near2 die

The first example retrieves citations where the terms drug abuse
appear side by side in a sentence.- The second example retrieves
records containing the terms within 2 words of each other in a
sentence.

   NOT   retrieves all records containing one term but not another.

            Ex. drug not abuse

This will retrieve records on drug but not abuse.

```
SilverPlatter v1.3       MEDLINE (R) 1985-1987 DISC 3
ΙΜΜΜΜΜΜΜΜΜΜΜΜΜΜΜΜΜΜΜΜΜΜΜΜΜΜΜΜΜΜΜΜΜΜΜΜΜΜΜΜΜΜΜΜΜΜΜΜΜΜΜΜΜΜΜΜ:
: No.  Request                                     Records  :
:                                                           :
: #1:  DRUG                                         56846   :
: #2:  ABUSE                                         1446   :
: #3:  #1 or #2                                     57535   :
: #4:  #1 and #2                                      557   :
: #5:  #1 near #2                                     223   :
: #6:  #1 not #2                                    56009   :
:                                                           :
:                                                           :
:                                                           :
:                                                           :
:                                                           :
:                                                           :
:                                                           :
```

To Limit Your Search Retrieval

If your strategy produces a large number of citations, you may
want to limit your retrieval by:

LANGUAGE - You can request all English language records.

             EX. #(previous request) and english in la

MJME - You can search for articles indexed as MJME or Major MeSH
headings, meaning that the main emphasis of the article will be
the MeSH heading.

             EX. hepatitis-antibodies-* in mjme

TITLE - You may ask that your term appears in the article's
title.
             EX. hepatitis in ti

DATE - = equals   py=1987
         < less than   py<1987
         > greater than   py>1987
         <= less than or equal to   py<=1987
         >= greater than or equal to   py>=1987

SilverPlatter v1.3   MEDLINE (R) 1985-1987 DISC 3
IMMMMMMMMMMMMMMMMMMMMMMMMMMMMMMMMMMMMMMMMMMMMMMMMMMMMMMMMMMMMMMMMMMMMMMMMMMMMMM;
: No. Request   Records :
:   :
: #1: HEPATITIS-ANTIBODIES-*   >76   :
: #2: HEPATITIS-ANTIBODIES-* in MESH   84   :
: #3: #2 and LA=ENGLISH   74   :
: #4: HEPATITIS-ANTIBODIES-*   >76   :
: #5: #3 and (HEPATITIS-ANTIBODIES-* in MJME)   26   :
: #6: HEPATITIS   2139   :
: #7: #5 and (HEPATITIS in TI)   13   :
: #8: #7 and PY=1987   10   :
:   :
:   :
:   :
:   :
:   :
:   :
:   :
:   :
HMMMMMMMMMMMMMMMMMMMMMMMMMMMMMMMMMMMMMMMMMMMMMMMMMMMMMMMMMMMMMMMMMMMMMMMMMMMMMM<
FIND:

Type a search request, then press RETURN. To SHOW records found, press F4.

To Display Your Search

Hit the **F4** key to display the records your search retrieves.
The computer responds with the following:

SHOW Fields: ALL   Records: ALL

You may ask for **CITN** rather than **ALL** fields to be displayed. By
typing **CITN** at the SHOW Fields: prompt, the computer will display
the ti, au, so, la, and an fields. By using the tab key, you can
move the cursor to the Records field and enter the number of
references you would like displayed.

To Print Your Search

Hit the **F6** key to print the records retrieved by your search.
The computer responds with the following:

PRINT Fields: CITN   Records: ALL
separate pages: (No) Yes   searches: (No) Yes

The **CITN** command will print the ti, au, so, la, and an fields.
By using the tab key, you can move the cursor to the Records
field and enter the number of references you would like printed.

To Exchange Compact Discs

SilverPlatter MEDLINE comes on several compact discs. Each disc
covers different dates.

Disc Label	Coverage Dates
1985-1987, disc 3	1986-1987
1985-1987, disc 2	1985-1986
1985-1987, disc 1	1985
1984-1983, disc 2	1983-1984
1984-1983, disc 1	1983-1984

To change discs, hit the **F2** key to return to the **FIND:** prompt.
Next, hit the **F8** or **XCHANGE** key. This will allow you to change
the compact discs. Follow the instructions as they appear on the
screen.

To End Your Search

Hit the **F7** key to restart the system for the next user.

Appendix C-1

```
                 Himmelfarb Health Sciences Library
            The George Washington University Medical Center


               RESULTS OF MEDLINE ON CD-ROM SURVEY

                                   # of Responses    % of Total
    1.   Respondents status:

         GWU Medical Center:
              Faculty, patient care            2
              Faculty,research or teaching     10
              Faculty, allied health           0
              Intern/Resident/Fellow           4
                (I - 2/R - 1/F - 1)
              Nursing staff                    0
              Staff of
                Pharmacy                        4
                Immunochemistry                 3
                Cardiology                      1
                Pathology                       1
                Physiology                      1
              Student, medical               13
              Student, graduate               4
              Student, allied health          2
                                             ----
                                               45           85.0


         GWU Non-Medical:
              Faculty                          0
              Student, graduate                4
              Student, UG                      0
                                             ----
                                                4            7.5


         Non-GWU:
              Faculty                          0
              Student                          2
              Law firm                         1
              Other (NIMH)                     1
                                             ----
                                                4            7.5

         Status total                        54          100.0

    Purpose of search:
              Research                        26           66.7
              Patient care                     5           12.8
              Education                        8           20.5
                                             ----         ------
                                               39          100.0


    2.   Which product used:  Silver Platter
```

437

	# of Responses	% of Total
3. Able to find relevant references:		
Yes	48	100.0
No	0	0.0
	48	100.0
4. Did you search for references by:		
Author	10	16.4
Title words	22	36.1
Medical Subject Heading	26	42.6
Journal	1	1.6
Other	2	3.3
	61	100.0
5. Sources checked prior to searching CD-ROM:		
Index Medicus	14	29.1
miniMEDLINE	23	47.9
Other		
Biosis	1	2.1
BRS-PsychInfo	1	2.1
Chemical Abstracts	1	2.1
Iowa	2	4.2
MEDLINE	1	2.1
Science Citation Index	4	8.3
Other	1	2.1
	48	100.0
6. Was database easy to search:		
1 (Easy)	35	70.0
2	11	22.0
3	2	4.0
4	2	4.0
5 (Difficult)	0	0.0
	50	100.0
7. Were prompts clear and easy to follow:		
1 (Clear)	25	49.0
2	16	31.4
3	5	9.8
4	5	9.8
5 (Not Clear)	0	0.0
	51	100.0
8. Did CD-ROM cover sufficient years:		
Yes	39	81.3
No	9	18.7
	48	100.0

Appendix C-3

	# of Responses	% of Total
9. Like to see in library permanently:		
Yes	49	100.0
No	0	0.0
	49	100.0
Would you pay to use service:		
Yes	28	62.2
No	14	31.1
Depends on cost	3	6.7
	45	100.0
10. Ever had library run a MEDLINE search:		
Yes	24	48.0
No	26	52.0
	50	100.0
11. Ever used miniMEDLINE:		
Yes	38	74.5
No	13	25.5
	51	100.0
If yes, which system preferred:		
miniMEDLINE	6	17.1
Silver Platter	29	82.9
Cambridge	0	0.0
	35	100.0
12. How often used this system:		
First time	24	47.0
1-2 times	10	19.6
3-5 times	8	15.7
6+ times	9	17.6
	51	100.0

System preference comments:

SILVERPLATTER MEDLINE
ON CD-ROM

EVALUATION AT UCLA LOUISE DARLING
BIOMEDICAL LIBRARY

By Julie Kwan

Louise Darling Biomedical Library
University of California, Los Angeles
10833 LeConte Avenue
Los Angeles, California 90024-1798

SilverPlatter Medline
on CD-ROM:
Evaluation At UCLA Louise Darling
Biomedical Library

Introduction

As part of the National Library of Medicine's CD-ROM evaluation project, the Louise Darling Biomedical Library at UCLA conducted a field test of MED-LINE® on CD-ROM from SilverPlatter Information, Inc. SilverPlatter's MEDLINE on CD-ROM was available for users in the library's Reference Reading Room beginning on April 14, 1988. MEDLINE on CD-ROM was available to users from 8:30 a.m. to 8:30 p.m. Monday through Thursday, 8:30 a.m. to 5:30 p.m. Friday, and 9:30 a.m. through 4:30 p.m. on Saturdays. The system was available to users through August 31, 1988.

The Biomedical Library Environment

The Louise Darling Biomedical Library at UCLA is a large and busy academic health sciences center library. The Biomedical Library serves the Schools of Medicine, Dentistry, Nursing, and Public Health, the UCLA Medical Center, and the Departments of Biology and Microbiology as well as related research institutes. We have a unique online catalog, ORION, which provides access to holdings information for materials in all campus libraries; a circulation module for ORION was introduced in July 1988 for Biomedical Library materials. Our collection includes over 450,000 volumes and 7,000 serial titles. In 1986/87, almost 3 million photocopies were made and over 60,000 reference inquiries answered. On a daily basis we may have 2,500 persons using the library.

MELVYL MEDLINE: A Local Subset

The University of California medical school libraries, working with the UC Division of Library Automation, have made a subset of the MEDLINE database available for public use. The subset, which includes two to three years of the complete MEDLINE file, first became available for general use in the five

---

*Registered trademark designation will not be repeated hereafter. - Ed.

University of California medical school libraries in November 1987. The complete MEDLINE file has been made available since close to 90% of the journals covered in MEDLINE are available within the University of California library system. At the Biomedical Library, ten MELVYL® terminals provide access to the MELVYL Catalog, the online catalog of the nine University of California campus libraries, and to MELVYL MEDLINE. MELVYL terminals are accessible all hours the Biomedical Library is open, even when reference service is not available. In July, 1988, access to the MELVYL MEDLINE database was provided through any MELVYL terminal in any campus library. In September 1988, dial-up access to MELVYL MEDLINE was instituted for UC faculty, staff, and students.

MELVYL MEDLINE provides access to users through a menu-driven mode, the Assist Mode, as well as a expert-mode, the Command Mode. Training documents, handouts and manuals were prepared by a task force of library staff members from the San Diego and Los Angeles campuses. Currently, MELVYL MEDLINE provides quite sophisticated search techniques. For example, author initials are automatically truncated so that users do not need to learn how to input variant name forms. Keyword searching provides access to terms which appear in article titles, abstracts, or as any word within a Medical Subject Heading. MeSH headings may be browsed so that users can see postings for the term in its totality or for the term with each subheading applied. MeSH headings may be exploded with or without subheadings. All cross-references within the MeSH file automatically map to the appropriate MeSH heading. The system software provides context sensitive help for incorrect responses as they are made by the user.

Prior CD-ROM Experience

At the Louise Darling Biomedical Library, we have had two prior experiences with MEDLINE on CD-ROM products. The first experience occurred in 1986, before the availability of MELVYL MEDLINE. The second began in December 1987, when MELVYL MEDLINE was available but during which time the MELVYL system was down for almost two weeks for software reconstruction. The third, this most recent experience with SilverPlatter's MEDLINE on CD-ROM, began five months after MELVYL MEDLINE became available. Having had experience with CD-ROM versions of MEDLINE on previous occasions, we were interested in incorporating our previous experience into this evaluation. We wanted to evaluate the system with a minimum of instruction for users. Therefore we consciously did not provide sponsored instructional programs to introduce the system to users. Instead, we relied on the manual, a sheet of brief instructions, and the help screens for the majority of user training. Reference Desk staff also provided on-the-spot assistance when requested to help users with specific problems.

CD-ROM Versus a Local Online Subset

We were also interested in assessing the utility of MEDLINE on CD-ROM in light of the fact that we also provide access for users to MEDLINE through the online subset, MELVYL MEDLINE. The MEDLINE subset was exceptionally popular with users from its first inception. It was so popular in fact that we decided to disable MELVYL MEDLINE printing on weekends to discourage off-campus users from printing lengthy bibliographies. Consequently, SilverPlatter's MEDLINE on CD-ROM became our only mechanism for users to print MED-LINE citations on weekends.

The CD-ROM Evaluation

Library staff mounted and tested the software prior to placing the workstation in the Reference Reading Room. Instructions for users and for Reference Desk staff were prepared (See Appendix A and B). Staff evaluations were primarily qualitative in nature. A special questionnaire was used to gather data.

Equipment and Databases

SilverPlatter provided the library with the following equipment for this evaluation project: an IBM PC/AT compatible personal microcomputer with 80286 processor, a Phillips CD-ROM external drive (CM100/22), and a Hewlett Packard ThinkJet printer. Two additional CD-ROM drives were provided late in the evaluation to test a new software development, daisy-chaining several discs at one time. The following databases were provided by SilverPlatter: MEDLINE (5 disks), 1983-1987; Cancer-CD; OSH-ROM, and ChemBank.

We obtained a locking Stelex desk to provide security for the processing unit, monitor and keyboard. The printer and CD-ROM drives were locked each night in drawers at the Reference Desk. The CD-ROM workstation was located in the Reference Reading Room approximately fifteen feet away from the Reference Desk. The CD-ROM workstation was visible to users who were passing through the library to the journal reading room. On the other side of the Reference Desk, against a wall, are located ten terminals which are used to access MELVYL MEDLINE.

Above the workstation was mounted a large sign announcing the Silver-Platter MEDLINE on CD-ROM with hours of availability. A brief list of instructions, the SilverPlatter manual, and a diagram explaining the function keys were placed for easy access.

The Evaluation Questionnaire

A user evaluation form was developed based on the questionnaire distributed to test sites by NLM staff (See Appendix C). A few additional questions were incorporated to seek information on issues of local interest, specifically:

1) comparison of use with MELVYL MEDLINE,
2) frequency with which users downloaded references to diskette, and
3) subject being searched.

Given the objective of completing 100 evaluation forms before the end of June, we only did a very small pre-test of the evaluation form. The pre-test evaluations were included in the final results. A total of 105 questionnaires were completed; the last questionnaire was collected on June 17, 1988. A copy of the questionnaire with a tally of responses is attached (Appendix C).

Summary of User Questionnaires

User Demographics, Search Purpose, and Search Capabilities

The following demographics describe the users of CD-ROM during this test:

Departmental Affiliation
Medicine	53
Dentistry	4
Nursing	7
Public Health	13
Allied Health	3
Other	26

Profession:
Physician	29
Nurse	6
Dentist	5
Other health care professional	3
Educator	4
Scientist/Researcher	36
Student	32
Librarian	2
Other	6

The majority of users were looking for articles by subject (93 responses), 12 responses were for works by a particular author, and 7 responses for materials in a particular journal. Search topics were understandably quite diverse; subjects were supplied by 103 respondents, one indicated "confidential" and one gave no answer. Most of the usage was for MEDLINE (96 responses); 7 used OSH-ROM.

Information was primarily gained for papers or reports (44 responses) or research projects (59 responses). The vast majority were satisfied with their searches, 46 responses indicating they found what they were looking for, 33 found some of what they needed. Only 11 found too much information and 11 found the search not useful.

The number of citations retrieved by users ranged from 0 to 1018. The average number of citations retrieved from all responses was 83. Those respondents who indicated that they found what they were looking for averaged 88 citations per search; those who found some of what they were looking for averaged 35. Among those users who found too much information or found the search not useful, several preferred working with printed indexes. At least two use MEDLINE from NLM. One was in a hurry to complete the evaluation and possibly in a hurry to conduct the search. Several included very positive comments, one saying "I wish we had one in our lab." The fact that they were not satisfied with their searches may indicate that they were primarily exploring the system rather than really needing the information on this occasion or that they just needed more experience or better instructions to perform an acceptable search.

Most users were experienced in using the printed indexes (77 responses), and 48 of these found the printed indexes harder to use than CD-ROM. Twenty four respondents indicated that they preferred searching online with other systems, including Grateful Med, MELVYL MEDLINE, and BRS.

Interestingly enough, most of the users used only a small part of the database since they indicated that they had only used one or two disks. Ten respondents indicated that they had downloaded citations. Most of the evaluation forms were filled out by first time users of SilverPlatter MEDLINE (78 responses), with 10 respondents indicating that they had used the system one time before, eight used it three to five times, and one respondent used the system six or more times.

User Evaluation of SilverPlatter Software

Respondents indicated a high level of satisfaction with the software. The levels of software satisfaction were graded by respondents in five categories, including: strongly agree, agree, neutral, disagree, and strongly disagree. The following figures represent the number of respondents who answered in the "strongly agree" or "agree" categories that the following were satisfactory:

Screen instructions:	81
Computer response rate:	75
Helpfulness of manual:	41

Ease in changing disks:	29
Time span covered:	61
Ease of use of overall system:	87

The fact that a majority of responses indicated that they had used only one or two discs and that 61 responses indicated that the time span covered was satisfactory seems to indicate that these users only needed a few quick references to materials or were satisfied because they viewed this as a test of a new system.

The two areas with the lowest level of satisfaction, i.e., helpfulness of the manual and ease in changing discs, in fact correlate with two weaknesses of the system as perceived by library staff. The SilverPlatter manual is a generic one, covering system commands without detailed descriptions and search strategy hints for specific databases. Changing discs, before the implementation of daisy- chaining software late in the evaluation period, required the user to request assistance from staff at the Reference Desk. Given the busy nature of our desk environment, this meant that users frequently had to wait in line just for this kind of assistance.

Staff Evaluation

Staff Observations of CD-ROM Use

In the report of our first experience in testing CD-ROM (Glitz, 1988), it was emphasized that librarians need to be closely involved in the development and testing of CD-ROM systems to create appropriate user- friendly systems which will be popular and useful with end-users. Our first experience with CD-ROM involved an early product; our second involved a product in beta-testing. Our most recent experience, with SilverPlatter, represents a product which had been tested and in use for a significant period of time. Consequently, the product had already benefited from the experience and expertise of many previous librarians and end-users. The active solicitation of involvement of libraries and end-users in this development by the producers has resulted in products of significantly higher quality than would have been possible otherwise.

Another change we have witnessed since our first test of CD-ROM is the increased computing power which is now available in personal computers. Accessing CD-ROM with the 8088 or 8086 processors is inadequate at best. The 80286 processor finally allows for acceptable response rates. As the 80386 processor becomes more widely available, we should see increased benefits in working with these systems. Developments in CD-ROM drives will also affect the success of these systems.

Staff Evaluation of the SilverPlatter System

In general, library staff felt that the SilverPlatter MEDLINE CD-ROM product was a very good one, providing reasonably speedy response time and good search software. SilverPlatter software considers each search term a separate set which can make a complex search quite lengthy, but which offers advantages for other searches. Some users who are already familiar with DIALOG, BRS, ELHILL, or other systems which use sets, seemed to prefer using SilverPlatter. As an example, when swapping discs it is very easy to request that a particular set number be executed on a new disc. In other cases, the use of sets provided easy access to subjects which involve numbers or initials. However, like many end-user systems, at the time of this test, SilverPlatter software did not allow for exploding MeSH headings. In fact, this has not been a great problem since even with MELVYL MEDLINE, users only infrequently have used the explode capability (Hubble, 1988).

A new search feature, lateral searching, also became available on the SilverPlatter software during the evaluation. Lateral searching allows the user to select additional search terms directly from the screen while examining database records. This search capability was extremely helpful in searching OSH-ROM which uses a numerical coding system for chemicals. When a user did a preliminary search using a textword for a specific chemical, the lateral search capability allowed further searching through the numeric code for the chemical which appeared in the record.

Comparison with MELVYL MEDLINE

Many CD-ROM users, at least during the initial part of the evaluation project, were unaware that MELVYL MEDLINE was available behind them on the other side of the Reference Desk. It is becoming more and more common to see ten simultaneous users at MELVYL terminals, especially during afternoons and early evenings. At the end of the evaluation project (and as can be seen from the evaluation responses), more users with MELVYL MEDLINE experience tried using the SilverPlatter MEDLINE. Unfortunately, the questionnaire did not rigorously discriminate between SilverPlatter and MELVYL MEDLINE use. It would have been advantageous to have included a question specifically asking if the user had ever used MELVYL MEDLINE. Instead, questions 12 and 13 alluded to using SilverPlatter versus MELVYL MEDLINE, but not specifically enough to make any valid comparisons.

As mentioned previously, MELVYL MEDLINE has proven extremely popular in our library since its inception in November 1987. A recent study (Hubble, 1988) analyzed user response to this system and concluded that users are satisfied with their searches although they have not yet realized its full potential. A long bank of terminals is certainly attractive to users as they are usually able to gain access to MELVYL MEDLINE, if not immediately, then with only a short wait. One comment on the user questionnaire for MEDLINE on CD-ROM lamented, "Don't advertise it, if everyone knows it's here, I'll never get online!"

A few sophisticated MELVYL MEDLINE users found instances when the SilverPlatter software handled their inquiries in a more satisfactory way.

Specifically, questions which require searching for single characters or numbers worked better with the SilverPlatter software, for example, M-CSF or CSF-1.

In general, staff preferred the online subset, MELVYL MEDLINE, which offers the following advantages:

1) more terminals, therefore multiple access sites
2) no need to swap disks for users (the local subset includes the complete MEDLINE database from January 1986 to present in one file)
3) MELVYL MEDLINE is more current since it is updated monthly
4) MELVYL MEDLINE software provided more power and flexibility with the MeSH vocabulary

Staff found problems with printing to be similar with MELVYL MEDLINE, including requests for additional paper and new ink cartridges. Swapping discs did present difficulties for users and staff alike; users needed to request assistance to search other discs and staff had to fit these requests into the already busy reference desk workloads.

Daisy Chaining CD-ROM Discs

On June 7, 1988, a new version of the SilverPlatter software was made available to users; this software allowed users to select three separate CD-ROM discs from an opening menu. Consequently we were able to make available three discs at one time. This obviated the need for users to request that Reference Desk staff swap discs for them. It also allowed users to select from some of the additional databases available to them. Staff are now perceiving higher use of databases such as OSH-ROM and Cancer-CD which we have mounted on the workstation along with the current MEDLINE file. Alternatively, MEDLINE coverage prior to that included in MELVYL MEDLINE could also be mounted for users.

Licensing Agreements

We have recently entered into purchase agreements for three CD-ROM systems. MELVYL MEDLINE provides the best access to the current MEDLINE file for our busy environment. However, we view CD-ROM as the best means to provide electronic access to users from disciplines for which MEDLINE does not provide adequate coverage. We decided to purchase the Life Sciences Collection, Science Citation Index, and PsycLit to meet the needs of our biology users and nursing students. Another obvious choice for the future are MEDLINE backfiles.

These purchase agreements have emphasized to us, that although CD-ROM products are priced for the library community, the licensing agreements are currently designed for departmental use rather than for large and active libraries. Proprietary databases provide restrictions for use by a single user on a single machine or only for staff and students of the primary institution. These restrictions preclude the use of CD-ROM in a networked environment even though we can guarantee, through network software, that only one user may use the CD-ROM product at one time.

Documentation

Staff were also acutely aware that database-specific documentation needs to be provided for both end-users of the database and for the library staff. SilverPlatter is planning to provide such documentation separate from the help screens contained within the system. We wholeheartedly support this effort since it will strengthen everyone's understanding of the database and its contents. As an example, the documentation which has been developed for MELVYL MEDLINE has added immeasurably to encouraging use of that system.

Non-MEDLINE Databases

Since we were testing the SilverPlatter CD-ROM system, we were able to work with several databases, including not only MEDLINE, but OSH-ROM, Cancer-CD, and eventually ChemBank, which includes RTECS. We found it quite valuable to have one software system to access a number of databases. In fact, we had a number of individuals since the last evaluation form was completed using OSH-ROM and Cancer-CD. Specialized files such as these, however, often include documents which are not readily available, and we must evaluate our service and collection development policies in light of increased interest in this type of material.

We were especially interested in the ChemBank file which includes the Registry of Toxic Effects of Chemical Substances (RTECS). This is a resource which we use on a regular basis for ready reference work. It also serves as a key to our collection since some of the document series are not analyzed in our library. The print copy, however, is too out-of-date to rely on, and the abbreviated references are time- consuming to explain to users at the Reference Desk. The microform version is also difficult to use and shares the problem of abbreviated references and data. To use RTECS online through NLM at the Reference Desk, however, can tie up a reference librarian and microcomputer for more time than is available in this environment. With RTECS via the ChemBank file, the user may spend as much time as is necessary; therefore, we believe that CD-ROM is an excellent alternative for this type of information.

Recommendations

Certainly, the development of CD-ROM has come a long way in the past two years. Software has developed considerably and the equipment with which this technology is best interfaced is more readily available. What is needed now are mechanisms for strengthening these products through "jukeboxes" capable of handling a reasonably high number of discs at one time and licensing agreements which will allow us to use these tools in the best possible way. Still to be determined are the balance points between the population size which can be served by CD-ROM versus the point at which an institution decides that an online subset with multiple access points is the best solution.

References

Glitz, Beryl. Testing the new technology: MEDLINE on CD-ROM in an academic health sciences library. *Spec Lib* 1988 Win;79(1):28-33.

Hubble, Ann B. MELVYL-MEDLINE: An end-user study. Los Angeles, UCLA Graduate School of Library and Information Science, May 20, 1988.

Appendix A

Reference Division
Louise Darling Biomedical Library
April 18, 1988

SilverPlatter MEDLINE CD-ROM
Instructions for Reference Desk Staff

We are providing public access to the SilverPlatter MEDLINE CD-ROM during the Spring Quarter as part of a CD-ROM evaluation project conducted by the National Library of Medicine. We plan to collect 100 completed evaluation forms for this project. The results Of the questionnaire will be tabulated for reporting to the National Library of Medicine.

Brief instructions, which explain the basic commands for the SilverPlatter software, are available by the machine and on the Reference Desk clipboard. A copy of the manual is also available for users to consult. A second copy of the manual is available in the Reference Office should replacement pages be needed (they will be photocopied if necessary). The SilverPlatter on screen instructions (use the F1 key) are quite good; direct users to them when they encounter problems or questions.

SilverPlatter MEDLINE is available on five discs covering 1983-1987. Supplements for 1988 will be available as received. We also have Cancer-CD (a cancer database) and OSH-CD (an occupational health database). These discs will be kept in the second right drawer of the Stelex microcomputer desk in the Reference Reading Room. Reference Division staff will swap discs for users when needed.

SilverPlatter MEDLINE CD-ROM should be attractive to users for three reasons:

1) Years of coverage extend earlier than those years available on MELVYL MEDLINE.

2) Printing will be available on Saturdays.

3) Downloading is an option with the SilverPlatter software. Users will need to supply their own formatted floppy disks.

Since we will need to collect 100 completed evaluation forms, we should strongly encourage users to use SilverPlatter MEDLINE. The sooner we collect the required number of forms, the sooner we will be able to complete our evaluation.

Search hints, with updates as we encounter specific problems, will be added to this instruction package at the Reference Desk. Copies will also be distributed to staff.

Appendix B-2

OPENING PROCEDURES

*   When the Reference Desk is opened in the morning, the Reference Assistant will set up the compact disc drive and the printer and turn on the machine.

*   The two black cords go to the printer. The two beige cords go to the compact disc drive.

*   The keys to the machine will be in the second drawer of the Stelex desk. The round key locks the disc drive. The square key turns the computer on and off. Until further notice, we will keep the disc drive locked so that no one can walk away with a disc.

*   The system will automatically boot from the autoexec.bat file.

RESPONSIBILITIES OF REFERENCE DESK STAFF

*   Reference Desk staff will assist users with questions while encouraging them to seek help directly from the system using the F1 key.

*   When users want to change discs (either to get different years of MEDLINE or to use either the cancer or occupational health discs), they will need to get assistance at the Reference Desk. You will need to unlock the disk drive, insert the new disc, and relock the drive before returning the key and the old disc to the drawer.

*   Reference Desk staff should encourage users to fill out evaluation forms so that we can get our required total evaluations.

*   If at any time, the system crashes and returns to the C: prompt, type in SPIRS to return the the SilverPlatter system.

*   Users may download citations if they so desire. Reference Desk staff may, at their discretion, suggest that users purchase a disk at the Health Sciences Student Store; Reference Desk staff may format the disk for the user using the Reference Desk microcomputer. This will facilitate our evaluation regarding user interest/experience in downloading from CD-ROM.

CLOSING PROCEDURES

*   When the Reference Desk is closed, the reference librarian on duty will turn off and disconnect the printer and the CD-ROM drive, lock them in the Stelex desk in the Reference

    Reading Room, and make sure that all discs are locked up as well. The monitor and computer should be turned off as well.

*   The reference librarian will also put completed evaluation forms in the Reference Assistant's in-box. He will number and date the evaluation forms.

Reference Division
Louise Darling Biomedical Library
April 18, 1988

SEARCH INSTRUCTIONS FOR SILVERPLATTER
Reference Desk

Help
Use the F1 key for help at any time in the search process.

Database Guides
Use the F3 key for a guide to the database including a
description of fields.

Search Structure and Logic
SilverPlatter software creates sets and gives you specific
postings for each set. Sets are numbered with a # preceding the
number. To recall a specific set be sure to include the # before
the set number. For example:
    #4

Searching
The F2 key is used to search (FIND).

Author Searching
Enter names as follows:
    Bunting-A*
    Bunting-A* in au (to qualify the specific field)

Year Limiting
Qualify years by using:
    YR=1985

Boolean Logic
SilverPlatter software assumes a logical "and" between any terms
strung together. Parentheses are used to construct complex
search statements.

Printing
The F4 key displays information on the screen. The F6 key prints
citations on the printer. Note that the user is prompted for
print options. The default print format is the citation (CITN).
The user can specify other formats, for example, ALL for the full
record, and CITN,AB for citation plus abstract. Note that search
terms which have retrieved results are highlighted on the
printout as well as on the screen.

Changing discs
When the user presses F8, the system will prompt for operator
assistance in changing discs. The Reference Librarian will
unlock the drive and change discs for the user. At this time,
encourage the user to complete and evaluation form.

SILVER PLATTER MEDLINE CD-ROM EVALUATION QUESTIONNAIRE
SPRING 1988

Instructions

This MEDLINE CD-ROM Silver Platter system is being tested by the
Louise Darling Biomedical Library. We would like you to complete
this questionnaire in order to help us find out who is using the
system, and how useful it is to you. Thank you!

*Please place your completed evaluation in the "Completed
Evaluation" box.*

1. My primary affiliation is: (Circle ONE only)

    a. Medicine [53]   d. Public Health [13]
    b. Dentistry [4]   e. Allied Health [3]
    c. Nursing [7]   f. Other [26]

2. My profession is: (Circle ALL that apply)

    a. physician [29]   f. scientist/researcher [36]
    b. nurse [6]   g. student [32]
    c. dentist [5]   h. librarian [2]
    d. other health care   i. other [6]
       professional [3]
    e. educator [4]

3. I was looking for articles: (Circle ALL that apply)

    a. by an author [12]   d. in a specific journal [7]
    b. under a title [6]   e. other [3]
    c. on a subject [93]

4. What was your search topic?

5. Which databases did you search: (Circle ALL that apply)

    a. MEDLINE [96]   c. OSH-CD [7]
    b. CANCER-CD [1]   d. Other [3]

6. I needed the information for: (Circle ALL that apply)

    a. patient care [8]   e. to check a reference [6]
    b. a paper or report [44] f. teaching/planning a course [5]
    c. a research project [59] g. not needed, just curious [4]
    d. keeping current [16]   h. other [3]

7. How many articles did your search retrieve? _____

8. The information I found was: (Circle ONE only)

    a. what I was looking for [46]   d. not useful [11]
    b. more than I needed [11]   e. other [1]
    c. some of what I needed [33]

*Answer questions 9 - 15 if you used SilverPlatter MEDLINE.
Otherwise, go to question 16 to complete the evaluation.*

9. Have you used any of the following printed publications:
INDEX MEDICUS, the INTERNATIONAL NURSING INDEX, the INDEX TO
DENTAL LITERATURE, or the HOSPITAL LITERATURE INDEX? (Circle
ONE only)

    a. yes [77]   b. no [15]   c. don't know [2]

10. If yes, you've used printed versions, how do they compare to
Silver Platter MEDLINE? (Circle ONE only)

    a. easier to use [18]   c. about the same to use [7]
    b. harder to use [48]   d. other [8]

11. Have you used an online version of MEDLINE (either yourself
or by having a librarian process a search for you)? (Circle
ALL that apply)

    a. yes, by myself [64]   c. no [13]
    b. yes, librarian search [31] d. don't know [2]

12. If yes, you've used online MEDLINE, which system do you
prefer? (Circle ONE only)

    a. online, by myself. Which system? [24]
    b. Silver Platter MEDLINE [50]
    c. online, librarian run [4]
    d. don't know [9]

13. If this CD-ROM system had not been available today, what would
you have done? (Circle ALL that apply)

    a. used a printed version [33] e. asked a friend or colleague [7]
    b. used MELVYL/MEDLINE [38]   f. browsed through the stacks [8]
    c. used another online   g. nothing [15]
       version [18]   h. other [6]
    d. asked a library staff
       member [11]

14. Next time you need this sort of information, what will you
do? (Circle ALL that apply)

    a. use Silver Platter   c. use another online version [23]
       MEDLINE [84]   d. use another option [8]
    b. use a printed version [16]

15. Silver Platter MEDLINE contains material on five discs covering 1983 to present. How many discs did you use today? _____

16. Did you download citations to diskette? (Circle ONE only)

    a. yes [10]   b. no

17. How often have you used the Silver Platter system? (Circle ONE only)

    a. first time [78]   c. 3-5 times [8]
    b. once before [10]   d. 6 or more times [1]

Choose ONE answer only (on the following 5 point scale) for questions 18 through 23.

SCALE: A   B   C   D   E

       Strongly   Agree   Neutral   Disagree   Strongly
       Agree   Disagree

	A	B	C	D	E
18. Instructions on Silver Platter screens were sufficient for my use.	27	54	6	14	1
19. The rate at which the computer responds is satisfactory.	40	35	13	13	0
20. The Silver Platter manual helped me to use the system.	12	29	31	6	5
21. Changing Silver Platter discs is easy.	15	14	31	3	3
22. The time span covered by Silver Platter was sufficient for my needs.	27	34	13	14	5
23. Overall, I found the Silver Platter system easy to use.	47	40	4	5	3

If you have any additional comments, please use the back of this questionnaire. THANK YOU!

Louise Darling Biomedical Library, UCLA   4/88

PART III

Appendixes

MEDLINE® ON CD-ROM:
Features Checklist

This checklist*indicates the various features in the MEDLINE® CD-ROM products currently available. It is meant as a starting point when gathering information about the products. In preparing the chart, a feature was considered present if it could be accomplished using any mode (novice or expert). Features indicated were available as of August 1, 1988. CD-ROM products are under constant development and most producers indicate that they are preparing new releases. For the most complete picture of these products and their current features, the producers should be contacted.

September 1988
Prepared by Joyce E.B. Backus, Reference Section, NLM
For the National Library of Medicine CD-ROM Evaluation Forum
September 23, 1988
Adapted from "Evaluation of CD-ROM version of MEDLINE database"
By Nancy S. Hewison, Life Sciences Library, Purdue University

*Editor's Note:
   A features Checklist is not intended to provide any assessment of the desirability of any feature or of the ease of execution of any feature on a particular system. All such a checklist can do is indicate the presence or absence of a wide range of features. The reader is referred to the bibliography in this volume of articles where such qualitative assessments can be found.

CONTENTS OF DISKS
Number of disks and time coverage

BiblioMed	BRS Colleague Disc	Compact Cambridge MEDLINE	Compact Med-Base	DIALOG OnDisc MEDLINE	MEDLINE/EBSCO CD-ROM	MEDLINE Knowledge Finder	Silver Platter MEDLINE	
●	●	●		●	●	●	●	Subscription for most recent file is one disk
	●	●					●	Latest subscription covers one year or less
							●	Latest subscription covers more than 1 yr but less than 2 yrs
●			●	●	●	●		Latest subscription covers 2 years or more

MEDLINE coverage

BiblioMed	BRS Colleague Disc	Compact Cambridge MEDLINE	Compact Med-Base	DIALOG OnDisc MEDLINE	MEDLINE/EBSCO CD-ROM	MEDLINE Knowledge Finder	Silver Platter MEDLINE	
	●	●	●			●	●	Entire MEDLINE for time period
●	●							English language only
●						●	●	Selected journals only

ADMINISTRATIVE/TECHNICAL

BiblioMed	BRS Colleague Disc	Compact Cambridge MEDLINE	Compact Med-Base	DIALOG OnDisc MEDLINE	MEDLINE/EBSCO CD-ROM	MEDLINE Knowledge Finder	Silver Platter MEDLINE	
		●	●	●				Option for passwords
			●	●				Store journal holdings
				●				Store ILL partners/suppliers
				●				Maintains ILL billing information
		●	●		●			Multiple disk players
●		●		●	●	●		Local Area Network Access
		●		●	●	●		Concurrent network use by more than one user
		●	●			●	●	Change disks without exiting to DOS

RECORD SEARCHING & PRINTING

BiblioMed	BRS Colleague Disc	Compact Cambridge MEDLINE	Compact Med-Base	DIALOG OnDisc MEDLINE	MEDLINE/EBSCO CD-ROM	MEDLINE Knowledge Finder	Silver Platter MEDLINE	
●	●	●	●	●	●	●	●	Author *searchable*
●	●	●	●	●	●	●	●	Author *printable*
●	●	●	●	●	●	●	●	Title *searchable*
●	●	●	●	●	●	●	●	Title *printable*
		●	●	●	●	●	●	Transliterated/vernacular title *searchable*
			●	●	●	●	●	Transliterated/vernacular title *printable*
●	●	●	●	●	●	●	●	Abstract *searchable*
●	●	●	●	●	●	●	●	Abstract *printable*
●	●	●	●	●	●	●	●	MeSH terms *searchable*
●	●	●	●	●	●	●	●	MeSH terms *printable*
		●	●					Tree numbers *searchable*
								Tree numbers *printable*
●	●			●	●	●	●	Personal name as subject *searchable*
			●	●	●	●	●	Personal name as subject *printable*
			●	●	●	●	●	Language *searchable*

BiblioMed	BRS Colleague Disc	Compact Cambridge MEDLINE	Compact Med-Base	DIALOG OnDisc MEDLINE	MEDLINE/EBSCO CD-ROM	MEDLINE Knowledge Finder	Silver Platter MEDLINE	
		•		•	•	•	•	Language *printable*
•		•		•	•			Year of publication *searchable*
•		•		•		•	•	Year of publication *printable*
•	•	•	•	•	•	•	•	Journal *searchable*
•	•	•	•	•	•	•	•	Journal *printable*
		•	•	•	•			Unique identifier *searchable*
		•	•		•	•	•	Unique identifier *printable*
			•		•			Entry month *searchable*
			•		•	•	•	Entry month *printable*
•			•					Author address *searchable*
•							•	Author address *printable*
		•	•	•	•	•		Registry number *searchable*
		•	•	•		•		Registry number *printable*
		•	•	•	•		•	Name of substance *searchable*
		•	•	•	•	•	•	Name of substance *printable*
		•	•	•		•		ISSN *searchable*
		•			•	•	•	ISSN *printable*
			•				•	Country of publication *searchable*
•			•			•	•	Country of publication *printable*
			•	•			•	Number of references *printable*

MeSH
MeSH features

BiblioMed	BRS Colleague Disc	Compact Cambridge MEDLINE	Compact Med-Base	DIALOG OnDisc MEDLINE	MEDLINE/EBSCO CD-ROM	MEDLINE Knowledge Finder	Silver Platter MEDLINE	
•		•	•	•	•		•	View MeSH display
			•	•	•		•	Scope notes displayable
•			•	•	•		•	Non-MeSH terms display
			•	•	•		•	Non-MeSH terms explodable
•			•	•	•		•	Select from MeSH display
•			•	•	•		•	View MeSH trees
			•	•				View tree numbers
•			•	•	•		•	Select from tree display
			•		•		•	Explode using MeSH term (multi and single word)
			•				•	Explode using term/subheading
			•	•				Explode using tree number
•			•				•	"Offers" subheadings
			•				•	"Offers" check tags

BiblioMed	BRS Colleague Disc	Compact Cambridge MEDLINE	Compact Med-Base	DIALOG OnDisc MEDLINE	MEDLINE/EBSCO CD-ROM	MEDLINE Knowledge Finder	Silver Platter MEDLINE	
								Treatment of MeSH terms
●		●	●	●	●	●	●	Single-word terms protected (liver without liver abscess)
●	●	●	●	●	●	●	●	Multi-word terms bound for precision (just liver abscess, not liver extracts and lung abscess)
●	●	●	●	●	●	●	●	Correct treatment of stopword and commands in multi-word terms (wounds *and* injuries)
●			●	●	●		●	MeSH cross references searchable (autotransfusion for blood transfusion, autologous)
								Major/minor MeSH headings
●	●	●	●	●	●	●	●	Indicated in records
●	●	●	●	●	●	●	●	Search both at once
●	●	●	●	●			●	Restrict search to major
●			●	●			●	Major MeSH terms posted to minor MeSH terms
								Subheadings
	●	●				●	●	Main heading/ no subheadings
●	●	●	●	●	●	●	●	Main heading/ one specific subheading
●	●	●	●	●	●	●	●	Main heading/ several specific subheadings
●	●	●	●	●	●	●	●	Main heading/ all possible subheadings
●					●	●	●	Main heading/ all possible subheadings plus with none
		●				●	●	Subheading without main heading
		●	●			●	●	Subheading in full or abbreviated format
								SEARCH FUNCTIONS
								Field searching
	●	●		●	●	●	●	Unqualified term searched in all searchable fields
●	●	●	●	●	●			Qualification to specific field
●	●	●	●	●	●			Qualification to more than one field at a time
●				●				Post qualification
●	●	●	●	●	●	●	●	Stopwords used
								Limiting
●				●	●	●	●	Human
●				●	●	●	●	Review
		●		●	●		●	Abstract available
●	●	●	●	●	●		●	English
			●				●	AIM list
		●		●			●	Special list indicator
		●		●				User's journal set

Feature comparison matrix for MEDLINE CD-ROM search products.

BiblioMed	BRS Colleague Disc	Compact Cambridge MEDLINE	Compact Med-Base	DIALOG OnDisc MEDLINE	MEDLINE/EBSCO CD-ROM	MEDLINE Knowledge Finder	Silver Platter MEDLINE	Feature
								Boolean logic
•	•	•	•	•	•		•	AND
•	•	•	•	•	•		•	OR
	•	•	•	•	•		•	NOT/AND NOT
								Order of precedence for evaluating operators
	•			•				AND before OR
•					•			OR before AND
		•	•				•	Left to right
•		•	•	•		•	•	Can control by nesting
								Proximity searching
•	•			•	•			Same field, any order, adjacent
	•				•			Same field, any order within # words
	•	•	•				•	Same field, same order, adjacent
				•				Same field, same order, within # words
								Combining search capabilities
•			•	•	•	•	•	Truncation and phrase/adjacency searching
•	•	•	•	•	•			Truncation and field qualification
•		•	•					Nested logic and field qualification
•		•	•	•				Phrase/adjacency searching and field qualification
								Truncation/wild card
•	•	•	•	•	•	•	•	Right
	•							Left
		•	•	•				Within word
								Search helps and timesavers
						•		Retrieves other than exact match
•		•	•	•		•	•	Display database text word index
•		•	•	•	•		•	Display particular index
•	•	•	•	•	•			Display search history
•	•	•	•	•		•		Save searches permanently
•		•	•	•		•	•	Erase prior search statements
•	•	•	•	•				Combine sets in any order
		•	•	•				Update topics/SDI on disk
				•				Transfer search to online

OUTPUT CAPABILITIES

Feature	BiblioMed	BRS Colleague Disc	Compact Cambridge MEDLINE	Compact Med-Base	DIALOG OnDisc MEDLINE	MEDLINE/EBSCO CD-ROM	MEDLINE Knowledge Finder	Silver Platter MEDLINE
Display formats								
Title only		●	●	●	●	●	●	●
Bibliographic citation	●	●	●	●	●	●	●	●
Bibliographic citation and abstract	●	●	●	●	●	●	●	●
Full record	●	●	●	●	●	●	●	●
Tagged fields	●	●	●	●	●	●	●	●
Title and descriptors	●	●	●	●	●	●	●	●
User-defined	●	●	●	●			●	●
Display capabilities/flexibility								
Specify which set to display	●	●	●	●	●		●	●
Specify which records to display	●	●			●		●	●
Specify how or if field labels are displayed				●				
Records last input are displayed first	●	●	●	●	●			
Highlights terms searched	●	●			●		●	●
Display order/sort								
Author			●	●				
Title				●				
Journal title			●	●				
Relevance to request				●			●	
Print formats								
Title only	●	●	●	●				●
Bibliographic citation	●	●	●	●	●	●	●	●
Bibliographic citation and abstract	●	●	●	●	●	●	●	●
Full record	●	●	●	●	●	●	●	●
Tagged fields					●	●	●	●
Title and descriptors	●	●	●	●	●	●	●	●
User-defined	●	●	●	●			●	●
User annotation							●	
Print capabilities/flexibility								
Specify which set to print	●	●	●	●	●		●	●
Specify which records to print	●	●	●	●	●	●	●	●
Specify how or if field labels are printed				●				
Records last input print first	●	●			●		●	●
Highlights terms searched		●					●	

	BiblioMed	BRS Colleague Disc	Compact Cambridge MEDLINE	Compact Med-Base	DIALOG OnDisc MEDLINE	MEDLINE/EBSCO CD-ROM	MEDLINE Knowledge Finder	Silver Platter MEDLINE
Print order/sort								
Author			•	•				
Title				•				
Journal title			•	•				
Relevance to request				•			•	
Downloading formats								
Title only	•		•	•			•	•
Bibliographic citation	•		•	•	•		•	•
Bibliographic citation and abstract	•		•	•	•		•	•
Full record	•	•	•	•	•	•	•	•
Tagged fields	•	•	•	•	•	•	•	•
Title and descriptors	•	•	•	•	•	•	•	•
User-defined	•		•	•			•	•
Downloading capabilities/flexibility								
Specify which set to download	•		•	•	•	•	•	•
Specify which records to download	•	•	•	•	•	•	•	•
Specify how or if field labels are downloaded				•				
Records last input download first	•	•			•	•	•	•
User annotation							•	
Downloading order/sort								
Author			•	•				
Title				•				
Journal title			•	•				
Relevance to request				•			•	
MODE OF USE								
One search mode	•	•			•	•	•	
Menu	•	•			•	•	•	
Function keys	•				•	•	•	
Commands					•			
Command abbreviations							•	
Undo last action	•				•	•	•	
Novice mode			•	•	•			
Menu			•	•	•			
Function keys			•	•	•			
Undo last action			•	•				

BiblioMed	BRS Colleague Disc	Compact Cambridge MEDLINE	Compact Med-Base	DIALOG OnDisc MEDLINE	MEDLINE/EBSCO CD-ROM	MEDLINE Knowledge Finder	Silver Platter MEDLINE	
		•	•	•				Expert mode
		•	•					Function keys
		•	•	•				Commands
		•	•	•				Command abbreviations
								Undo last command

USER ASSISTANCE
Processing

BiblioMed	BRS Colleague Disc	Compact Cambridge MEDLINE	Compact Med-Base	DIALOG OnDisc MEDLINE	MEDLINE/EBSCO CD-ROM	MEDLINE Knowledge Finder	Silver Platter MEDLINE	
•	•	•	•	•	•	•	•	Indicates when processing occurs
						•	•	Indicates amount of processing completed
		•	•	•	•	•	•	Can interrupt processing

On screen help

BiblioMed	BRS Colleague Disc	Compact Cambridge MEDLINE	Compact Med-Base	DIALOG OnDisc MEDLINE	MEDLINE/EBSCO CD-ROM	MEDLINE Knowledge Finder	Silver Platter MEDLINE	
•	•		•	•	•	•	•	Independent tutorial
•	•		•	•	•	•	•	Contextual/point of need help screens
	•		•	•	•	•	•	Table of contents for help or instructions
•	•	•	•	•	•	•	•	Error messages explain and help correct error

Other producer support

BiblioMed	BRS Colleague Disc	Compact Cambridge MEDLINE	Compact Med-Base	DIALOG OnDisc MEDLINE	MEDLINE/EBSCO CD-ROM	MEDLINE Knowledge Finder	Silver Platter MEDLINE	
	•		•	•	•	•	•	Indexed user's manual
•	•	•	•	•	•	•	•	Telephone support

SBS No. 1988-3

CD-ROM:
COMPACT DISC -- READ ONLY MEMORY

July 1988

371 Selected Citations

Compiled by Alvin J. Barnes

**U.S. Department of Health
and Human Services**
Public Health Service
National Institutes of Health

National Library of Medicine
Public Services Division
8600 Rockville Pike
Bethesda, Maryland 20894

CD-ROM: COMPACT DISC - READ ONLY MEMORY

This bibliography was prepared expressly for the *Evaluation Forum: MEDLINE on CD-ROM* held at the National Library of Medicine on September 23, 1988. The Forum was organized by the Library, and featured representatives of biomedical library and clinical sites that participated in the evaluation of seven commercially-available CD-ROM products containing subsets of the MEDLINE database. MEDLINE is the National Library of Medicine's bibliographic database covering the fields of medicine, nursing, dentistry, veterinary medicine, and the preclinical sciences; it contains about six million records from 1966 forward.

CD-ROM has emerged as an important alternative access medium for scientific, technical, business, and a host of other informational databases. The subjects in this publication, therefore, are broader than the specific theme of the Forum and are intended to address the needs of various user groups with an interest in this technology and its applications. In addition to MEDLINE on CD-ROM, for example, it contains citations to articles about public access library catalogs, economic issues, specific databases, and standards. In gathering references, the MEDLINE and Health Planning & Administration databases of the National Library of Medicine were searched as well as ERIC, Information Science Abstracts, INSPEC, and LISA. The majority of the material comes from the non-NLM databases, and is not available in the National Library of Medicine's collection.

This bibliography is not intended to be exhaustive, and the exclusion of a particular item is no reflection on its quality or usefulness. The purpose is to indicate to the audience the type and range of materials available and to provide a starting point for further investigation.

This bibliography has been divided into four sections. The first section includes journal articles subdivided by topical area. Citations may appear under more than one topic. The second and third sections contain citations for monographs and serial titles. An author index comprises the final section, in which each author's name is followed by the page number on which his or her citation appears.

SAMPLE CITATIONS

Citations in this bibliographic series are formatted according to rules established for *Index Medicus*. Sample journal and monograph citations appear below.

Journal Article:

Authors   *Article Title*

Kuhlman JR ; Lee ES. Data-power to the people.
        Am Libr 1986 Nov;17(10):757-8, 760, 778

Abbreviated Journal   *Date* *Volume* *Issue* *Pages*
        Title

Monograph:

Author   *Title*

Intner, Shiela S. Microcomputer environment: management issues.
        Phoenix, AZ: Oryx Press, 1987. 248p.

Place of Publication   *Publisher*   *Date*   *No. of Pages*

471

TABLE OF CONTENTS

I. JOURNAL ARTICLES

GENERAL

Abeytunga PK. CD-ROMs on the job--one organization's experience. CIPS Rev 1986 Nov;10(6):17-9

Alberico R. Print and CD-ROM: we need them both. Small Comput Libr 1987 Jun; 7(6):8-12

Anderson DT ; Seiter C. Managing sequence data on a CD-ROM. Am Biotechnol 1988; 6(3):54

Archer D ; Rawsthorn S ; Robinson B. What is CD-ROM? Libr Info Res News 1986; 9(34):29-32

Arnold SE. A baker's dozen of CD-ROM myths. Electron Opt Publ Rev 1987 Jun; 7(2):58-63

Arnold SE. Electronic information on CD--a product or a service. Online 1987 Nov; 11:56-60

Baldwin C. CD-ROM services and products. In: Stanford-Smith B ; Hendley T ; Walsh R, editors. Report on the Intensive Workshop on CD-ROM. A Joint Project by the CEC (DG XIIIB) and EURIPA, 12-13 Feb 1987, Luxembourg. Wilmslow, Cheshire, UK: Europe Information Industry Assoc., 1987. p.68-70

Bardes D'E. Attention novices: friendly intro to shiny disks. Libr Software Rev 1986 Jul-Aug;5(4):240-5

Bartenbach B The impact of optical disc publishing on the information community (CD-ROM-Read Only Memory). Inspel 1986;20(4):205-20

Borgman D. Information retrieval from CD-ROM: status quo or a revolution in end-user access. Can J Inf Sci 1987;12(3-4):43-53

Biesel D. Old books - new technologies. Ref Libr 1986 Fall;(15):209-15

Bovey JD ; Brown PJ. Interactive document display and its use in information retrieval. J Doc 1987 Jun;43(2):125-37

Bowers RA. Opportunities in application design using optical technology. Electron Opt Publ Rev 1987 Dec;7(4):182-5

Bristow A. Reference sources on CD-ROM at Indiana University. Electron Libr 1988 Feb;6(1):24-9

Brito CJ. Pan-American Health Organization CD-ROM pilot project. Inf Dev 1987 Oct; 3:208-13

Bunnell D. The challenge of CD-ROM. PC World 1986 Jun;4(6):13-28

CD-ROM special. Commun Technol Impact 1986 Aug;8(5):1-12

Chen PPS. The compact disk ROM: how it works. IEEE Spectrum 1986 Apr;23(4):44-9

Co F. CD-ROM and the library: problems and prospects. Small Comput Libr 1987 Nov;7(10):42-4, 46-9

Collier H. Optical publishing: a who-is-doing-what appraisal. Electron Publ Rev 1985 Dec;5(4):245-56

Compact discs: the state of the art. Bookseller 1986 Mar 1;(4184):844-6

Crane N. Entering uncharted territory: putting CD-ROM in place. Wilson Libr Bull 1987 Dec;62(4):28-30

Danziger PN. CD-ROM: is the future now? Bull Am Soc Inf Sci 1987 Oct-Nov;14:19-20

de Gooijer J. Much ado about CD-ROM. LASIE 1987 Jan-Feb;17(4):78-86

Desmarais N. Buying and selling laserbases. Electron Opt Publ Rev 1986 Dec;6(4):184-8

Desmarais N. Information management on a compact silver disc. Opt Inf Syst 1987 May-Jun;7(3):193-204

Discussion: the videodisc, CD-ROM, downloading, and the future of online. Infotecture Eur 1985 Apr 2; (67):1-2

Durr WF. CD-ROM and information precision. In: National Online Meeting. Proceedings of the Eighth Annual Meeting, 5-7 May 1987, New York. Medford, NJ: Learned Information, 1987. p.119-20

Dysart JI. Content critical for CD-ROM products: a user's view. In: National Online

Meeting. Proceedings of the Eighth Annual Meeting, 5-7 May 1987, New York. Medford, NJ: Learned Information, 1987. p.121-3

Eaton NL. Receptivity of librarians to optical information technologies and products. Electron Opt Publ Rev 1986 Dec;6(4):190-2

Ekengren B. Information retrieval-databases online or on CD-ROM-a question of today and tomorrow. In: Online Information 87. 11th International Online Information Meeting, 8-10 Dec 1987, London. Oxford, Eng.: Learned Information, 1987. p.313-17

Gale JC. Current trends in the optical storage industry. Bull Am Soc Inf Sci 1987 Sep-Aug; 13(6):12-4

Gale JC ; Brownrigg EB ; Lynch CA. The impact of optical media on information publishing. Bull Am Soc Inf Sci 1986 Aug-Sep;12(6):12-4

Glossary of CD-ROM-related technical terms and acronyms. Opt Inf Syst 1986 May-Jun; 6(3):230-4

Harvey FA. Emerging digital optical disc technologies: an opportunity and a challenge for educational researchers. AECT-RTD 1987 Fall;12(1):2-10

Hatvany BR. Comparison of CD-ROM and online. In: Online Information 87. 11th International Online Information Meeting, 8-10 Dec 1987, London. Oxford, Eng.: Learned Information, 1987. p.285-90

Hatvany BR. Criteria for converting to CD-ROM. In: National Online Meeting. Proceedings of the Seventh Annual Meeting, 6-8 May 1986, New York. Medford, NJ: Learned Information, 1986. p.163-6

Helgerson LW. CD-ROM: a revolution in the making. Libr Hi Tech 1986 Spring;4(1):23-7

Helliwell J. Innovations: the hand-held encyclopedia. Can Bus 1987 Feb;60(2):37, 40, 42

Hendley T. An introduction to CD-ROM (Compact Disc Read Only Memory). Inf Media Technol 1986 Summer;19(3):103-6

Herther NK. CD-ROM and information dissemination: an update. Online 1987 Mar;11(2):56-64

Herther NK. CD ROM technology: a new era for information storage and retrieval. Online 1985 Nov;9(6):17-28

Hickey TB ; Handley JC. Interactive display of text and graphics on an IBM PC. In: Helal, AH ; Weiss JW, editors. Impact of new information technology on international library cooperation. Essen Symposium, 8-11 Sep 1986, Essen, Germany. Essen: Essen University Library, 1987. p137-49.

Hlava M. CD-ROM vs. online. Bull Am Soc Inf Sci 1987 Oct;14(1):14-27

Jack RF. Oh, say can you CD-ROM. Bull Am Soc Inf Sci 1987 Oct-Nov;14:17-8

Janke RV. Where is online headed? Library science students speak out. Online 1987 Jan;11(1):53-5

Knerr L ; Nelson F ; Zuck G. CD-ROM: several subspecies. Tex Libr J 1986 Fall;62:158-9

Kolin D. CDROM-deja vu? Database 1987 Jun;10:6-7

Kollegger J. Approaching the markets for CD-ROM. In: National Online Meeting. Proceedings of the Seventh Annual Meeting, 6-8 May 1986, New York. Medford, NJ: Learned Information, 1986. p.251-5

Kuhlman JR ; Lee ES. Data-power to the people. Am Libr 1986 Nov;17(10):757-8, 760, 778

Kuhn C. Questions and answers about CD-ROM. CALICO J 1987 Sep;5(1):73-6

Lopez TM. CD-ROM: sweet music for information distribution? Int J Microgr Video Technol 1987;6(1-2):5-10

Macmillan A. CD-ROMs and after. Indexer 1988 Apr; 16(1):17-21

McGinty T. Three trailblazing technologies for schools. Electron Learn 1987 Sep;7(1): 26-30

Miller DC. Text as image: graphic data on CD-ROM. Inform 1987 Feb;1(2):27-7

Moore B. An introduction to CD-ROM technology. Show-Me Libr 1987 Aug;38:12-4

2

Mortensen E. The CD-ROM debate: what is its potential value? Office 1988 May; 107(5):71-2

Nelson NM. The CD-ROM industry: a library market overview. Wilson Libr Bull 1987 Dec;62(4):19-20

Nelson NM. CD-ROM: fad or fashion? Colo Lib 1987 Dec;13:20-5

Newhard R. Converting information into knowledge: the promise of CD-ROM. Wilson Libr Bull 1987 Dec;62(4):36-8

Newhard R. Social/public library implications of CD-ROM. Technicalities 1987 Sep;7:3-5

Norman-Watt R. Patents and CD-ROM. World Pat Info 1986;8(3):175-6

O'Connor MA. CD-ROM versus erasable compact disc. Videodisc Opt Disk 1985 Nov-Dec;5(6):464-7

O'Connor MA. Education and CD-ROM. Opt Inf Syst 1986 Jul-Aug;6(4):329-31

Paisley W ; Butler M. The first wave: CD-ROM adoption in offices and libraries. Microcomput Inf Manage 1987 Jun; 4(2):109-27

Peischl TM. Back to the warehouse. Or some implications on end user searching in libraries. In: National Online Meeting. Proceedings of the Seventh Annual Meeting, 6-8 May 1986, New York. Medford, NJ: Learned Information, 1986. p.347-52

Peters CM. Acceptance of optical publishing by libraries. In: National Online Meeting. Proceedings of the Eighth Annual Meeting, 5-7 May 1987, New York. Medford, NJ: Learned Information, 1987. p.397-400

Pooley CG. The CD-ROM marketplace: a producer's perspective. Wilson Libr Bull 1987 Dec;62(4):24-6

Preschel BM. Social science information on CD-ROM: concerns of database producers, libraries and end-users. In: Online Information 87. 11th International Online Information Meeting, 8-10 Dec 1987, London. Oxford, Eng: Learned Information, 1987. p.253-8

Price JW. The Library of Congress use of microcomputers in the Optical Disk Pilot Program. Microcomput Inf Manage 1985 Dec;2(4):241-50

Price N ; Flatley J. Opting for high tech: implementing optical disk technology for government agencies. J Inf Image Manage 1986 Oct;19(10):22-3, 25

Price-Wilkin J. OPTEXT: government publications on CD-ROM. Ref Serv Rev 1987 Summer;15(2):9-14

Remmer D. Information image of the future (fileless hospital). Health Serv J 1988 Apr 21;98(5097):5

Review: a hi-tech training selection. Bank Technol 1988 Mar;5(3):32-4

Saviers S. Reflections on CD-ROM: bridging the gap between technology and purpose. Ser Libr 1987 Fall;78(4):288-94

Schaefer MT. CD-ROM arrives in the library: powerful databases marketed. Inf Retr Libr Autom 1986 Mar;21(10):1-5

Schwerin JB. Microsoft and CD-ROM. Electron Opt Publ Rev 1987 Mar;7(1):22-5

Siitonen L. Advancing optical disc technology for social sciences in non-high tech societies. INSPEL 1988; 22(1):70-83

Sippings G. The use of information technology by information services: the Aslib information technology survey 1987. Electron Libr 1987 Dec; 5(6):354-7

Slonin J ; Mole D ; Baues M. Write-once laser disc-technology. Libr Hi Tech 1985;3(4):27-42

Smith SS ; Ryland JN. Applications that really work--fulfilling the promise of laser optic technology for information distribution. In: National Online Meeting. Proceeding of the Seventh Annual Meeting, 6-8 May 1986, New York. Medford, NJ: Learned Information, 1986. p.421-5

Stillger J ; Hartung V. Use of CD-ROM for patent information. World Pat Inf 1988; 10(1):37-40

Sy KJ. CD-ROM and related technologies: challenges for federal information policy. Bull Am Soc Inf Sci 1987 Aug-Sep; 13(6):26-7

Tenopir C. Publications on CD-ROM:

3

librarians can make a difference. Libr J 1987 Sep 15;112:62-3

Van Hartevelt J. Advantages of CD-ROM for local access to computerized databases in developing countries, in comparison with traditional bibliographic services: suggested pilot projects. Q Bull Int Assoc Agri Libr Doc 1987;32(2):161-8

Venkataraman SR. A new phase in publication and information retrieval. Can J Inf Sci 1986;11(3):48-57

Wertz RK. CD-ROM. A new advance in medical information retrieval. JAMA 1986 Dec 26; 256(24):3376-8

White MS. Impact of optical disc technologies on the storage and distribution of patent and trademark information. World Pat Inf 1986;8(3):177-81

Williams BJS. Implications for preservation of the newer information media. Inf Media Technol 1985-86 Winter;19(1):13-5

Williams ME. Highlights of the online database field: CD-ROM and new technologies vs. online. In: National Online Meeting. Proceedings of the Seventh Annual Meeting, 6-8 May 1986, New York. Medford, NJ: Learned Information, 1986. p.1-4

Wilson B ; Hubbard A. Redefining the role of school media specialists-bridging the gap. Online 1987 Nov;11(6):50-4

ONLINE PUBLIC ACCESS CATALOGS

Akeroyd J. CD-ROM as an online public access catalogue. Electron Libr 1988 Apr;6(2):120-4

Beiser K. Microcomputing. Wilson Libr Bull 1987 Apr;61(8):40-1

Bills LG ; Helgerson LW. CD-Rom public access catalogs: database creation and maintenance. Libr Hi Tech 1988;6(1):67-86

Cassel RE. Pennsylvania's CD-ROM statewide union catalog. In: SCIL 1987. The Second Annual Software/Computer/Database Conference and Exposition for Librarians and Information Managers, Conference

Proceedings, 30 Mar-1 Apr 1987, Arlington, Va. Westport, CT: Meckler, 1987. p.34-5

CD-ROM leads the way at ALA. Libr Syst Newsl 1987 Feb;7(2):9-14

Chen CC. Libraries and CD-ROM. Microcomput Info Manage 1985 Jun; 2(2):129-34

Epler DM ; Cassel RE. ACCESS PENNSYLVANIA: a CD-ROM database project. Libr Hi Tech 1987 Fall; 5(3):81-92

Harrison N ; Murphy B. Multisensory public access catalogs on CD-ROM. Libr Hi Tech 1987 Fall; 5(3):77-80

Helgerson LW. Acquiring a CD-ROM public access catalog system. I. The bottom line may not be the top priority. Libr Hi Tech 1987 Fall;5(3):49-75

Herther NK. LaserCat from WLN... an interview with David Andresen, Marketing Director for Lasercat. Online 1987 May; 11(3):135-8

Hildreth CR. CD-ROM public access library catalogues: uses, advantages, problems. In: Helal AN ; Weiss JW, editors. Impact of New Information Technology on International Library Cooperation. Essen Symposium, 8-11 Sep 1986, Essen, Germany. Essen: Essen University Library, 1987. p.151-77

Hoffmann J. Strengthening small library service with WLN's LaserCat CD-ROM. In: Optical Publishing and Storage: Products that Work. Proceedings of Optical Publishing and Storage '87 - The Conference on the Applications of Optical Information Systems in Publishing, 11-13 Nov 1987, New York. Medford, NJ: Learned Information, 1987. p.57-65

Schaub JA. CD-ROM for public access catalog. Libr Hi Tech 1985; 3(3):7-13

Watson PD. CD-ROM catalogs - evaluating LePac and looking ahead. Online 1987 Sep;11(5):74-80

Watson PD. Distributing an online catalog on CDROM...The University of Illinois experience. Online 1987 Mar;11(2):65-74

Wilsondisc: Readers Guide to Periodical Literature. Booklist 1987 Dec 1;84:609-10

Webber SAE. Are you suffering from blinkered
    front ends? In: Proceedings, 10th
    International Online Information Meeting,
    1986, London. Oxford, Eng: Learned
    Information, 1986. p.185-98

MEDLINE

Broering NC ; Larson RH ; Bagdoyan HE. An
    enhanced miniMEDLINE SYSTEM:
    abstracts, more journals, and CD-ROM.
    Ser Rev 1986 Summer-Fall;12(2-3):33-9

Capodagli JA ; Mardikian J ; Uva PA.
    MEDLINE on compact disc: end-user on
    searching Compact Cambridge. Bull Med
    Libr Assoc 1988 Apr;76(2):181-3

Compact Cambridge-Medline. A review of the
    Medline CD-ROM. Electron Opt Publ Rev
    1987 Mar;7(1):26-31

Glitz B. Testing the new technology:
    MEDLINE on CD-ROM in an academic
    health science library. Spec Libr 1988
    Winter;79(1):28-33

Kemp R. Compact Cambridge-MEDLINE: a
    review of the MEDLINE CD-ROM.
    Electron Opt Publ Rev 1987 Mar;7(1):26-9

Purcell R. MEDLINE on micro. Small
    Comput Libr 1987 Jul;7:16-8

Silver H. Managing a CDROM installation: a
    case study at Hahnemann University.
    Online 1988 Mar;12(2):61-6

Tennenhouse M. MEDLINE on CD-ROM at
    the University of Manitoba Medical Library.
    Bibl Med Can 1987;8(4):209-11

Whitsed N. Compact Cambridge: Running
    MEDLINE on CD-ROM. Comput Libr
    1988 Mar;1(7):4-5

BIBLIOGRAPHIES/DIRECTORIES

Connolly B. Laserdisk directory. Part 1.
    Database 1986 Jun;9(3):15-26

Connolly B. Laserdisk directory. Part 2. Online
    1986 Jul;10(4):39-49

Connolly B. Laserdisk directory. Part 3.
    Database 1986 Aug;9(4):34-9

Connolly B. Laserdisk directory. Part 4. Online
    1986 Sep;10(5):54-8

Connolly B. Laserdisk directory. Part 5.
    Database 1986 Dec;9(6):46-8

Nazim Ali S. Directory of databases on optical
    discs. Electron Opt Publ Rev 1986
    Dec;6(4):198-208

Rechel M. How to keep up: absolutely essential
    CD-ROM reading. Wilson Libr Bull 1987
    Dec;62(4):41-2

Roose T. The new papyrus: CD-ROM in your
    library? Libr J 1986 Sep;111(14):166-7

Tenopir C. Databases on CD-ROM. Libr J
    1986 Mar 1;111:68-9

Swora T ; Fischer A. Technical services in 1984
    and 1985: micrographs, optical disk
    technology, and fair use. Libr Res Tech Serv
    1986 Jul-Sep;30(3):183-217

HARDWARE/SOFTWARE

Alberico R. Search hardware: latest and
    greatest. Database Searcher 1988 Mar;
    4(3):13-24

Allen RJ. The CD-ROM Services of
    SilverPlatter Information, Inc. Libr Hi Tech
    1985;3(4):49-60

Bonta BD. CD-ROM in the social science
    reference room. INSPEL 1988;22(1):44-7

Brandis R. CD-ROM review: PC-SIG public
    domain library. PC Consult 1987 Jul;
    3(4):4-5, 9

Brunell D. Comparing CD-ROM products.
    Act Libr 1987 Nov;13(11):1-2

Brunell D. Comparing CD-ROM products. Pt.
    2. Act Libr 1987 Dec;13(12):1-2

Cichocki EM ; Ziemer SM. Design
    considerations for CD-ROM retrieval
    software. J Am Soc Info Sci 1988
    Jan;39(1):43-6

5

Coolidge RC. The software factor. I. Making software: the case for CASE. Inform 1988 Feb;2(2):19-22

Davies DH. The CD-ROM medium. J Am Soc Info Sci 1988 Jan;39(1):34-42

Desmarais N. An evaluation of the PC-laser Library from the Library Corporation. Opt Inf Syst 1988 Jan-Feb;8(1):14-8

Fenichel CH. The linear file. For optical disks and information retrieval the time is now: a librarians view from the NFAIS meeting. Database 1986 Jun;9(3):6-8

Ferrell MS ;Parkhurst CA. Using LaserQuest for retrospective conversion on MARC records. Opt Info Syst 1987 Nov-Dec; 7(6):396-400

Goldstein CM. Optical disk technology and information. Science 1982 Feb;215(4534): 862-8

Goldstein CM. Storage technology: present and future. Microcomput Inf Manage 1984 Jun;1(2):79-93

Greenberg E. INFOTRAC-a case study-a research library dilemma. In: Optical Publishing and Storage: Products that Work. Proceedings of Optical Publishing and Storage '87 - The Conference on the Applications of Optical Information Systems in Publishing, 11-13 Nov 1987, New York .Medford, NJ: Learned Information, 1987. p.41-4

Hamilton FK. Company model: from online to CD-ROM: database design. Bull Am Soc Inf Sci 1987 Oct-Nov;14:25-6

Helgerson LW. CD-ROM search and retrieval software: the requirements and realities. Libr Hi Tech 1986 Summer;4(2):68-77

Herther NK. Apple, computers, and CD-ROM. Database 1987 Dec;10(6):91-6

Herther NK. The silver disk-access software for optical/laser information packages. Database 1986 Aug;9(4):93-7

Hurley G. Considering a compact disc system? OCLC Micro 1987 Jun;3(3):23-4

McCarthy P. CD ROM-an alternative information distribution medium. In: Online Information 85. 9th International Online Information Meeting, 3-5 Dec 1985,

London. Oxford, Eng: Learned Information, 1985. p.163-9

McQueen J. Hardware decisions for CD-ROM. Bull Am Soc Inf Sci 1987 Oct-Nov;14:26-7

Melin N. Cutting edge. Wilson Libr Bull 1987 Apr;61(8):36-7

Murphy B. CD-ROM and libraries. Libr Hi Tech 1985;3(2):21-6

Myers E. Big Blue and the optical disc market (IBM). Inform 1988 April;2(4):39-41

Newhard R. A shoppers guide to CD-ROM. Pub Libr 1987 Winter;26:149-50

Nugent RW. Lots of information please: the world of optical discs. In: Stead WW. editor. Proceedings of the Eleventh Annual Symposium on Computer Applications in Medical Care, 1-4 Nov 1987, Washington, DC. Los Angles: IEEE Computer Society Press, 1987. p.10-11

OCLC search software enhanced. Inf Retr Libr Automn 1987 Dec;23(7):1-2

Oren T. The compact disk ROM: applications software. IEEE Spectrum 1986;23(4):49-54

Pooley CG. SilverPlatter brings CDROM to the reference desk. Database 1986 Aug; 9(4):40-2

Rivett M. Videodiscs and digital optical disks. J Inf Sci 1987;13(1):25-34

Schaefer MT. New hardware, software debut in CD-ROM technologies geared for libraries and information centers. Inf Retr Libr Automn 1986 Apr;21(11):1-5

Schwerin JB. Optical systems for information delivery and storage. Electron Publ Rev 1985 Sep;5(3):193-8

Seddon G. CD-ROM services and products (BRS/Search). In: Stanford-Smith B ; Hendley T. ; Walsh R, editors. Report on the Intensive Workshop on CD-ROM. A Joint Project by the CEC (DG XIIIB) and EURIPA, 12-13 Feb 1987, Luxembourg. Wilmslow, Cheshire, UK: Europe Information Industry Assoc.,1987. p.58-60

Silver H. Managing a CDROM installation: a case study at Hahnemann University. Online 1988 March;12(2):61-6

6

Steinbrecher D. Optical disks go head to head with traditional storage media. Today's Off 1987 Oct; 22(5):24-6, 28-30

Tally RD. Case study: creating a CD-ROM with the help of a simulator. Bull Am Soc Inf Sci 1987 Aug-Sep;13(6):21-2

Tiampo JM. Update on retrieval software products. Opt Inf Syst 1988 Mar-Apr; 8(2):86-8

Welsh J ; Martin S. Public domain software on compact disc: an instant software collection for libraries. Small Comput Libr 1988 Feb;8(2):29-30

Williams I. CD-ROM products and services (CD/Guide). In: Stanford-Smith B ; Hendley T ; Walsh R, editors. Report on the Intensive Workshop on CD-ROM. A Joint Project by the CEC (DG XIIIB) and EURIPA. 12-13 Feb 1987, Luxembourg. Wilmslow, Cheshire, UK: Europe Information Industry Assoc., 1987. p.50-7

Zoellick B. CD-ROM software development. Byte 1986 May; 11(5):177-88

COST/ECONOMICS

Alberico R. Justifying CD-ROM. Small Comput Libr 1987 Feb;7(2):18-20

Berry J. The economy of library automation. Libr J 1986 Nov 1;111(18):LC3, LC8, LC20, LC25, LC30

Biesel D. Old books - new technologies. Ref Libr 1986 Fall;(15):209-15

Cohen E ; Young M. Cost comparison of abstracts and indexes on paper CD-ROM, and online. Opt Inf Syst 1986 Nov-Dec; 6(6):485-90

Desmarais N. Buying and selling laserbases. Electron Opt Publ Rev 1986 Dec;6(4):184-8

Eaton NL ; Crane NB. Integrating electronic information systems into the reference services budget. Ref Libr 1987;(19):161-77

Gatten JN. Purchasing CD-ROM products: considerations for a new technology. Libr Acq 1987;11(4):273-81

Gibbons P. Pricing software and information on CD-ROM. Electron Opt Publ Rev 1987 Dec;7(4):176-80

Gray E. To film or not to film: that is the question! an essay. Int J Microgr Video Technol 1986;5(3-4):177-83

Herther NK. Market projections for CDROM. Database 1987 Aug;10(4):114-8

Jayatilleke R. CD-ROM: implications of the emerging technology for academic information services. In: Optical Publishing and Storage: Products that Work. Proceedings of Optical Publishing and Storage '87 - The Conference on the Applications of Optical Information Systems in Publishing, 11-13 Nov 1987, New York. Medford, NJ: Learned Information, 1987. p.93-101

Kotick AR. CD-ROM conference spotlights an evolving market. Libr Hi Tech 1987 May; (38):1-6

McLagan DL. The end of the rainbow: products that work. In: Optical Publishing and Storage: Products that Work. Proceedings of Optical Publishing and Storage '87 - The Conference on the Applications of Optical Information Systems in Publishing, 11-13 Nov 1987, New York. Medford, NJ: Learned Information, 1987. p.117-21

Oppenheim C. CD-ROM-panacea or hype? Aslib Inf 1986 Mar 14;(3):50

Peters CM. Databases on CD-ROM: comparative factors for purchase. Electron Libr 1987 Jun; 5(3):154-60

Rosen TH. The impact of emerging technologies upon the economics of database production. In: National Online Meeting. Proceedings of the Seventh Annual Meeting, 6-8 May 1986, New York. Medford, NJ: Learned Information, 1986. P.389-92

Schwerin JB. CD-R0M: potential markets for information. J Am Soc Inf Sci 1988 Jul; 39(1):54-7

Schwerin JB. CD-ROM market opportunities: highlights of a major market research study. In: National Online Meeting. Proceedings of the Seventh Annual Meeting, 6-8 May 1986, New York. Medford, NJ: Learned

Information, 1986. p.415-20

Tenopir C. Costs and benefits of CD-ROM.
Libr J 1987 Sep 1;112:156-7

Van Arsdale WO. The rush to optical discs.
Libr J 1986 Oct 1;111(16):53-5

Van Hartevelt J. Advantages of CD-ROM for
local access to computerized databases in
developing countries, in comparison with
traditional bibliographic services: suggested
pilot projects. Q Bull Int Assoc Agri Libr
Doc 1987;32(2):161-8

Van Ommeslaghe BJ. CD-ROM versus online:
economic issues the case of the database of
the National Bank of Belgium. In: Online
Information 87. 11th International Online
Information Meeting, 8-10 Dec 1987,
London. Oxford, Eng.: Learned
Information, 1987. p. 291-311

Watson PD. Cost to libraries of the optical
information revolution. A survey shows
diverse funding methods. Online 1988
Jan;12(1):45-50

White MS. The market for CD-ROM and CD-
I products and services in the USA and
Europe. In: Proceedings, 10th International
Online Information Meeting, 1986, London.
Oxford, Eng.: Learned Information, 1986.
p.263-70

DATABASES

Barney R. Consumer laserbooks? A compact
disc Encyclopedia. EPB 1985 Sep;3(7):4-5

Beltran AB. Use of InfoTrac in a university
library. Database 1986 Jun;9(3):63-6

Bezanson D. Integrating CD-Rom with printed
and online services: a SilverPlatter end-user
perspective. Opt Inf Syst 1987 Nov-Dec;
7(6):387-90

Bloechle MK. Streamlining book ordering
through the use of BIP+ in the CD-ROM
medium. Tex Libr J 1987 Summer;63:56-7

Brandhorst T. Distributing the ERIC database
on compact disc: a case history of private
sector involvement in the distribution of
public sector data. Gov Publ Rev 1987;
14(5):541-57

Carney RD. InfoTrac vs. the confounding of
technology and its applications. Database
1986 Jun;9(3):56-61

Case D ; Powers R. Databases and text files on
optical media: a survey of publishers and
products. Int J Microgr Video Technol
1986;5(3-4):199-212

Chiang KS. A question of format: the Census
of Agriculture on compact disk. Database
1987 Oct;10(5):85-8

Datext on CD-ROM. Online Bus Inf 1987
Jul;9:1-4

Demas S. Comparing BIG bibliographies on
CD ROM. Am Libr 1987 May;18(5):332-5

Desmarais N. End-user's report on
LaserSearch. Opt Inf Syst 1987 Mar-
Apr;7(2):125-31

Dunman S. ERIC: an essential online tool for
educators. Electron Learn 1988 Jan;
7(4):45-7

Ferraro AJ. Ulrich's PLUS: a new serials
reference technology. Serials Rev 1987
Fall;13:19-23

Fries JR; Brown JR. Business information on
CD-ROM: the Datext service at Dartmouth
College, New Hampshire. Program 1987
Jan;21(1):1-12

Fries JR ; Brown JR. DATEXT-using business
information on CD ROM. Online 1986
Sep;10(5):28-40

Gallinger S. CD-Rom technology expands
information delivery in public libraries:
using INfoTrac II. Opt Info Syst 1987
Nov-Dec;7(6):391-5

Garrett T. Datext offers users online historical
financial information with CD/NewsLine.
Electron Publ Bus 1986 Dec;4(11):11-12

Hagan DL. The Tacoma debut of Books in
Print Plus. Libr J 1987 Sep 1;112(14):149-51

Halperin M. Company and industry
information: online and ondisc. Bus Info
Rev 1987 Jul;4(1):12-7

Halperin M ; Pagell RA. CD/CorpTech:
making use of hi-tech. Online 1987
Mar;11(2):78-80

8

Halperin M ; Pagell RA. Compact disclosure: realizing CDROM's potential. Online 1986 Nov;10(6):69-73

Hendley T. LISA on compact ROM disc: an option for heavy users? Inf Media Technol 1985-86 Winter;19(1):23-6

Hlava MMK ; Reinke SP. CD-ROM user survey: impact of CD-ROM technology on searching AV Online. In: National Online Meeting. Proceedings of the Eighth Annual Meeting, 5-7 May 1987, New York. Medford, NJ: Learned Information, 1987. p.179-82

Hlava MMK ; Reinke SP. CD-ROM: how the users react (NICEM's database, A-V Online). Bull Am Soc Inf Sci 1987 Oct-Nov; 14:23-4

Holloway C. Books in Print and Ulrich's on CD-ROM: a preliminary review. Online 1987 Sep;11(5):57-61

Johnson J. CD-ROM databases thrive. Comput Commun Decis 1987;19(13):51-3

Johnstone JC. A-V Online now on compact laserdisk (CDROM). Database 1986 Aug;9(4):44-5

Kemp R. Compact Disclosure: a review of the new Disclosure CD-ROM. Electron Opt Publ Rev 1986 Dec;6(4):218-23

Lewis C. Lotus markets financial databases on CD-ROM. Electron Bank Finance 1987 Oct;4(8):11-4

Mays LE. CD-ROM and libraries: a natural pair. OCLC Micro 1987 Feb;3(1):16-7, 26

McLaughlin PW. New access points to ERIC: CD-ROM versions. Educ Libr 1987 Fall; 12(3):73-6

McSweeney L. Books in Print Plus. In: Optical Publishing and Storage: Products that Work. Proceedings of Optical Publishing and Storage '87 - The Conference on the Applications of Optical Information Systems in Publishing, 11-13 Nov 1987, New York. Medford, NJ: Learned Information, 1987. p.123-4

Minnich NP. Automated circulation: building the database. Libr Comput 1986 Nov; 33(3):LC5-LC11

Moore NL. LISA on CD-ROM-leading the

way. Libr Assoc Rec 1987 May;89(5):237-8

Moore NL. Searching LISA on the SilverPlatter CD-ROM system. Program 1988 Jan;22(1):72-6

Mullan NA ; Blick AR. Initial experiences of untrained end-users with a Life Sciences CD-ROM database: a salutary experience. J Inf Sci 1987;13(3):139-41

Olson L. Experiencing CD-ROM ERIC. Educ Libr 1987 Fall;12(3):77-80

Optical disc-based cataloguing support. Libr Syst Newsl 1985 Jul;5(7):51-3

Pantry S. HSELINE, NIOSHTIC and CISDOC on compact disc, read only memory (CD-ROM). State Libr 1987 Nov;35:33-4

Preschel BM. PAIS on CD-ROM. In: Online '87 Conference Proceedings, 20-22 Oct 1987, Anaheim, CA. Weston, CT: Online, 1987. p.178-82

Purcell R. Compact disc stores newspaper index. Small Comput Libr 1987 May;7:19-22

Purcell R. Wilson goes compact. Small Comput Libr 1987 Dec;7:17-21

Rawnsley LS. Making tracs: road-testing the INFOTRAC and LEGALTRAC video-disk databases. Leg Ref Serv Q 1986 Fall-Winter;6(3-4):169-80

Regazzi JJ. The silver disk WILSONDISC: WILSONLINE on CDROM. Database 1986 Oct; 9(5):73-4

Schipma PB. A CD-ROM database for oncology. J Am Soc Inf Sci 1988 Jan; 39(1):63-6

Schipma PB ; Cichocki EM ; Ziemer SM. Medical information on optical disc. In: Stead WW. editor. Proceedings of the Eleventh Annual Symposium on Computer Applications in Medical Care, 1-4 Nov 1987. Washington, DC. Los Angles: IEEE Computer Society Press, 1987. p.732-8

Scott T. Commercial databases on CD-ROM. The Digital Equipment Corporation! experience. In: Online '86 Conference Proceedings, 4-6 Nov 1986. Weston, CT. Weston, CT.: Online, Inc.,1986. p.224-6

Spigai F. Databases on floppy disks: new

9

publications for libraries. Libr Hi Tech 1985;3(4):11-9

Tenopir C. InfoTrac: a laser disc system. Libr J 1986 Sep 1;111(14):168-9

Tooey MJ. PsycLIT on CD-ROM: the UMAB experience, or serving Psychological Abstracts to library users on a SilverPlatter. In: Online '86 Conference Proceedings, 4-6 Nov 1986. Weston, CT. Weston, CT: Online, Inc., 1986. p.246-60

Van Auker R ; Frost S ; Klingberg S. Online bibliographic searching (SilverPlatter's ERIC). Ref Serv Rev 1987 Winter; (15):89-94

Van Hartevelt J. Advantages of CD-ROM for local access to computerized databases in developing countries, in comparison with traditional bibliographic services: suggested pilot projects. Q Bull Int Assoc Agri Libr Doc 1987;32(2):161-8

Van Ommeslaghe BJ. CD-ROM versus online: economic issues the case of the database of the National Bank of Belgium. In: Online Information 87. 11th International Online Information Meeting, 8-10 Dec 1987, London. Oxford, Eng.: Learned Information, 1987. p. 291-311

Wigton RS. The new knowledge bases: CD-ROM and medicine. MD Comput 1987 May-Jun;4(3):34-8

PUBLISHING

Bowers RA. Changing the publishing model with optical media. Electron Opt Publ Rev 1987 Mar;7(1):4-6

Klausmeier JA. The implications of CD ROM for database producers. In: National Online Meeting. Proceedings of the Seventh Annual Meeting, 6-8 May 1986, New York. Medford, NJ: Learned Information, 1986. p.245-9

Leach SS. Optical disk-the electronic library arrives. Ref Libr 1986 Fall;(15):251-67

Machovec GS. CD-ROM revolution for electronic publishing. Online Libr Microcomput 1985 Nov; 3(11):1-5

McCarthy P. CD-ROM products and services. In: Stanford-Smith B ; Hendley T : Walsh R, editors. Report on the Intensive Workshop on CD-ROM. A Joint Project by the CEC (DG XIIIB) and EURIPA, 12-13 Feb 1987, Luxembourg. Wilmslow, Cheshire, UK: Europe Information Industry Assoc., 1987. p.44-9

Paisley W. Optical publishing: the fourth revolution. In: Optical Publishing and Storage: Products that Work. Proceedings of Optical Publishing and Storage '87 - The Conference on the Applications of Optical Information Systems in Publishing, 11-13 Nov, 1987, New York. Medford, NJ: Learned Information, 1987. p.131-8

Richman B. Dense media and the future of publishing. Electron Publ Bus 1987 Feb; 5(2):12-5

Smith G. World movement towards in-house CD ROM publishing. In: Optical Publishing and Storage: Products that Work. Proceedings of Optical Publishing and Storage '87 - The Conference on the Applications of Optical Information Systems in Publishing, 11-13 Nov 1987, New York. Medford, NJ: Learned Information, 1987. p.155-9

Spigai F. Electronic publishing in the information age. Electron Publ Bus 1987 Feb;5(2):4-11

Vaughan K ; Barnfield L. The CD-ROM as a publishing medium: the Crystal Ball approach. In: Proceedings, 10th International Online Information Meeting, 1986, London. Oxford, Eng.: Learned Information, 1986. p.271-282

Weisenfeld MR. A manual on every desk: how CDROM solves the online documentation dilemma. In: Optical Publishing and Storage: Products that Work. Proceedings of Optical Publishing and Storage '87 - The Conference on the Applications of Optical Information Systems in Publishing, 11-13 Nov 1987, New York. Medford, NJ: Learned Information, 1987. p.193-7

Whitaker D. CD-ROM-the migration from print, or the 500 megabyte solution. Bookseller 1987 May 22; (4248):1969-71, 73

Williams BJS. CD-ROM a new medium for publishing. Inf Media Technol 1986 Summer;19(3):107-9

10

PRODUCTS

Baldwin C. CD-ROM services and products. In: Stanford-Smith B ; Hendley T ; Walsh R, editors. Report on the Intensive Workshop on CD-ROM. A Joint Project by the CEC (DG XIIIB) and EURIPA, 12-13 Feb 1987, Luxembourg. Wilmslow, Cheshire, UK: Europe Information Industry Assoc., 1987. p.68-70

Beiser K. WLN Previews CD-ROM product. Wilson Libr Bull 1986 Nov;61(3):41-2

Case D ; Powers R. Databases and text files on optical media: a survey of publishers and products. Int J Microgr Video Technol 1986;5(3-4):199-212

Collier H. Where is CD-ROM? Some brief product reviews. Electron Opt Publ Rev 1987 Jun;7(2):70-6

Cooke DF. Map storage on CD-ROM. BYTE 1987 Jul;12(8):129-30, 32, 34-6, 38

Dubashi J. Warp speed (CD-ROM systems). Financ World 1987 Sep 22;156(19):52, 54

Duggan MK. A look at Dialog's first CD-ROM product. Opt Inf Syst 1987 Nov-Dec; 7(6):401-5

Herther NK. Microsoft's Bookshelf. Online 1988 May;12(3):79-80

Hoffman J. Many CD-ROM products available to LaserCat users. PC Consult 1987 Jul; 3(4):8-9

Kesselman M. Online update. Wilson Libr Bull 1987 Apr;61(8):38-9

Labombarda P. Recording the Italian cultural heritage: a challenging area for optical memory systems. Electron Opt Publ Rev 1987 Sep;7(3):136-40

Machovec GS. OCLC optical disc products for reference, cataloging and resource sharing. Online Libr Microcomput 1987 May; 5(5):1-3

Miller T.SilverPlatter: dishing up data for libraries. Info Today 1986 Jun;3(6):23-5, 39

Nelson NM. 'Do you have any books about....?'. Inf Today 1987 Nov;4(10):13, 26

Private files on videodisc and CD-ROM. Libr Syst Newsl 1985 Jul;5(7):53-5

Rann LS ; Kuchta NE ; Winokur MG. The computerized clinical information system on CD-ROM (Compact Disk Read Only Memory). Opt Inf Syst 1986 Jul-Aug; 6(4):313-7

Stephens A. CD-ROMs at ALA: a review of product developments from the American Library Association midsummer exhibition. Program 1988 Jan;22(1):77-80

Tenopir C. CD-ROM database update. Libr J 1986 Dec 1;111(20):70-1

Tenopir C. What's new with WILSONLINE. Libr J 1986 Jun 1;111(10):98-9

Walker L. Medical information via CD-ROM technology. Healthc Comput Commun 1985 Dec 2;12:54-5

Walsh RV. CD-ROM market development. Commun Technol Impact 1987 Sep;9(6):1-8

Wilson BJ. CD-ROM for the trial lawyers: applications, markets and opportunities. In: Optical Publishing and Storage: Products that Work. Proceedings of Optical Publishing and Storage '87 - The Conference on the Applications of Optical Information Systems in Publishing, 11-13, Nov 1987, New York. Medford, NJ: Learned Information, 1987. p.9-12

Young J. Integrating a CD-ROM into an inhouse library system: Sirsi's Lasertap. Libr Hi Tech 1986 Summer;4(2):51-3

STANDARDS

Bardes D'E. Attention novices: friendly intro to shiny disks. Libr Software Rev 1986 Jul-Aug;5(4):240-5

Bardes D'E. Don't wait to adopt CD-ROM. Libr Software Rev 1987 Mar-Apr;6(2):94-6

Bardes D'E. Where are all the CD-ROM discs? Roll-outs stalled until drives are embedded. Libr Software Rev 1986 Sep-Oct;5(5):300-4

11

CD-ROM is 'an idea whose time has come'.
Tele/Contact (Netherlands) 1986;(3):8-12

Frank FHU. CD-ROM technology and
standards. In: Stanford-Smith B ; Hendley T
; Walsh R, editors. Report on the Intensive
Workshop on CD-ROM. A Joint Project by
the CEC (DG XIIIB) and EURIPA, 12-13
Feb 1987, Luxembourg. Wilmslow,
Cheshire, UK: Europe Information Industry
Assoc., 1987. p.29-33

Jacob M. CD-ROM standardization activities.
Bull Am Soc Inf Sci 1986 Feb-Mar;
12(3):19-20

Moes RJ. The CD-ROM/CD-I puzzle: where
do the pieces fit? Int J Microgr Video
Technol 1987;6(1):15-8

Morton B. Computer-based information:
online and on disc. Libr Hi Tech News 1987
Mar;(36):1, 8-10

New technology for the library
microcomputer. Libraries and CD-ROM: a
special report. Small Comput Libr 1985
Apr;5(4):7-10

Robertson B. CD-ROM comes of age. Comput
Graph World 1986 July;9(7):83-8

Schwerin JB. CD-ROM standards-extended.
Inf Today 1987 Jun;4(6):13-39

Trail J. Standardization and CD-ROM [letter].
JAMA 1987 Apr 3;257(13):1731-2

Zoellick B. CD-ROM software architecture to
promote interchangeability. J Am Soc Inf
Sci 1988 Jan;39(1):47-53

LIBRARIES

Bartenbach W. CD-ROM and libraries:
opportunities, concerns, challenges. In:
National Online Meeting. Proceedings of
the Eighth Annual Meeting, 5-7 May 1987,
New York. Medford, NJ: Learned
Information, 1987. p.9-19

Becker KA. CD-ROM: a primer. Coll Res Libr
News 1987 Jul-Aug;48(7):388-90, 92-93

Boulanger M. Online services at the reference
desk: new technologies vs. old problems.
Ref Libr 1986 Fall;(15):269-77

Campbell B. Whither the white knight: CD-
ROM in technical services. Database 1987
Aug;10(4):22-40

Co F. CD-ROM and the library: problems and
prospects. Small Comput Libr 1987 Nov;
7(10):42-4, 46-9

Connolly B. Looking backward - CDROM and
the academic library of the future. Online
1987 May; 11(3):56-61

Davis WP. Missouri libraries move into CD-
ROM world. Show-Me Libr 1987 Dec;
39:4-6

Desmarais N. Lasersbases for library technical
services. Opt Inf Syst 1987 Jan-Feb;
7(1):57-61

Drake MA. From print to nonprint materials:
library information delivery systems.
EDUCOM Bull 1988 Spring;23(1):28-30

Eaton NL. Receptivity of librarians to optical
information technologies and products.
Electron Opt Publ Rev 1986 Dec;6(4):190-2

Erickson LJ. CD-ROM in a sci-tech library?
Bull Am Soc Inf Sci 1987 Oct-Nov;14:18-9

Fenichel CH. Supporting users searching
CDROM: a comparison with online. In:
Optical Publishing and Storage: Products
that Work. Proceedings of Optical
Publishing and Storage '87 - The
Conference on the Applications of Optical
Information Systems in Publishing, 11-13
Nov 1987, New York. Medford NJ: Learned
Information, 1987. p.37-9

Gell MM. Technology, philosophy, and library
services. Coll Build 1986;8(1):30-1

Graves GT ; King BF ; Harper LG. Planning
for CD-ROM in the reference department.
Coll Res Libr News 1987 Jul Aug;48(7):
393, 395-96, 399-400

Horny KL. New turns for a new century:
library services in the information era. Libr
Res Tech Serv 1987 Jan-Mar;31(1):6-11

Lo Bue B. CD-ROM and the end-user. Colo
Libr 1987 Dec;13:29-30

Manns B ; Swora T. Books to bits: digital
imaging at the Library of Congress. J Inf
Image Manage 1986 Oct;19(10):26-32

12

484

Mays LE. CD-ROM and libraries: a natural pair. OCLC Micro 1987 Feb;3(1):16-7, 26

Meyer R. Strategies for libraries (when using CD-ROM). Bull Am Soc Inf Sci 1987 Oct-Nov;14:22-3

Miller DC. Laser disks at the library door: the Microsoft first international conference of CD-ROM. Libr Hi Tech 1986 Summer; 4(2):55-68

Miller DC. Online CD-ROM: moving graphic images. Inform 1987 Mar;1(3):28-33, 45

Miller DC. Runnning with CD-ROM. Am Libr 1986 Nov;17(10):754-6

Murphy B. CD-ROM and libraries. Libr Hi Tech 1985;3(2):21-6

Nelson NM. The CD-ROM industry: a library market overview. Wilson Libr Bull 1987 Dec;62(4):19-20

Nelson NM. CD-ROM: fad or fashion? Colo Lib 1987 Dec;13:20-5

Peters CM. Acceptance of optical publishing by libraries. In: National Online Meeting. Proceedings of the Eighth Annual Meeting, 5-7 May 1987, New York. Medford, NJ: Learned Information, 1987. p.397-400

Peters CM. CD-ROM: its potential in libraries. In: National Online Meeting. Proceedings of the Seventh National Online Meeting, 6-8 May 1986, New York. Medford, NJ: Learned Information, 1986. p.353-8

Peters CM. Optical information product purchases by libraries: cost justification. In: Optical Publishing and Storage: Products that Work. Proceedings of Optical Publishing and Storage '87 - The Conference on the Applications of Optical Information Systems in Publishing, 11-13 Nov 1987, New York. Medford, NJ: Learned Information, 1987. p.139-43

Rice J. The golden age of reference services: is it really over? Wilson Lib Bull 1986 Dec; 61(4):17-9

Rietdyk RJ. Creation and distribution of CD-ROM data bases for the library reference desk. J Am Soc Inf Sci 1988 Jan;39(1):58-62

Sabelhaus L. CD-ROM use in an association special library: a case study. Spec Libr 1988 Spring;79(2):148-51

Schaefer MT. CD-ROM in libraries and information centers. From avant-garde to advantageous. Inf Retr Libr Automn 1986 May;21(12):1-4

Silver H. Supporting CD-ROM users and its effect on library services. In: Optical Publishing and Storage: Products that Work. Proceedings of Optical Publishing and Storage '87 - The Conference on the Applications of Optical Information Systems in Publishing, 11-13 Nov 1987, New York. Medford, NJ: learned Information, 1987. p.151-4

Sweeney RT. CD-ROM publications and the library market. In: Optical Publishing and Storage: Products that Work. Proceedings of Optical Publishing and Storage '87 - The Conference on the Applications of Optical Information Systems in Publishing, 11-13 Nov 1987, New York. Medford, NJ: Learned Information, 1987. p.171-7

Tooey MJ. CD-ROM: a new technology for libraries. Med Ref Serv Q 1987 Fall;6:1-15

Vandergrift KE ; Kemper M ; Champion S ; Hannigan JA. CD-ROM: an emerging technology. Pt 2: Planning and management strategies. Sch Libr J 1987 Aug;33(11):22-5

Vandergrift KE ; Kemper M ; Champion S ; Hannigan JA. CD-ROM: perspectives on an emerging technology. Sch Libr J 1987 Jun-Jul;33(10):27-31

Vanderstar J. Optical storage. Int Libr Rev 1987 Apr;19(2):153-9

DOCUMENT DELIVERY

Befeler M. Combining image and text using a CD-ROM document delivery system. Int J Microgr Video Technol 1987;6(1-2):1-4

13

Campbell RM ; Stern BT. ADONIS-a new approach to document delivery. Microcomput Inf Manage 1987 Jun; 4(2):87-107

CD-ROM special. Commun Technol Impact 1986 Aug;8(5):1-12

Hickey TB ; Calabrese AM. Electro document delivery: OCLC's prototype system. Libr Hi Tech 1986 Spring;4(1):65-71

Hickey TB ; Love RA. Electronic document delivery of primary research journals. Chem Inf Bull 1986 Spring;38(1):22

Stern B. ADONIS--publishing on CD-ROM in mixed mode. In: Proceedings, 10th International Online Information Meeting, 1986, London. Oxford, Eng.: Learned Information, 1986. p.23-32

EVALUATION

Campbell B. Whither the white knight: CD-ROM in technical services. Database 1987 Aug;10(4):22-40

Day JM. LISA on CD-ROM-a user evaluation. In: Online Information 87. 11th International Online Information Meeting, 8-10 Dec 1987, London. Oxford, Eng: Learned Information, 1987. p.273-84

Desmarais N. End-user's report on LaserSearch. Opt Inf Syst 1987 Mar-Apr;7(2):125-31

Desmarais N ; Bailey E. Datext's CD/Corporate. Opt Inf Syst 1987 Sep-Oct;7(5):347-54

Demas S. Comparing BIG bibliographies on CD ROM. Am Libr 1987 May;18(5):332-5

Dodson C. CD-ROMs for the library. Spec Libr 1987 Summer;78(3):191-4

Hagan DL. The Tacoma debut of Books in Print Plus. Libr J 1987 Sep 1;112(14):149-51

Herther NK. Between a rock and a hard place: preservation and optical media. Database 1987 Apr;10(2):122-4

Herther NK. How to evaluate reference

materials on CDROM. Online 1988 Mar;12(2):106-8

Hilditch BM ; Schroeder EE. Pertinent comparisons between CD-ROM and online. Bull Am Soc Inf Sci 1987 Oct-Nov;14:15-6

Hlava M. CD-ROM vs. online. Bull Am Soc Inf Sci 1987 Oct;14(1):14-27

McConnell KS. Evaluating the potential of optical technology and its interaction with traditional data delivery media. In: SCIL 1987. The Second Annual Software/Computer/Database Conference and Exposition for Librarians and Information Managers, Conference Proceedings. 30 Mar-1 Apr 1987. Arlington, Va. Westport, CT: Meckler, 1987. p.106-7

Metcalfe JR ; Jones FG. CD-ROM in developing countries. Electron Opt Publ Rev 1987 Sep;7(3):132-4

Miller DC. Evaluating CD-ROMs: to buy or what to buy? Database 1987 Jun;10:36-42

Miller T. Early user reaction to CD-ROM and videodisc-based optical information products in the library market. Opt Inf Syst 1987 May-Jun;7(3):205-9

Mullan NA ; Blick AR. Initial experiences of untrained end-users with a Life Sciences CD-ROM database: a salutary experience. J Inf Sci 1987;13(3):139-41

Mutter D. The MicroVAX II and CD-ROM-an evaluation. Inf Media Technol 1987 Jan;20(1):30-3

Nelson NM. Libraries test PsycLIT on CD-ROM. Info Today 1987 Feb;4(2):13, 35

Preschel BM. Social science information on CD-ROM: concerns of database producers, libraries and end-users. In: Online Information 87. 11th International Online Information Meeting, 8-10 Dec 1987, London. Oxford, Eng.: Learned Information, 1987. p.253-8

Quint B. How is CD-ROM disappointing? Let me count the ways. Wilson Libr Bull 1987 Dec;62(4):32-4, 102

Reese J. A comparison and evaluation of 3 CD-ROM products. Opt Inf Syst 1988; 8(3):123-6

Reese J ; Steffey R. ERIC on CD-ROM: a

14

comparison of DIALOG onDisc, OCLC'S Search CD450 and Silver Platter. Online 1987 Sep;11(5):42-54

Reich VA ; Betcher MA. Library of Congress staff test optical disk system. Coll Res Libr 1986 Jul;47(4):385-91

Schaefer MT. CD-ROM update: developments impact information community. Inf Retr Libr Automn 1986 Nov;22(6):1-4

Schwarzkopf LC. United States Census Bureau CD-ROM evaluation project. a news note. Gov Publ Rev 1987;14(3):353-4

Snow B. Life science sources on laserdisk. Online 1987 Mar;11(2):113-6

Stewart L. Picking CD-ROMs for public use. Am Libr 1987 Oct;18(9):738-40

Stewart L ; Olsen J. Compact disk databases: are they good for users? Online 1988 May;12(3):48-52

WORK STATIONS

Alberico R;. Workstations for reference and retrieval: Pt. 1 : The scholars workstation. Small Comput Libr 1988 Mar;8(3):4-12

Alberico R. Workstations for reference and retrieval. Pt. 2. Small Comput Libr 1988 April;8(4):4,6,8,10

Gale JC. The information workstation: a confluence of technologies including the CD-ROM. Inf Technol Libr 1985 Jun;4(2):137-9

Groundwater NP ; Bodick N ; Marquis, A. A SunView user-interface for authoring and accessing a medical knowledge base. In: EUUG Autumn '87 Conference Proceedings, 21-25 Sep 1987, Dublin, Ireland. Buntingford, UK: Europe UNIX Systems User Group, 1987. p.93-104

Micco M ; Smith I. Designing an integrated system of databases: a workstation for information seekers. Libr Software Rev 1987 Sep-Oct;6(5):259-62

15

487

II. MONOGRAPHS

Davis, Susan. CD-ROM: technology and applications. White Plains, NY: Knowledge Industry, 1986. 170p.

Hendley, Tony. CD-ROM and optical publishing systems. Westport, CT: Meckler Publishing, 1987. 150p.

Information Systems Consultants Inc. Videodisc and optical digital disk technologies and their applications in libraries. A report to the Council of Library Resources. Washington, DC: Information Systems Consultants, Inc., 1985. 200p.

Intner, Sheila S. Microcomputer environment: management issues. Phoenix, AZ: Oryx Press, 1987. 248p.

Lambert, Steve ; Ropiequet, Suzanne, editors. CD-ROM: the new papyrus: the current and future state of the art. Redmond, WA: Microsoft Press, 1986. 630p.

Myers, Patti. Publishing with CD-ROM: a guide to compact disc optical storage technologies for providers of publishing services. Westport, CT: Meckler Publishing, 1987. 98p.

Nelson, Nancy Melin. CD-Roms in print. Westport, CT: Meckler, 1987. 102p.

Optical disk initiatives at the National Technical Information Service. Springfield, VA: National Technical Information Service, June 1986. 137p. (PB86-868536)

Rasdall, Mark ed. The international directory of information products on CD-ROM 1986/87. London, Alan Armstrong & Associates Ltd, 1986, 125 leaves;

Roth, Judith P,Editor. Essential guide to CD-ROM. Westport, CT: Meckler Publishers, 1986. 189p.

Schwerin, Julie.CD-ROM standards: the book. Medford, NJ: Learned Information, 1986. 53p.

16

III. SERIAL TITLES

CD DATA REPORT
McLean, VA.: Langley Publications.
Monthly.
1N1,Nov 1987--

CD-ROM LIBRARIAN
Westport, CT.: Meckler Publishing.
(Continues Optical Information Systems
Update/Library & Information Center
Applications. Bimonthly.
2N4,Jul-Aug 1987--

**CD-ROM REVIEW: THE MAGAZINE OF
COMPUTER DISK DATA STORAGE.**
Peterborough, NH: CW Communications.
Bimonthly.
2N1,Mar-Apr 1987--

CD-ROM SOURCEBOOK.
Falls Church, VA.: Diversified Data
Resources. Monthly.
1986--

**ELECTRONIC AND OPTICAL
PUBLISHING REVIEW: AN
INTERNATIONAL JOURNAL**
Medford, NJ.: Learned Information.
Quarterly.
6N4,Dec 1986--

**INTERNATIONAL JOURNAL OF
MICROGRAPHICS & VIDEO
TECHNOLOGY.**
New York: Pergamon Press. Quarterly.
1N1,1982--

**OPTICAL INFORMATION SYSTEMS
UPDATE.**
Westport, CT.: Meckler. (Continues:
Videodisc and Optical Disk Update). Semi-
monthly.
5N7,Apr 1986--

SMALL COMPUTERS IN LIBRARIES
Westport, CT.: Meckler. Monthly.
1,Apr 1981--

VIDEO DISC MONITOR
Falls Church, VA.: Future Systems, Inc.
Monthly.
1,1982--

IV. AUTHOR INDEX

INDEX

by Helen Webbink

The entries in this index are filed word by word. When formal and informal names are used for a given evaluation site, it is entered under each of these. Parentheses have been used for scope notes that clarify the meaning of the entries. Personal proper names have been inverted; however, a proper name has not been inverted if it is part of the name of a library.